ADVANCED IMMUNOASSAYS IN RHEUMATOLOGY

Edited by

Marius Teodorescu, M.D., Ph.D.

Professor of Microbiology, Immunology, and Medicine
and Director, Rheumatology/Immunology Laboratory
University of Illinois College of Medicine
Chicago, Illinois

Christopher J. Froelich, M.D.

Associate Professor of Medicine
Northwestern University Medical School
and Head, Rheumatology Research Laboratory
Evanston Hospital
Evanston, Illinois

CRC Press
Boca Raton Ann Arbor London Tokyo

Library of Congress Cataloging-in-Publication Data

Advanced immunoassays in rheumatology/edited by Marius Teodorescu, Christopher J. Froelich.
p. cm.
Includes bibliographical references and index.
ISBN 0-8493-5974-0
1. Joints — Diseases — Immunodiagnosis. 2. Connective tissues--Diseases — Immunodiagnosis. 3. Immunoassay. I. Teodorescu, Marius. II. Froelich, Christopher J.
[DNLM: 1. Immunoassay — methods. 2. Enzyme-Linked Immunosorbent Assay. 3. Rheumatic Diseases — immunology. WE 544 A2442 1994]
RC932.A39 1994
616.7′230756 — dc20
DNLM/DLC
for Library of Congress 93-28311
CIP

Direct all inquiries to CRC Press, Inc., 2000 Corporate Blvd., N.W., Boca Raton, Florida 33431.

International Standard Book Number 0-8493-5974-0
Library of Congress Card Number 93-28311
Printed in the United States of America 1 2 3 4 5 6 7 8 9 0
Printed on acid-free paper

PREFACE

To reduce costs and increase throughput without sacrificing accuracy and precision, modern clinical chemistry laboratories perform multiparametric testing with sophisticated acute analyzers. Unfortunately, due to the perceived absence of appropriate technology, the director's preferences, and tradition, most Clinical Immunology laboratories have not yet adopted this approach. Consequently, a laboratory frequently may have protocols that detect antinuclear antibody and anti-dsDNA by immunofluorescence, anti-RNP and anti-Sm by hemagglutination, anti-SSA and SSB by agar gel double diffusion and rheumatoid factor by latex agglutination. Further complicating the situation, the protocols do not incorporate external standards and the results are reported semiquantitatively (e.g., the titer and pattern of the F-ANA).

The trend in Clinical Immunology laboratories, however, is changing. If the present pace continues, in the next few years most laboratories will implement solid phase immunoassays such as ELISA. The simplicity and versatility of ELISA allow the office and small hospital laboratory as well as the large, high volume, reference laboratory to attain similar precise and accurate results. Therefore, we have chosen to focus on the value of ELISA testing as the prototype of the solid phase immunoassays in the diagnosis and management of rheumatic diseases.

The book represents an integrated approach that will interest both clinical and laboratory immunologists. The clinical significance of the test results is brought to life by illustrative case presentations, where the true integration takes place. After an introductory chapter on methodology, each type of analyte (e.g., antinuclear autoantibodies, rheumatoid factors, cytokines) is described in three parts, each in at least one chapter. The three parts are: 1. the theoretical and experimental basis for the detection of the analyte; 2. details of specific techniques usually based on ELISA; and 3. the interpretation of the tests results in clinical context with case presentations. The impact that different techniques, including multiparameter ELISA testing, can have on clinical diagnosis is emphasized. Special attention is given to issues of quality control and trouble shooting; the techniques described have been routinely practiced by the authors of various chapters.

The book is the result of a collective effort of scientists with very busy schedules. We thank all of them for their dedicated efforts. We also thank Jeanette Wallman, B.S. and Katherine L. Russo, B.S. for their support in the development of several ELISA tests described in this book.

Marius Teodorescu
Christopher J. Froelich

THE EDITORS

Marius Teodorescu, M.D., Ph.D.
Professor of Microbiology, Immunology, and Medicine
and Director, Rheumatology/Immunology Laboratory
University of Illinois College of Medicine
President and CEO, TheraTest Laboratories, Inc.
Chicago, Illinois

Dr. Teodorescu received his M.D. and Ph.D. degrees in Microbiology from the Institute of Medicine and Pharmacy in Bucharest, Romania. After a four-year period as a general practitioner, he worked for ten years as a research scientist in Bucharest's Cantacuzino Institute in the fields of Viral Immunology and Vaccine Preparation. Since 1974 he has been on the faculty at the University of Illinois College of Medicine where he has taught Immunology and practiced Clinical Rheumatology. He has also been on the faculty of the Institute for Graduate Medical Education in Chicago.

He has published 100 papers including one on the discovery of bacterial adhesion to lymphocytes–a method of defining functionally distinct subpopulations in which lectins on lymphocytes interact with carbohydrates on other cell surfaces; another dealing with the original work on the α_2-macroglobulin as a carrier for cytokines such as IL-1; and a third about the concept of clinical value of simultaneous multiparameter solid phase immunoassay for autoantibodies.

For the past several years he has focused on the clinical laboratory needs of the rheumatologist. He founded and is still directing the Rheumatology/ Immunology Laboratory at the University of Illinois and at TheraTest Laboratories, Inc. in Chicago.

Christopher J. Froelich, M.D.
Associate Professor of Medicine at
Northwestern University Medical School
Head of Clinical and Basic Research Laboratory at Evanston Hospital
Consultant in Regulatory Affairs for TheraTest Laboratories, Inc.

Dr. Froelich received his B.A. degree in Chemistry from the University of Colorado (Boulder) in 1973. He obtained his M.D. degree from Loyola University-Stritch School of Medicine in 1976. At the University of New Mexico, Dr. Froelich completed Internal Medicine Residency Training and a Fellowship in Rheumatology (1976–1980). Thereafter, he was appointed Assistant Professor of Medicine at the University of New Mexico. In 1984, he moved to the University of Illinois at Chicago where he was appointed Associate Chief of Rheumatology at University Hospital and Chief of Rheumatology at the Westside Veteran's Administration Medical Center. In 1988, he was promoted to the rank of Associate Professor of Medicine. In 1990, he assumed his present position.

Dr. Froelich is a member of the American Association of Immunologists, the Central Society for Clinical Research, the American Society for Clinical Investigation, the American College of Rheumatology, and the Clinical Immunology Society. He has served on the Medical and Scientific Committee of the Arthritis Foundation, Illinois Chapter and on the Medical Advisory Board of Lupus Foundation of Illinois.

He was elected to the Alpha Omega Alpha Honor Society in 1975 and was the recipient of the Veteran's Administration Career Development Award and the Research Fellowship Award from the National Arthritis Foundation.

In addition to receiving research support from numerous philanthropic trusts, Dr. Froelich has been funded by the Veteran's Administration Merit Review, the National and Illinois Arthritis Foundation, the National and Illinois Lupus Foundation, and the American Cancer Society.

Dr. Froelich has presented more than 20 invited lectures at various universities and institutes. He has published more than 50 research and clinical papers. His current major research interests include the study of the biological and pathologic roles of lymphocyte serine proteases and the clinical utility of laboratory testing in the rheumatic diseases.

CONTRIBUTORS

Ronald A. Asherson, M.D.
Lupus Arthritis Research Unit
The Rayne Institute
St. Thomas Hospital
London, U.K.

Ricard Cervera, M.D., Ph.D.
Department of Internal Medicine
Hospital Clinic
Barcelona, Spain

Linda Cook, Ph.D.
Department of Hospital Laboratories
Lahey Clinic Medical Center
Burlington, Massachusetts

Christopher Froelich, M.D.
Rheumatology Research Laboratory
Evanston Hospital
Evanston, Illinois

James S. Grober, M.D.
Department of Medicine/Rheumatology
Evanston Hospital
Evanston, Illinois

Mona L. Hall, Ph.D.
Genzyme Corporation
Cambridge, Massachusetts

E. Nigel Harris, M.D.
Department of Medicine
University of Louisville
Louisville, Kentucky

William F. Koopman, M.D.
Department of Medicine/Rheumatology
University of Alabama at Birmingham
Birmingham Veterans Administration Medical Center
Birmingham, Alabama

Robert G. Lahita, M.D., Ph.D.
Department of Medicine/Rheumatology
St. Luke's-Roosevelt Hospital
New York, New York

Velta A. Lazda, Ph.D.
Histocompatibility Laboratory
Regional Organ Bank of Illinois
Chicago, Illinois

Mariana Linker-Israeli, Ph.D.
Department of Medicine
Cedars-Sinai Medical Center
Los Angeles, California

Martin Lotz, M.D.
Department of Medicine
University of California, San Diego
La Jolla, California

Silvia Pierangeli, Ph.D.
Department of Medicine
University of Louisville
Louisville, Kentucky

Elizabeth G. Posillico, Ph.D.
Genzyme Corporation
Cambridge, Massachusetts

John D. Reveille, M.D.
Department of Medicine/Rheumatology
University of Texas Health Science Center
Houston, Texas

Ralph E. Schrohenloher, Ph.D.
Department of Medicine/Rheumatology
University of Alabama at Birmingham
Birmingham, Alabama

Marius Teodorescu, M.D., Ph.D.
Department of Microbiology/Immunology
University of Illinois College of Medicine
Chicago, Illinois

CONTENTS

I. Introduction

Chapter 1

ELISA and Other Immunologic Techniques in Rheumatology

Marius Teodorescu and Christopher J. Froelich

CONTENTS

0-8493-5974-1/94/$0.00 + $.50

I. OVERVIEW OF IMMUNOLOGIC TECHNIQUES IN RHEUMATOLOGY

A. INTRODUCTION

Our understanding of the biochemical nature of autoantigens and the development of thermoplastics technology has lead to the development of new *in vitro* diagnostic (IVD) tests. The consequent availability of diverse IVDs presents clinical laboratories with the task of deciding which tests are most suitable for their particular circumstances. The superimposition of issues such as cost containment and quality assurance clearly shifts the focus toward computerized test systems that offer automation, high throughput, and the potential to monitor performance. The recent tendency, therefore, has been to adopt solid-phase immunoassays, the most versatile being the 96-microwell enzyme-linked immunoadsorbent assay (ELISA). The practical application of ELISA-based IVDs will be discussed primarily. The theoretical aspects of ELISA and other solid-phase assays have been extensively reviewed.[1-3] Many laboratories continue to use "classic" immunologic methods (immunodiffusion, latex agglutination, and immunofluorescent slide testing). These techniques, which have been extensively described elsewhere,[4] will be briefly summarized.

Immunoassays relevant to rheumatology focus on products of immune system activation (e.g., antibodies and cytokines). Gene typing, on the other hand, may directly identify factors that contribute to abnormal immune function. The techniques will likely become routine and therefore may provide significant diagnostic and prognostic insight (see Chapters 17–20).

B. DETECTION OF ANTIBODIES BY CELL STAINING

Antibodies directed toward cellular antigens are often detected with cells fixed to a glass slide. This technique is used for most nuclear antigens (ANA test), DNA (*Crithidia luciliae* kinetoplast), neutrophil cytoplasmic antigens (ANCA test), and others (e.g., smooth muscle). Glass microscope slides that have multiple tissue sections or spots of cultured cell suspensions are incubated with increasing dilutions of test sera in parallel with positive and negative controls. Standards may be incorporated to "quantify" antibody binding. After washing the unbound immunoglobulins, a fluorescent anti-human immunoglobulin antibody is added and the reactivity is assessed by ultraviolet (UV) light microscopy. An enzyme-coupled antibody may function as an alternate reporter; subsequent addition of a substrate which precipitates at the sites of antibody–antigen complex provides a permanently stained specimen. The laboratory reports the endpoint dilution that produces a positive reaction, as well as the distribution of nuclear/cytoplasmic stain (homogeneous, speckled, rim, nucleolar, centromere, etc.).

To determine the phenotypic characteristics of relevant cell populations (e.g., mononuclear cells), various membrane-associated structures on suspended viable cells undergo labeling with the appropriate probe. For example, to determine if a patient's cells displays a certain histocompatibility gene product, the individual's cells are mixed with fluorescent antibody of the desired specificity and subsequently analyzed either by UV light microscopy or by flow cytometry. This technique accurately determines the proportion of lymphocytes that bear certain cluster determinants (CD), class I MHC antigens (e.g., HLA B27) and class II antigens (e.g., DR 3) (see Chapter 18).

The use of cells to detect antibodies may take the form of complement-mediated killing. This method is standard for histocompatibility testing (e.g., HLA B27, see Chapter 18). Antiserum that contains the desired specificity is incubated with the patient's viable lymphocytes. Complement is added, and cell death is visualized microscopically by trypan blue staining. This method, although widespread, may be replaced in time by the combination of monoclonal antibody staining and flow cytometry.

C. IMMUNOPRECIPITATION AND AGGLUTINATION

Double diffusion, which relies on precipitation in gel, has been used extensively to detect clinically relevant analytes (autoantibodies). To detect autoantibodies (e.g., anti-Sm, -RNP, or -SSA), the antigen (usually a crude extract) and the test sample are dispensed into adjacent wells made in a lawn of agar gel. The antigen and the antibody diffuse radially from the wells and form a visible precipitate at the point of equivalence (Figure 1). The antibody specificity of the specimen is validated by simultaneously testing a control serum that contains the desired antibody specificity. The precipitation lines formed between the positive control and the unknowns represent lines of identity, non-identity, or partial identity. Gel double diffusion offers relatively high diagnostic specificity, but the concomitant reduction in test sensitivity decreases the value of immunodiffusion for screening studies. Furthermore, since the data are subject to observer bias and the results are usually reported as positive and negative, the technique has limited value to diagnose and manage patients with autoimmune disease.

For the radial-diffusion technique, the reactant (e.g., antibody) that is used to identify the analyte (e.g., C3) is mixed in the gel. Serum is placed in a well in agar gel and the analyte diffuses radially until a ring of precipitation forms at point of equivalence. The diameter of the ring is directly proportional to the concentration of analyte and is compared to a standard.

Immunodiffusion may be performed in an electric field, i.e., counter-immunoelectrophoresis (see Figure 1). The antigen and dilutions of serum are placed in agar gel wells on a slide. The electric field causes the antigen to migrate toward the diluted serum specimen. Since the various antigenic proteins migrate differentially in the gel, antibody molecules with distinct specificities in the specimen form discrete precipitation bands. For example, the lines of precipitation for RNP and Sm are slightly separated and may be identified based on coincident use of a positive control.

A variant of immunoprecipitation is based on the use of radiolabeled antigen to quantify the reaction. Although any radiolabeled protein may act as the reactant, this assay has been used primarily to measure levels of anti-DNA antibody (see Chapter 6). Radiolabeled ^{125}I-DNA is incubated with serum and forms immune complexes with the anti-DNA antibody. These complexes and irrelevant immunoglobulin are precipitated with hypertonic ammonium sulfate (Farr assay), and a gamma counter measures the radioactivity in the precipitate. The results are expressed as percent DNA bound (precipitated) or as I.U.

Agglutination is used to detect either antigens or antibodies with the help of particles or red blood cells coated with either one of the reactants. The agglutination reaction may be monitored visually, and the results are expressed as positive/negative or at an endpoint dilution. Red blood cells coated with antigen are used mainly in passive agglutination, which has relatively high sensitivity. However, inasmuch as coupling efficiency of the reactant to the red cells varies markedly, hemagglutination is particularly prone to imprecision. In addition, when the analyte is an antibody, the methods preferentially detect IgM class. Therefore, the techniques are particularly useful to detect IgM rheumatoid factor, but are less likely to reliably measure other clinically relevant IgG autoantibodies (e.g., anti-DNA).

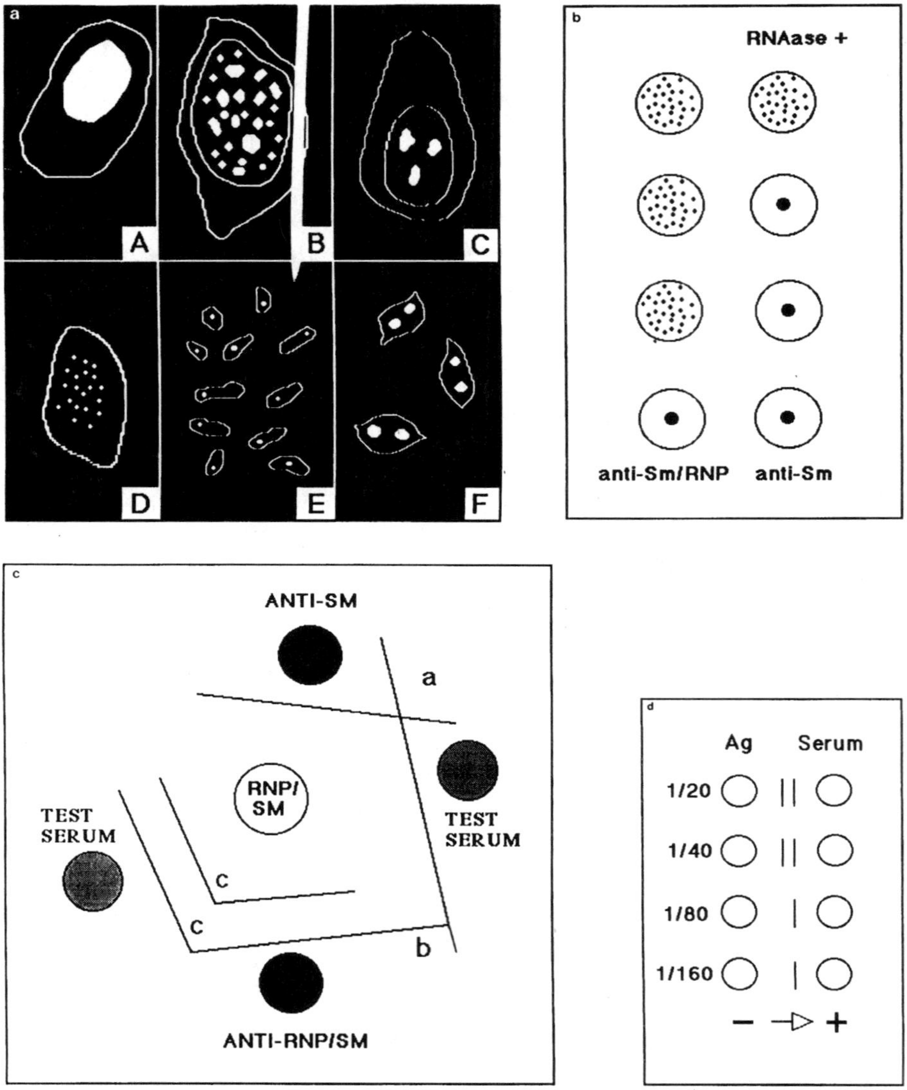

Figure 1 Schematic representation of immunoassays used in clinical rheumatology laboratory. Explanations in the text. (a) Immunofluorescence: A, B, C, and D are patterns (homogeneous, speckled, nucleolar, and fine-speckled) inappropriately considered to predict antibody specificities responsible for the staining; E and F are kinetoplast (anti-DNA) and nuclear plus kinetoplast fluorescence on *Crithidia luciliae.* (b) Passive hemagglutination. (c) Immunodiffusion (a: lines of non-identity; b: partial identity; c: identity). (d) Counter immunoelectrophoresis. (e) Enzyme immunoassay: EIA in microwell represents indirect ELISA. (f) Immunoblotting. (g) Radioimmunoassay for anti-dsDNA antibody (Farr assay): A: ammonium sulfate precipitation for high-affinity antibody; B and C: assays for all anti-dsDNA antibody (low and high affinity).

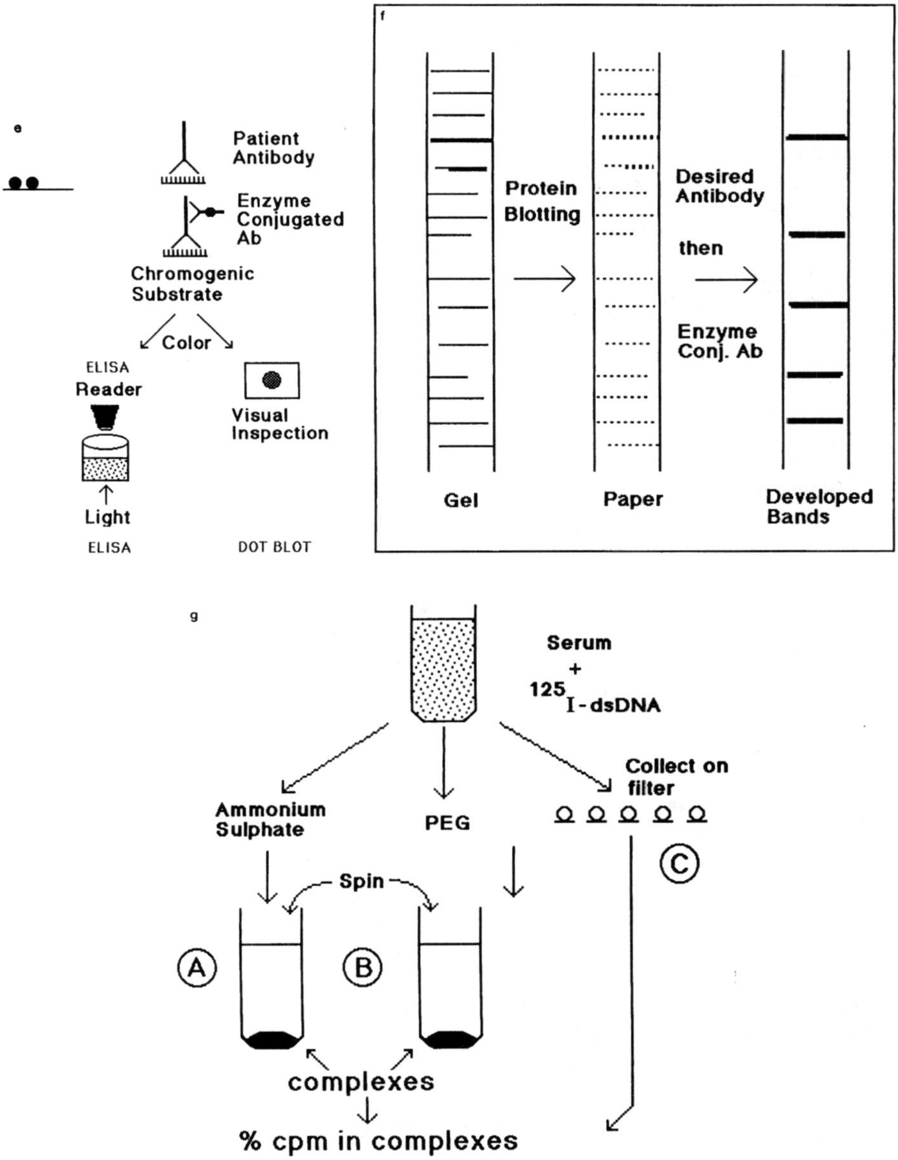

Figure 1 (continued).

Quasi-equilibrium nephelometric methods measure light scatter at the beginning of the reaction and after a constant time interval. Rate (kinetic) nephelometry obtains data based on constant monitoring of the reaction over time. Nephelometry is used to detect and/or quantify either antigen (e.g., C3) or antibody (e.g., rheumatoid factor) in test serum (see Appendix at the end of this volume). Based on the Tyndall effect, nephelometry measures the scattering of a light beam that traverses a solution containing a lattice of antigen-antibody complexes. The amount of light scattered depends on the size of the complexes, which makes the relationship between analyte concentration and light scatter sigmoidal. The complexes consist of the analyte and the detection molecule (e.g., IgG antibody). Some nephelometric instruments base the measurement on microagglutinates by having one of the reactants (e.g., IgG for rheumatoid factor) antigen-coated onto small particles. To obtain quantitative results, the reaction is monitored at multiple time points and the data are compared with standard curves. Although rate nephelometry offers high sample throughput and quantitative results, it has several limitations: (1) it is relatively insensitive, (2) sample turbidity reduces accuracy, (3) the instrumentation is relatively expensive, (4) if the analyte is an antibody, a high serum concentration may produce a prozone phenomenon, and (5) the antibody class in the immune complex is not identified — an issue that is particularly relevant to the analysis of autoimmune sera.

D. IMMUNOBLOTTING AND IMMUNOFILTRATION

Western blotting represents a variant of the solid-phase immunoassay in which an antigen is separated by polyacrylamide gel electrophoresis and then undergoes electrotransfer to a membrane support (see Figure 1). In this manner, complex antigenic mixtures are separated (e.g., into 68-, 27-, and 21-kDa components of RNP). The antigen fixed on this solid phase reacts with serum antibody. A second antibody — usually class-specific anti-Ig antibody coupled to an enzyme — is added, followed by a substrate. A visible precipitate forms a band at the site of antibody reaction with the separated membrane-bound antigen. The difference between immunoblotting and ELISA is that the former provides a visual estimate of antibody binding, while the latter offers quantitative analysis by spectrophotometry. Using various sandwich configurations, the sensitivity of Western blot may equal or exceed that of standard ELISA. However, the process is laborious and expensive for the clinical laboratory and is limited to special investigations.

For dot blotting, the purified antigen is either directly dried on the membrane or immobilized by vacuum suction (Figure 1). Similar to the Western blot method the presence of reactive antibody is determined with an enzyme-conjugated antibody and substrate. Depending on the intensity of the color reaction, the result is scored visually as positive or negative. To reduce false positives, the assay sensitivity is markedly attenuated.

Enzyme immunofiltration assay (EIFA) represents another variant of ELISA that entails (1) microporous membrane to bind the reactant and (2) filtration to hasten contact of the test analyte and the reporter system with the solid phase. Quantitative assays based on EIFA have reproducibility and sensitivity comparable to the ELISA format.

II. SOLID-PHASE IMMUNOASSAYS

A. PRINCIPLES AND TYPES OF ELISA

ELISA and related solid-phase methods (fluorometry, EIFA, magnetic bead assays chemiluminescence) are sufficiently versatile that a laboratory is able to use a single technique to measure many distinct immunologic parameters: (1) antibodies to nuclear antigens, IgG, phospholipids, and arthritogenic pathogens, and (2) antigens such as complement activation fragments, cytokines, and C reactive protein. Due to availability of relatively inexpensive reagents and instrumentation, ELISA-based assays have been preferentially adopted by many clinical laboratories. Nevertheless, the theoretical and practical aspects of ELISA discussed below apply to any sensitive solid-phase immunoassay.

The theoretical and technical facets of ELISA have been reviewed extensively.[1-3,5,6] Here, the basic principles and practical applications relevant to the clinical rheumatology laboratory will be described. ELISA can be separated into three operations:

1. Binding or capture of an analyte to a reactant that has been immobilized on a solid phase
2. A signal-generator (or reporter) system that identifies bound analyte
3. The detection system

Although the solid phase is either plastic microwells (96-well format), microparticles, or tubes, microwell ELISA has the potential for automation; therefore, this format has been adopted to produce a variety of clinical laboratory tests (see Appendix). The signal generator that recognizes the analyte consists of an antibody that provides test specificity and an enzyme that signals detection. The enzyme degrades a substrate to yield a stoichiometric color reaction. The detection system — often called an ''ELISA plate reader'' — is a spectrophotometer that ''reads'' the 96-well plate. Ideally, the reader interfaces with a computer containing the software to facilitate rapid data reduction.

To detect the desired analyte in the test sample, the reactant is either directly immobilized or captured indirectly onto a solid-phase support. In many instances the analyte is an antibody and the immobilized reactant is its antigen (indirect ELISA format). The purified antigen is nonspecifically coated to the microwells by hydrophobic interaction (Figure 2). Alternately, a spacer molecule with a reactive group for the coating protein may provide a covalent linkage. After blocking unreacted hydrophobic sites, serum that contains the antibody is incubated in the antigen-coated well, and specific antibody remains attached after washing. An enzyme-labeled antibody directed against the immunoglobulin of interest is added, followed by the substrate that produces a color change that is proportional to the amount of bound analyte.

The antigen-capture technique (see Figure 2) has a design comparable to the indirect ELISA, except that an antibody is used to immobilize the desired reactant. The wells are coated with antibody that binds to one epitope of the reactant (e.g., SSA). The reactant or antigen is added to the well and remains attached after washing. This antigen-capture method is particularly valuable to selectively remove the antigen from a mixture. Furthermore, since the direct binding of the antigen to the plastic material may result in significant denaturation, the capture technique is desirable if the intent is to detect antibodies that react with conformational epitopes (e.g., neutrophil cytoplasmic antigen for ANCA test) (see Chapter 6).

When the analyte is a non-antibody macromolecule, two designs, sandwich and competitive (see Figure 2), are most often employed. In principle, the sandwich method is similar to the antigen-capture system. In this instance the reactant — often a monoclonal antibody that binds one epitope of the analyte — is attached to the solid phase (see Figure 2). The sample containing the analyte (e.g., C5a) is incubated in the well, and unbound material is washed away. A second antibody that carries the enzyme binds to an unrelated epitope of the immobilized analyte. Specific binding is determined by addition of the substrate followed by the detection of the resultant color reaction (see Chapter 15).

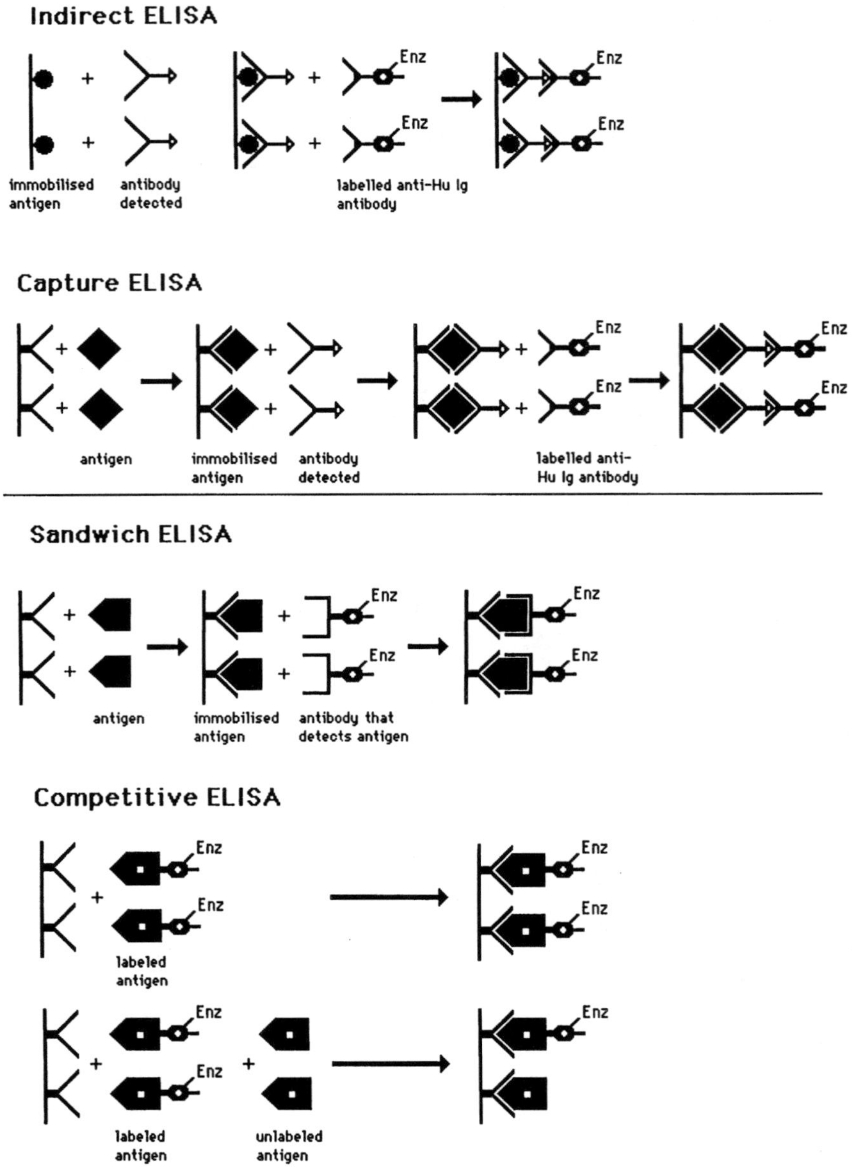

Figure 2 Schematic representation of different types of ELISA for the detection of antibodies and antigens: indirect, capture, sandwich (two site), and competitive ELISA (explanations in the text).

Competitive ELISA (see Figure 2) indirectly detects the unknown antigen by measuring its ability to compete for the binding to the solid phase with known amounts of enzyme-labeled antigen. Therefore, the enzymatic activity is inversely proportional to the amount of antigen present in the test sample. A standard curve is obtained by adding various amounts of free antigen. This method is suitable to measure very low concentrations of analyte (e.g., cytokines in serum) (see Chapter 15).

B. MECHANISM OF SOLID-PHASE COATING

The development and manufacture of solid-phase materials that serve to immobilize proteins for ELISA testing have been extensively reviewed.[3,5] Thermoplastics such as polystyrene are polymer resins that maintain their physical characteristics when heated and cooled; these materials are ideal for the manufacture of various configurations by the injection mold technique. Polystyrene is a particular favorite because it retains clarity and it is inexpensive and easy to process. Although polystyrene has many attributes required for injection mold manufacture, additives such as flow agents, plasticizers, and mold-release agents are often used to facilitate fabrication. These additives may alter the binding characteristics of the polystyrene by changing the surface chemistry or by diffusing to the surface of the plastic during storage.

Protein immobilization occurs by adsorption or by covalent binding to the plastic through a spacer. The adsorption of proteins, carbohydrates, and lipids depends primarily on the hydrophobic interactions with the plastic. These interactions are in turn influenced by the pH and salt concentration of the buffer as well as by concentration of the solid-phase reactant and irrelevant proteins in the coating solution. Most often the protein solution is simply incubated in the microwell. High-pH buffers, such as carbonate/bicarbonate, although frequently employed, do not provide a singular advantage. In some instances the alkaline pH favors denaturation of the reactant and markedly impairs binding (see below).[7] However, the pH may facilitate binding when the coating is done at the PI of the protein; under this condition, the protein is more likely to coaggregate with the solid phase. The salt concentration of the coating buffer may temporarily denature the antigen, producing additional hydrophobic sites that enhance binding. Too high a concentration of reactant in the coating solution may lead to the formation and binding of aggregates that may detach from the solid phase and be free to compete for the analyte during the assay.

Adsorption may alter the conformation of the coated protein. The consequence is a possible loss of epitopes or functional groups reactive with the analyte. Therefore, when the conventional indirect ELISA is used to measure serum antibody, it strongly favors the selection of antibodies that recognize unfolded antigen.[8] This issue is particularly important when the intent is to measure antibodies that bind conformational epitopes. For the capture ELISA, the method of passive adsorption at pH 9.6 significantly denatures the capture antibody. For example, less than 3.0% of the binding sites of a monoclonal capture antibody and 5 to 10% of polyclonal antibodies could capture antigen after passive adsorption to plastic.[3] Nevertheless, despite the complexity and inefficiency of protein adsorption, the simplicity of the coating process makes it a popular choice for the preparation of the solid-phase immunoassays. For each reactant, the choice of plastic and coating conditions (temperature, incubation period, buffer, and antigen concentration) must be determined empirically (see below). Nevertheless, the obvious vagaries of the adsorption process emphasize the need to develop new methods to immobilize reactants.

Efforts to improve the binding efficiency and biologic activity of reactants have led to the development of plastic materials that allow covalent binding through spacers with amino and carboxyl groups attached. Homobifunctional reagents, such as glutaraldehyde and carbodiimide, are routinely used for amino and carboxyl group coupling, respectively. However, the ideal coupling agent should be heterobifunctional, consisting of a spacer molecule with two reactive groups: one that attaches preferentially to the desired reactant and another that attaches to the solid phase. Although covalent coupling will likely replace standard adsorption, each antigen will have to be experimentally tested to determine if covalent binding is advantageous. In most instances the covalent bond is followed by a hydrophobic interaction, resulting in the same distortion of the antigen as the noncovalent attachment.

After coating the reactant, a blocking step is performed to saturate residual hydrophobic sites. This process is necessary to reduce nonspecific binding of the reporter molecules and the attendant amplification of background signal. Although nonionic detergents (Tween 20 or Triton X-100) commonly serve this function, we have observed that protein-rich solutions (horse serum, fetal bovine serum, or bovine serum albumin) offer superior performance. Most adsorbed proteins do not uniformly coat the solid phase.[7] Large areas of the solid phase, therefore, must be saturated with the blocking agent. Nonionic detergents, although highly hydrophobic, may be washed away; this provides sites that react with the reporter molecules, which results in a reduction in the signal-to-noise ratio (i.e., increased background).

The blocking solution should maximally fill the microwells (200 to 400 μl), beyond the maximum level of specimen (e.g., 100 μl). This strategy will ensure that all exposed hydrophobic sites are blocked. Blocking occurs for 3 to 6 h at room temperature or 1 to 2 h at 37°C and is followed by three to four washes. If the washing process is ineffective, residual blocking proteins may obscure or "cover up" the reactant, or aggregated reactant may detach during the assay and compete with bound material. The plates coated with antigen are stable when sealed in metalized pouches that contain a dessicant. The pouches may be packaged in an inert gas to further prolong shelf life. Plates prepared "in house" may be stored frozen at −20°C in sealed pouches containing a dessicant.

C. PREPARATION OF SOLID PHASE

The development of an ELISA test is highly empiric. The desired analytical sensitivity and specificity are attained by adjustment of the following parameters:

1. Incubation time of each reactant
2. Concentration of reactant for coating
3. Concentration of enzyme conjugate
4. Concentration of substrate

For an indirect ELISA, the overall goal is to produce an assay that yields low absorbance values (e.g., <0.2) when normal specimens are tested, while a potent reaction (e.g., >1.5) occurs with specimens known to contain the analyte.

The substrate concentration and its incubation time for the assay are dictated by the sensitivity of the enzyme to the inhibitory effects of degradation product and to the stability of the accumulating chromogenic product. The commercial availability of standardized substrates facilitates the establishment of these two parameters. The incubation

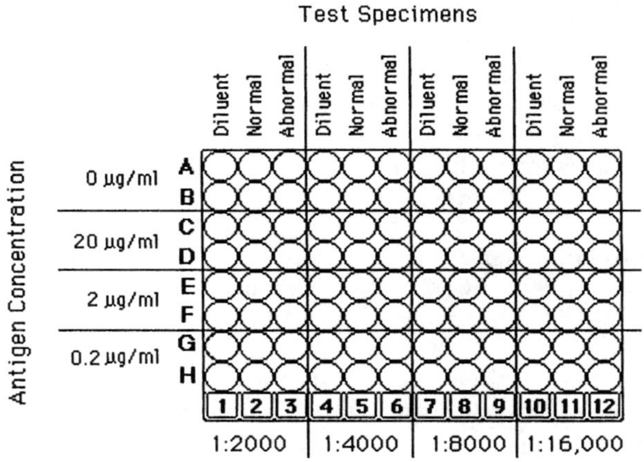

Figure 3 Checkerboard arrangement of reagents to determine optimal concentration of enzyme and antigen. Explanation in the text.

time for the specimens and enzyme conjugate may be initially set at 15 to 30 min and later modified during final optimization of the assay. Consequently, two parameters remain to be ascertained experimentally: (1) the concentration of coating material (antigen or antibody), and (2) the concentration of enzyme. A checkerboard design is arranged on a 96-well plate (Figure 3). Duplicate rows are coated with various concentrations of antigen, for example, as follows: rows A and B — "zero antigen", rows C and D — 20 μg/ml, rows E and F — 2 μg/ml, and rows G and H — 0.2 μg/ml. The plate is coated, blocked, dried, and tested with a normal specimen, an abnormal specimen, and specimen diluent (conjugate blank). Starting with a concentration recommended by the manufacturer and continuing with fivefold dilutions, the enzyme conjugate is added to microwells in each column. In subsequent experiments the dilution range is narrowed through interpolation.

For preliminary analytical verification of the assay, approximately 20 specimens that are shown by an independent method to have "abnormal analyte levels" are tested in the newly devised ELISA (see Section IV.C in this chapter). This comparison should demonstrate, as a minimum, equivalent analytical sensitivity. Whenever available, national and international controls and standards also warrant inclusion. Simultaneously, the results for 20 normals should be low (e.g., <0.2 absorbance value for indirect ELISA).

The final step of the process entails the standardization, calibration, and validation of the assay (see below). Additional adjustments in the analytic sensitivity are frequently performed by modifying one or two parameters of the test.

D. REPORTER SYSTEMS: ENZYME CONJUGATES AND SUBSTRATES

The reporter molecule, either antigen or antibody, is directly coupled to an enzyme or connected by bridging molecules (e.g., biotin-avidin). The latter approach reduces steric hindrance and enhances analytic sensitivity (see Chapter 15). The signal amplification, cost, stability, and endogenous enzymatic activity of the analyte influence the choice of enzyme/substrate system. For example, immobilized myeloperoxidase may degrade substrates used with horseradish peroxidase (HRP).

The most widely used enzyme/substrate systems are HRP/3,3′,5,5′-tetramethyl benzidine (TMB) and alkaline phosphatase/*para*-nitrophenyl phosphate (pNPP); urease, β-galactosidase, glucose oxidase, and carbonic anhydrase are also used in enzyme conjugates. HRP, the smallest of the three with a molecular weight of 40,000, has eight glycosylation sites, which renders it less hydrophobic and thus less likely to produce background noise.

To avoid nonspecific binding or background "noise", polyclonal (goat or rabbit) affinity-purified antibodies or their $(Fab')_2$ fragments are used at a relatively high dilution (1:6,000 to 1:50,000). Mouse monoclonals are used primarily for two-site and competitive ELISA.

The signal generated by fluorogenic substrates is 10 to 1000 times greater than the chromogens. However, test sensitivity generally increases by only a factor of 2 to 10.[9] This apparent paradox emphasizes that the major determinant that enhances sensitivity of the assay at the level of the reporter is the affinity of the antibody and the signal/noise ratio.

E. DILUENTS AND WASH SOLUTIONS

1. Specimen Diluent

Simple salt buffers (e.g., phosphate-buffered saline [PBS]), buffers with nonionic detergents, and complex protein solutions containing animal serum are suitable specimen diluents. The specimen diluent should contain all potentially immunoreactive constituents that are used during the coating process, except the reactants. For example, if fetal calf serum was used to saturate the plastic during manufacture of an indirect ELISA for antigen X, it should also be present in the specimen diluent to act as a competitor for patient antibodies that may react against bovine proteins on the solid phase.

In a sandwich ELISA that employs murine monoclonal antibodies, heterophile antibodies in the human test specimen may cause a false-positive test. In the absence of analyte, the heterophile reacts with mouse IgG and causes bridging between the two parts of the sandwich. Again, the presence of mouse IgG in the diluent effectively prevents the heterophile antibody from interacting with the solid phase.

2. Wash Solution

The design of the wash solution should result in the effective removal of nonspecifically bound analyte and enzyme conjugate. This is achieved through empirical manipulation of salt concentration and, whenever possible, by inclusion of a nonionic detergent. Washing efficiency is reflected by a low absorbance value for the conjugate blank (<0.1) and specimen blank (<0.2). If TMB is used with HRP, deionized water (CAP Type 1, USP or equivalent) devoid of interfering agents (e.g., trace metals) is mandatory.

F. SPECIMENS, STANDARDS, AND CONTROLS

1. Specimens

Although serum is most frequently used as the specimen, whole blood, plasma, and serosal and joint fluids may be subject to testing. A lipemic or hemolyzed sample may alter the results; therefore, procedures should be available to clarify the sample and to minimize red cell damage. The influence of storage conditions of blood or serum may significantly influence the performance of the assay. For example, for antibody testing the blood may clot at room temperature, and the serum can be stored at room temperature for as long as 5 days. Unless the serum sample will be tested within 30 days, the sample is frozen. The lab may store serum samples at −20°C for prolonged periods (12 months), or at −70°C. However, the level of certain autoantibodies may decrease significantly after thawing.

Cryoglobulins may distort test results. Rheumatoid factor activity, as well as other autoantibodies (anti-DNA), may be lost during cryoprecipitation; therefore, if cryoglobulins are suspected, clot formation should occur in a water bath (37°C) and the serum should be immediately tested. Sodium citrated or heparinized plasma is also acceptable as long as the temperature is maintained near 37°C.

The influence of IgM rheumatoid factor (RF) on the performance of ELISAs that detect IgG antibodies warrants comment. Theoretically, if the patient has serum IgM RF and the intent is to detect IgG antibody, IgM RF may bind to the IgG antibody immobilized by the reactant. The IgM RF could block binding of the enzyme conjugate, producing a false-negative result. On the other hand, when the goal is to measure IgM class antibody, IgM RF becomes attached to the IgG antibody on the solid phase and causes a falsely abnormal IgM antibody test result. It has been suggested that pepsin digestion of the serum sample to produce $F(ab')_2$ fragments may eliminate this problem. However, in our experience, antibodies of IgM and IgG class against various antigens can be measured without interference in sera of patients with very high levels of RF. Nonetheless, to ensure that RF does not alter the performance of a newly implemented ELISA test, serum samples from patients with high levels of IgM RF should be tested to provide assurance that the system is not altered by IgM RF.

2. Standards and Controls

A standard is a material that has been established by a recognized national or international authority as the rule for the measurement of the analyte in the test specimen. For example, antibody standards are either individual or pooled sera that have been characterized empirically against a defined antigen preparation for quantity, quality, and specificity. A certain number of units, such as 100 or 1000, are assigned arbitrarily. These standards differ from control sera, which lack assigned unit activity.

To enhance accuracy, the standard is used to determine the quantity of analyte in the unknown either by heterologous interpolation of a standard curve or by one-point calibration. The characteristic sigmoidal shape of a linear standard curve may be transformed to extend the linear portion of the curve that is subsequently available for interpolation.[3,5] Since the multipoint standard curve offers more accurate results than the one-point calibration method, the former approach should be used when the goal is to study levels of an analyte longitudinally in patient serum.

Inasmuch as implementation of the one-point calibrator reduces operational costs, it is often used by the clinical laboratory. Nevertheless, this approach results in an assay that is prone to greater systematic error (bias). If one-point calibration is implemented, the laboratory should generate a multipoint curve to determine the interval wherein the slope of the calibrator is linear. To obtain reasonably accurate results, the absorbance values for the unknowns should fall in this region of the curve.

The World Health Organization (WHO) and Centers for Disease Control (CDC) (Atlanta, GA) provide various standards and positive controls (see Appendix). Commercial sources also offer standards (or calibrators), but the designated units may not correspond to the international system of units. Thus, an internal laboratory standard may be prepared by sufficiently diluting a known reactive specimen with normal serum until it matches the unit value observed for the external standard. The working standard should be validated against a stored standard (external or internal) at predetermined intervals that are defined by test sample volume (e.g., every 3 to 12 months). Generally, the activity of a working standard for ELISA (expressed as units) should vary by no more than 15% of the value obtained for the original stored standard (tested in triplicate). If the deviation exceeds this value, the following parameters may be adjusted: (1) the amount of reactant on the solid phase, (2) the concentration of enzyme conjugate, and (3) the amount of analyte in the working standard (calibrator).

Normal and abnormal controls ensure that the assay functions as intended for clinical specimens; they are available from CDC (AF/CDC ANA Reference Laboratory, Center for Disease Control, Immunology Branch, 1600 Clifton Road, 1-1202 A25, Atlanta, GA), from commercial sources, or may be prepared in the lab as internal controls.

G. STEPS IN ELISA PROCEDURES

The following are steps for an indirect ELISA procedure. Other specific applications will appear in subsequent chapters.

1. Dilution of specimens and controls — Specimens, controls, and calibrators are usually diluted in specimen diluent (1/50, 1/100, or 1/200). To obtain a standard curve three to four dilutions of the calibrator (standard) are prepared. If a large number of specimens and/or multiple antigens are tested, dispensing all the specimens and standards in a timely fashion improves precision. A relatively simple solution is to use 96-well formatted racks of minitubes. The specimen is added to the minitubes containing the diluent; caps, available as strings, are placed on all minitubes. With pressure exercised on the caps with a rigid surface the tubes are turned upside-down four to five times for a complete mix. An effective mix may also be obtained with a multichannel pipettor. Poor mixing results in aberrant results.

2. Incubation with specimen — To avoid incubation time differences between standards, controls, and specimens, all diluted samples (100 μl) should be added within a short period of time. Premixed specimens are dispensed with an 8- or 12-channel pipettor in less than 1 min. The plates are incubated (30 min) at room temperature. If multiple plates are used loading of the antigen should be staggered at intervals equal to the washing time (4 to 6 min/plate). After incubation the plates are washed three to four times with 200 to 400 μl of wash solution.

3. Incubation with enzyme conjugate — The anti-Ig enzyme conjugate is added and the plates are incubated again at room temperature (e.g., 30 min), washed three to four times, and thoroughly blotted on absorbent paper to remove residual wash buffer.

4. Addition of substrate and reading the absorbance — The substrate is dispensed and the reaction is terminated by adding a stop solution (e.g., sulfuric or phosphoric acid) after a predetermined time (e.g., 10 or 15 min) and the absorbance determined. For kinetic analysis readings are taken at various time intervals until the color reaction reaches a predetermined value, usually the highest for which the reaction is still linear (e.g., 1.2) (see Instrumentation, below).

III. INSTRUMENTATION AND MEASUREMENTS FOR ELISA

A. THE ELISA READER: DETERMINATION OF ABSORBANCE VALUES

The intensity of the color (light absorbance) that a degraded chromogenic substrate generates is measured at the appropriate wavelength (color filters) with an ELISA reader (see Appendix, commercial sources). The absorbance level (or optical density) depends on the concentration of product and the height of the fluid column. Consequently, if the fluid volume is doubled with colorless diluent (e.g., water), the absorbance value in the well does not change significantly. For example, if wash solution is accidentally added instead of stop reagent (acid), the test run may be salvaged by the addition of the stop reagent.

The absorbance value for a microwell is the sum of the absorbance value contributed by the color change plus any light-absorbing material in the path of the beam (e.g., incidental scratches or smudges on the bottom of the well). To correct for spurious absorbance, a dual reading spectrophotometer is set at the specific wavelength to measure the color reaction (e.g., 450 nm yellow) and at an unrelated wavelength (e.g., 630 nm blue). The value obtained at 630 defines nonspecific absorbance and is automatically subtracted.

The selection of a reader (manual, semiautomated, or robotic) is influenced primarily by the needs of the laboratory. A small office lab that infrequently performs a limited variety of tests may prefer a manual reader, a hospital laboratory with moderate volume may use a semiautomated reader, and a large regional or national reference lab that has high sample throughput and desires flexible formatting of the plates may need a robotic or automated system. Semiautomated readers measure the absorbance values in sequential rows or scan the entire plate. Many readers contain microprocessors that perform such manipulations as blank well subtraction and basic data reduction tasks. However, the increased availability of powerful personal computers combined with specialized software facilitates sophisticated data analysis (see Appendix) and thereby minimizes the necessity for readers to have advanced microprocessors.

To ensure that the measured absorbance value for a test sample is reliable, the value should be obtained from the linear portion of the "color versus absorbance" curve specified for the instrument. Although the upper limit of the linear range for absorbance may vary from 1.2 to 4.0, most instruments offer a linear range up to 2.0. Inasmuch as the absorbance value for a specimen may exceed the linearity of the instrument, various strategies have been suggested to determine minimum absorbance value without resorting to the retesting of a more dilute specimen. For a substrate whose maximum absorbance occurs at 450 nm, the sample may be measured at a different wavelength.[10] In this instance the value is significantly lower (e.g., 0.8 instead of 2.4) and well within the linear range of the instrument. Another approach is to replace 50% of the microwell volume with a clear fluid (water or an acid solution). The observed absorbance value is then multiplied by a factor of two. Another procedure is the kinetic reading at preset time intervals. Subsequently time is used as a factor in the equation for the calculation of total absorbance. Computer programs, such as Kineticalc™ from Biotek (see Appendix), keep track of the values in all wells, facilitating data generation.

Modern ELISA readers are configured to perform self-check of their linear range. Validation by manual technique, however, may be required by government agencies or professional regulatory groups. Analysis may be performed with a set of manufactured plates that have different color intensities. Preferably, the accuracy of instrument readings is determined with various dilutions of the working substrate. A small amount of enzyme conjugate and the substrate are mixed and, when the absorbance value reaches a value between 1.0 and 2.0, the reaction is terminated with acid solution (1 *M* sulfuric). The solution is diluted with deionized water to approximately 1.0. To perform the calibration, twofold dilutions of the stock solution are prepared in water and pipetted into microwells. After setting up the blank (water), the wells are read and the blank is subtracted to provide net values that are tabulated:

Expected Absorbance	Measure Absorbance	Ratio
1.20	1.20	1.00
0.60	0.58	0.96
0.30	0.31	1.03
0.15	0.14	0.93

At low absorbance values (<0.2) the effect of the noise created by the blank may affect the ratio more than at the high values. Ratios that range from 0.9 to 1.1 are acceptable for most clinical assays.

Most ELISA plate readers are interfaced with a computer that uses software to facilitate data reduction (see Appendix). The report to the clinician should include the normal and abnormal ranges for each test value (see Chapters 3, 6, and 9). In addition, graphic display of data, particularly for multiple analytes, is desirable because the presentation facilitates rapid interpretation.

B. ACCURACY, PRECISION, AND BIAS

Accuracy is best defined by the absence of errors that are generated by bias and imprecision. Imprecision reflects the random errors that cause measurements to be scattered about a mean value that approximates the true value, whereas bias stems from systematic errors in which all measurements are equally deflected from the true value. Precision is estimated by determining the standard deviation or coefficient of variation (C.V.) of replicate measurements that span the range of analyte concentration (precision profile) (C.V.s <10% are acceptable for ELISA tests). Precision is influenced by the physical characteristic of the specimen (e.g., viscosity), quality of the pipettes and instruments, incubation time-dependent drift, the skill of the technologist, and the strategy for data transformation. On the other hand, the use of a standard (calibration) curve that contains an analyte which parallels the activity present in the unknown samples reduces bias. Under ideal conditions, the quantity and behavior of analyte in the specimen and the standard are identical and both are directly proportional to the measured absorbance value.

The following assumptions hold for measured absorbance: (1) the recorded value is directly proportional to the concentration of end product (see instrument linearity above);

(2) accumulated end product does not inhibit the enzymatic reaction; (3) the enzymatic reaction occurs in substrate excess; (4) the solubility of degradation products remains constant through-out the concentration range encountered in the assay; and (5) the quantity of analyte in the test sample is proportional to that attached to the solid phase. While the first four conditions are usually achieved by experimental manipulation of the chosen enzyme/substrate system, the fifth condition is partially fulfilled by generating a standard curve. The composition and behavior of the standard, however, are rarely identical to those of the analyte; therefore, the effect of standardization on test bias is relative.

Although a multipoint standard curve may minimize bias, for clinical testing certain compromises are necessary to ensure that the assay is accurate and reliable, but at the same time economical and practical. Therefore, a one-point standard (or calibrator) is substituted for the standard curve, even when the slope of the standard curve diverges significantly from the ideal value of 1.0. The general equation for a one-point standard is

$$\text{units in specimen} = \frac{\text{units in calibrator}}{\text{Abs. of calibrator}} \times \text{Abs. of specimen} \times \frac{\text{Dilution of specimen}}{\text{Dilution of calibrator}}$$

The first two parts of the equation are constant for the entire test run and are calculated first as the calibration factor.

C. ACCESSORY TOOLS AND MATERIALS

1. Washing devices

The effective removal of nonspecifically bound reactants enhances accuracy. Multi-channel single or repeat pipettors are commonly used to manually wash the 96-well plate. Fluid that remains after the wash may produce a dilution error by as much as 10% at each step. Therefore, the plate should be tapped vigorously on an absorbent material (e.g., paper towels) to remove residual fluid. If four or more plates are assayed simultaneously, devices that wash either the entire plate or individual rows are cost-effective alternatives.

2. Micropipettes, microtubes, and other accessories

Eight- to 12-channel pipettors (40 to 200 μl) facilitate the loading of multiple samples. Specimens may be diluted in microtubes (1 to 2 ml) racked in the format of 96-well ELISA plate and then transferred to the appropriate microwells with the multichannel pipettor. The microtubes have caps connected as strings and may be used to mix the specimens in their diluents by inverting the entire rack four or five times. Pipettors should be recalibrated periodically; they are a major source of error.

3. Robotics

Robotics that perform ELISA testing in the 96-microwell plate format are available from several manufacturers (see Appendix). The device performs dilutions, dispenses the specimens, conjugates, and the substrate, and reads the absorbance and calculates the results. For the average rheumatology laboratory available robotic instruments do not offer a significant advantage in labor costs or precision over a simple combination of a computer-controlled reader and a plate washer.

IV. IMPLEMENTATION, VALIDATION, AND QUALITY CONTROL OF ELISA TESTS

A. NORMAL REFERENCE RANGE AND ABNORMAL VALUES

Older immunoassays were often reported merely as "positive" and "negative". This nomenclature fostered the perception among clinicians that their patient was either absolutely positive or negative for the test, which carried the connotation of wellness or disease. For example, when the laboratory reports the result to the clinician that a patient is "ANA positive", the clinician casually relates the result to the patient, who then anxiously seeks further medical advice and treatment for being "positive". Obviously, these terms are applicable when the analyte is either present or absent (e.g., identification of HLA-B27). The results for most assays, however, are reported numerically and the patient's value is compared to a normal reference range. The clinician then is able to ascertain not only whether the patient is "positive" but how greatly the test value differs from the normal range (e.g., borderline vs. significant divergence). The clinician may then report the numeric value to the patient and interpret the result as normal, borderline, or abnormal. Throughout the text we shall substitute normal and abnormal for positive and negative.

For most immunoassay kits, the manufacturer identifies the normal reference range. This range, however, may vary in different populations; therefore, the laboratory should independently validate the reference range. The following guidelines, based on a recent review, provide the framework for such a protocol.[11]

The distribution of values for any detected autoantibody obtained from either a pool of normals or patients is inherently non-gaussian (i.e., nonparametric). Therefore, the upper limit of normal cannot be defined properly as the mean plus two or three standard deviations. The uppermost normal value, however, can be established by testing normals in multiples of at least 100. The upper limit is designated by a defined percentile value and should be accompanied by the confidence value. For example, the 95th percentile may be considered the cut-off for the normal range where a 0.90 confidence interval was used. The uppermost five values are then "potentially abnormal".

Despite defined confidence values, the cut-off percentile is frequently designated by convention (e.g., 95%). When an antibody is relatively prevalent in the "normal population", the number of false abnormal tests may be reduced by choosing a cut-off level that is likely to exclude a reasonable percentage of the normals. To facilitate the decision making, a distribution curve of antibody values (i.e., ranking) for the normals is generated (Figure 4). For autoantibody testing the curve will be significantly skewed to the right, inasmuch as a few normals will have values that are distinctly higher than the majority, which will cluster at a lower point on the scale. For an antibody that is relatively prevalent among normals (e.g., anti-SSA), exclusion of the values that are clearly disparate from the majority (e.g., uppermost five) would indicate that the 95th percentile is the normal limit. On the other hand, for relatively uncommon antibodies, such as anti-dsDNA, -Sm, -SSB, and -Scl70, the exclusion of the highest one value may be acceptable (99th percentile) (Chapter 6).

B. DIAGNOSTIC SENSITIVITY, SPECIFICITY, AND PREDICTIVE VALUE

An optimal diagnostic test should be interpreted as abnormal when applied to a patient known to have the disease and as normal when performed on an individual known to

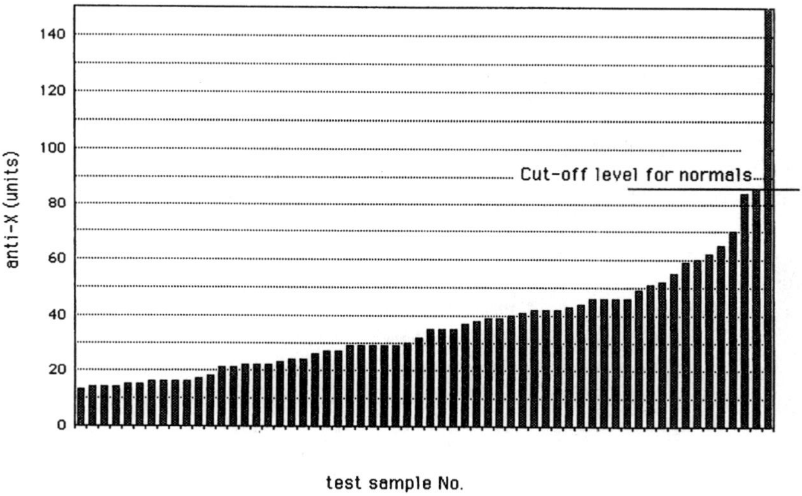

Figure 4 Distribution of autoantibody levels for an antigen in a control population used to determine the upper limits. Explanation in the text.

be free of the disease in question. The diagnostic sensitivity of a test is the proportion of true abnormal results in patients with the specific disease. Thus, a good diagnostic test should be highly sensitive; i.e., it should give abnormal values in patients with the disease of interest.

$$\text{Sensivity} = \frac{\text{True Abnormal}}{\text{True Abnormal} + \text{False Normal}} \times 100$$

Conversely, a good diagnostic test should also give normal values in non-diseased individuals. Specificity is the term applied to describe the frequency or proportion of true-normal.

$$\text{Specificity} = \frac{\text{True Normal}}{\text{True Normal} + \text{False Abnormal}} \times 100$$

For a test to have diagnostic utility, it must have a high predictive value (i.e., the proportion of all abnormal values that are true abnormal). The predictive value of a positive test calculates as follows:

$$\text{Predictive Value} = \frac{\text{True Abnormal}}{\text{True Abnormal} + \text{False Abnormal}} \times 100$$

The predictive value of a test varies according to the prevalence of the disease. For example, to determine the value of a diagnostic test, 30 patients with the disease and 30 age- and sex-matched controls are tested. In the study 26 patients had abnormal tests, one control was abnormal, and the remaining 29 were normal.

$$\text{Sensitivity} = \frac{26}{26 + 4} \times 100 = 86\%$$

$$\text{Specificity} = \frac{29}{29 + 1} \times 100 = 96\%$$

$$\text{Predictive Value} = \frac{26}{26 + 1} \times 100 = 96\%$$

Thus, the test appears to have relatively high sensitivity, specificity, and predictive values. This, however, is applicable if the prevalence of disease is 50% (i.e., 30 of 60 in the study have the disease). The test is now implemented by a clinical lab and performed on 300 patients. The prevalence of the disease is 1%, therefore three patients will have abnormal tests (i.e., true abnormals). Although the test is specific (96%), among the 300 patients, 12 individuals will test falsely abnormal. Therefore, the predictive value of the test at 1% disease prevalence becomes:

$$\text{Predictive Value} = \frac{3}{1 + 12} \times 100 = 23\%$$

As the prevalence of the disease decreases, the number of true abnormals, by definition, also decreases and the number of false abnormals is likely to increase. Therefore, a useful diagnostic test should have high clinical specificity and predictive value. These goals are sometimes achieved through a reduction in the diagnostic sensitivity of the assay (see the previous section).

C. VERIFICATION OF CLAIMS FOR THE ASSAY

An ELISA test may be adopted by the lab to measure a new clinical parameter or to replace an operative technique. In either case, the laboratory must verify the analytical claims of the manufacturer. Analytical parameters that should be verified are accuracy, precision, and the linear range of the assay.[12] To assess accuracy, at least 40 patient comparisons should be performed with an assay previously adopted by the lab. Although designed to determine if the two techniques have equivalent performance, the experiment may also provide information that the ELISA-based assay is more specific and has a greater predictive value. If a comparative assay is unavailable, accuracy is assessed with samples of known analyte value that are obtained from several sources (e.g., College of American Pathologists reference materials). Precision (within run) is evaluated with three different concentrations of analyte that span the linear range of the test. One level of analyte should be slightly above the reference range. Linearity is tested by analyzing dilutions of a specimen and plotting the data on xy graph paper.

D. QUALITY ASSURANCE (QA)

Quality assurance is generally described as a system in which quality control (QC) and proficiency testing (PT) are used to substantiate that routine tests conform to specified performance criteria. In this context the goals of a QA program are to ensure that the testing is performed in an accurate and reproducible manner and that the results generated provide information that significantly contributes to quality health care. For a given

Date____/____/____Kit Lot #__________#__________#__________#__________

Performed by _____Verified by _____[ ] New run [ ] Repeat run of: ____/____/____

TEST NAME (circle applicable): ____ ______ ______ ______
______ ______ ______ ______ ______ All as a panel

[_] ACCEPTABLE PERFORMANCE OF COMPONENTS

Blanks: Calibrators < ______[ ]OK Normal control <._____[ ]OK Abnormal control <______[ ]OK

Enzyme conjugate< ______[ ]OK Specimens < ________[ ]OK except #______________

Substrate blank < __________[ ]OK

Calibrators (standards) ([ ] name > absorbance) (e.g. anti-X Ab > 0.7)

[ ]______>______ [ ]______>______ [ ]______>______ [ ]______>______

[ ]______>______ [ ]______>______ [ ]______>______ [ ]______>______

Previous calibrator (s) used for: ____ ____ ____ ____ ____ ____ ____
Date calibrator (s) previously used: ____/____/____

[_] ACCEPTABLE LONGITUDINAL TREND

Tra nd of calibrator (absorbance) ________ **[ ] Acceptable** behavior
[ ] Downward shift for ________ [ ] Downward trend for ________
[ ] Upward shift for ________ [ ] Upward trend for ________

*Trand of Positive Controls (units)*________ **[ ] Acceptable**
[ ] Downward shift for ________ [ ] Downward trend for ________
[ ] Upward shift for ________ [ ] Upward trend for ________

Trand of Negative Control (units:) **[ ] Acceptable**
[ ] Downward shift for ________ [ ] Downward trend for ________
[ ] Upward shift for ________ [ ] Upward trend for ________

[_] ACCEPTABLE REPORTABLE RESULTS

Relationships between paired analytes detected simulataneously (see Table 1, #7):

______>______ [ ] YES [ ] NO= [ ] repeat OR **[ ] Acceptable**
______>______ [ ] YES [ ] NO = [ ] repeat OR **[ ] Acceptable**
______=______ [ ] YES [ ] NO = [ ] repeat OR **[ ] Acceptable**

Adjacent Specimens : have very similar unit values for particular analyte
[ ] NO: **acceptable**
[ ] YES: Specimen No. and tests________________________

Frequent abnormal values for a relatively rare analyte [ ] NO: **acceptable**

Specimen No. and tests________________________

[_] ACCEPTABLE RUN [_] REPEAT RUN : [ ] All Specimens **OR** only

[ ] Specimen No. and tests________________________

Figure 5 Model form for quality control for ELISA tests. Explanation in the text.

technique, the monitors for effective QC and PT generally focus on the behavior of the blanks, calibrators, controls, and test specimens. The observations are documented with a form that also ensures that personnel systematically evaluates each component of the assay. Although this review process may be computerized, professional regulatory agencies require periodic manual validation of computer-generated data. A general form is shown in Figure 5.

Applicability of the form — This form may be used for a single test, such as anti-dsDNA antibody, or for several related tests that form a panel. If the panel is assembled from different kits, all lot numbers are entered to ensure traceability.

Acceptability of results — After reviewing each section a check mark is placed in the box on the left side that signifies acceptable performance. If all categories are acceptable, the test results are reported.

Behavior of controls — The upper limit of absorbance for blanks are entered on the form: (1) the substrate blank tests reaction of the solid phase with the substrate; (2) the conjugate (specimen diluent) blank tests nonspecific binding of enzyme conjugate to the solid phase; (3) the specimen blank controls for nonspecific attachment of specimen material to a solid phase in the absence of the immobilized reactant. The substrate blank is useful to determine whether the substrate solution has been contaminated by enzyme. When the absorbance values for specimen blanks of multiple specimens are elevated, one or more of the following conditions may exist:

- Inefficient washing and/or blotting, i.e., residual enzyme conjugate in microwell
- Excess conjugate (inaccurate pipetting?)
- Contaminated washing buffer contains an exogenous source of enzyme
- Prolonged incubation time at any one of the steps
- Incorrect mixing of the specimen in diluent
- Substrate solution contaminated during previous run; substrate solutions that are a mixture of two reactants should be prepared immediately before each run

Inasmuch as patients with autoimmune diseases have hypergammaglobulinemia, the specimen blank controls for nonspecific binding of the patient's gammaglobulins. This control is particularly important for assays that measure levels of autoantibodies. An isolated high specimen blank value may be due to:

- Ineffective protein saturation of the solid phase
- Hydrophobic immunoglobulins in the specimens; repetition of the test will yield similar results
- Binding of material in the specimen to immobilized reactant
- Heterophile antibodies
- Accidental contamination of a microwell with a droplet of conjugate

Behavior of calibrators and controls — Most commercial immunoassays use one-point calibrators, with the caveat that the slope of the calibration curve rarely approaches 1.0. Consequently, a unit value that is twice as large as another should not be interpreted as a doubling of the unit value but rather as a significant increase. The performance of the calibrator is influenced by system noise. An elevation in the absorbance value of a specimen blank reduces the net value of the calibrator; this, in turn, increases the calibration factor. As a consequence, the unit values for the positive and negative controls will be greater than expected. Similarly, certain normal specimens may have abnormal values. Similarly, a minimum absorbance value for the calibrator is also monitored. The fluctuation in the absorbance values for calibrators and the unit values for positive and negative controls are visualized by sequential plotting of the data for each run. This approach offers immediate feedback for performance of the test system (e.g., a sudden shift in a value is noted) and facilitates the identification of anomalous trends in system components. For example, when the calibrator displays aberrant behavior, the following may exist:

A sudden upward shift in the absorbance value of the calibrator suggests:

- Inadequate dilution
- Inadequate protein saturation of a particular well
- Accidental contamination of a well with enzyme conjugate

A downward shift suggests:

- Excessive dilution
- Quality of the water for wash solution is poor

A downward trend suggests:

- Loss of analyte in the calibrator
- Poor storage or transport conditions

Repeat testing is generally the best approach when a plausible explanation for an aberrant result is not forthcoming. However, when the results for a large number of specimens are suspect, under certain conditions the run may be salvaged. For example, the absorbance value for the calibrator abruptly drops but the values for the controls are comparable to the previous run of the same lot. In this instance, the absorbance value for the calibrator may be "borrowed" from this run to calculate unit values for the specimens. This is recorded on a dated QC form. To ensure that the decision was valid, two or three specimens can be retested in the next run. Standard curves may be stored for multiple runs.

The behavior of unknown samples — In a particular disease, two or more analytes may frequently be abnormal (e.g., anti-SSA and anti-SSB antibody levels — see Chapters 5, 6, and 7). Thus, when the usual behavior is not displayed, a technical error is considered. Another common problem is that an autoantibody is frequently detected slightly above the reference range. In this instance if the antibody has a low prevalence, the solution is to adjust the reference range. Contiguous specimens may produce similar values for a particular analyte. The most likely explanation is that the same test sample was inadvertently pipetted into two adjacent wells. The organization of specimens and their diluent, therefore, warrants evaluation. The final decision may be to repeat the test run on some or all of the specimens. Inasmuch as ELISA is highly sensitive, it is advisable to repeat the test when the result is ambiguous.

In addition to monitoring the technical performance of the assay, the test should be continuously monitored to ensure that it provides clinically meaningful information. Some suggested procedures are

- Periodic chart review of sets of normal and abnormal results, particularly after the final diagnosis is established
- Documentation and review of inquiries by clinicians about specific cases
- Surveys of clinicians regarding the clinical relevance of test results
- Formal clinical studies

REFERENCES

1. **Carpenter, A. B.,** Enzyme linked immunoassays, in *Manual of Clinical Laboratory Immunology,* 4th ed., Rose, N. R., de Macario, J. L., Fahey, J. L., Friedman, H., and Penn, G. M., Eds., American Society of Microbiology, Washington, D.C., 1992, 2.
2. **Ternyck, T. and Avrameas, S.,** *Immuno-Enzymatic Techniques, Techniques in Immunology,* Vol. 1, Elsevier, Amsterdam, 1990, 1.
3. **Kemeny, D. M. and Challacombe, S. H.,** *ELISA and Other Solid Phase Immunoassays,* John Wiley & Sons, New York, 1988.
4. **Nakamura, R. M., Peebles, C., Rubin, R., Molden, D., and Tan, E. M.,** *Autoantibodies to Nuclear Antigens (ANA),* American Society of Clinical Pathologists, New York, 1985.
5. **Butler, J. E.,** *Immunochemistry of Solid-Phase Immunoassay,* CRC Press, Boca Raton, FL, 1991, 1.
6. **Kenney, J. S., Masasda, M. P., and Allison, A. C.,** Development of two-site ELISA for soluble proteins, in *Laboratory Methods in Immunology,* Zola, H., Ed., CRC Press, Boca Raton, FL, 1990, 230.
7. **Butler, J. E., Ni, L., Nessler, R., Joshi, K. S., Suter, M., Rosenberg, B., Chang, J., Brown, W. R., and Cantarero, L. A.,** The physical and functional behavior of capture antibodies adsorbed on polystyrene, *J. Immunol. Meth.,* 150, 77, 1992.
8. **Schwab, C. and Bosshard, H. R.,** Caveats for the use of surface-adsorbed protein antigen to test the specificity of antibodies, *J. Immunol. Meth.,* 147, 125, 1992.
9. **Porstmann, T. and Kiessig, S. T.,** Enzyme immunoassay techniques. An overview, *J. Immunol. Meth.,* 150, 5, 1992.
10. **Madersbacher, S. and Berger, P.,** Double wavelength measurement of 3,3′,5,5′-tetamethylbenzidine (TMB) provides a three-fold enhancement of ELISA measuring range, *J. Immunol. Meth.,* 158, 121, 1993.
11. **Young, D. S.,** Determination and validation of reference ranges, *Arch. Pathol. Lab. Med.,* 116, 704, 1992.
12. **Hartmann, A. E.,** The concept of establishing vs verifying analytic claims in methods evaluation, *Arch. Pathol. Lab. Med.,* 116, 714, 1992.

II. Rheumatoid Factor

Chapter 2

Rheumatoid Factor: Mechanisms of Production and Biological Significance

William J. Koopman and Ralph E. Schrohenloher

CONTENTS

I. INTRODUCTION

Autoantibodies directed against the Fc portion of IgG, commonly designated rheumatoid factors (RF), were initially identified in the sera of patients with rheumatoid arthritis (RA). In addition, however, it is clear that RF also may be present in the sera of ostensibly healthy individuals and patients with a variety of chronic infectious and inflammatory diseases. Considerable evidence suggests that RF, likely in the form of RF-IgG immune complexes, contributes to tissue injury in some of these diseases, particularly RA.

The observation that a significant fraction of paraproteins possesses RF activity prompted intensive investigation of these monoclonal proteins, with the belief that they were representative of RF present in other diseases. These studies have yielded important insights concerning the structure, binding specificity, and biologic functions of these molecules. Unexpectedly, it was shown that germline immunoglobulin variable region genes capable of encoding RF are highly conserved in the population, suggesting that RF (either fluid-phase or membrane-bound) subserve an important physiologic role(s). The results of these studies have provided a useful framework for approaching similar questions regarding the properties and origins of polyclonal RF present in diseases such as RA. While the molecular basis of RF production in human disease remains unclear, results obtained from the study of animal models indicate that exaggerated expression of RF in disease reflects an antigen-driven process rather than nonspecific polyclonal activation.

0-8493-5974-1/94/$0.00 + $.50

Table 1 **Major Human Rheumatoid Factors**

Immunoglobulin Isotype	Molecular Form	Approximate Mol Wt	Sedimentation Constant
IgM	Pentamer	900,000	19S
	Complexed with IgG	1,700,000	22S
IgA	Monomer	16,000	7S
	Polymer	32,000–~1,000,000	10S–20S
IgG	Monomer	150,000	7S
	Self-associated complexes	300,000–~600,000	9S–17S

A brief review of the structure and specificity of RF is presented elsewhere in this chapter, followed by a discussion of the mechanisms underlying RF expression and the biologic properties of these autoantibodies. Methods for the detection of RF are described elsewhere in this volume (see Chapter 3).

II. STRUCTURE AND SPECIFICITY

As depicted in Table 1, RF exhibits considerable immunochemical heterogeneity in the rheumatic diseases. In addition to IgM RF (readily detected by common serologic tests), the occurrence of IgA-RF and IgG-RF is well established[1-4] and IgE-RF has also been detected.[5] Structurally, IgM-RF consists of five identical subunits (molecular weight 185,000 Da each) joined by disulfide bonds to form a pentameric structure exhibiting a valence of 5. Complexes of IgM-RF and IgG, containing one molecule of IgM-RF and five molecules of IgG, occur in the sera of some patients with rheumatoid arthritis; these 22S complexes have a molecular weight of approximately 1,700,000 Da. IgA-RF present in RA and Sjögren's syndrome is also predominantly polymeric, although serum IgA is mostly monomeric.[6,7] Alternative assay procedures have also revealed the presence of some monomeric IgA-RF activity in both serum and synovial fluid from patients with RA.[7] While IgG-RF is exclusively monomeric, complex formation with itself and other IgG molecules can yield higher-molecular-weight forms.[8,9]

The binding specificity of RF found in the rheumatic diseases has not been completely delineated. Several allotypic and nonallotypic determinants distributed among all four subclasses if IgG have been identified among RF in RA.[10] All are located within the Fc portion (i.e., the C_H2 and C_H3 domains) of the molecule.

Most RF in the serum of RA patients appear specific for the nonallotypic Ga (or γ1-2-4) site present on IgG1, IgG2, and IgG4 molecules.[10,11] Studies with proteolytic cleavage fragments of IgG have revealed that this site is located in the C_H2 domain or C_H2-C_H3 interface region[10,12] and may overlap with the sites recognized by bacterial Fc-binding proteins.[13] Evidence that IgM-RF synthesized by rheumatoid synovial plasma cells has a greater reactivity and avidity for IgG3 than IgG1 suggests that one or more sites on IgG3 may also be important antigens for RF.[14,15] This site has been localized to the C_H3 domain of the molecule.[15]

RF reactive with the Gm(a) (Gm1) and Gm(x) (Gm2) allotypic groups present in the C_H3 region of IgG1 and Gm(b1) (Gm5) and Gm(g) (Gm21) groups present in the C_H2 region of IgG3 may also be present in the sera of RA patients.[16-19] In addition, specificities for the isoallotypic groups "non-a", "γ4-non-a", and "non-b1" have been identified.[20-22] Isoallotypic groups occur as genetic variants in one IgG subclass but they are present on all molecules of at least one other subclass. For example, non-a is an allotypic antigen antithetic to Gm(a) in IgG1 and is an isotypic antigen present on all IgG2 and IgG3 molecules. It is also present on IgG1 molecules positive for Gm(f) (Gm3).

RF in RA characteristically exhibit broad cross-reactivity with several mammalian IgG, including rabbit, bovine, and equine IgG.[23] Although most RF appear to react *in toto* with human IgG, differences in the extent of cross-reactivity have been described.[24] RF that cross-react with rabbit IgG are specific for the Ga site or closely related structures of human IgG together with the ''non-a'' antigen.[25]

III. MOLECULAR BASIS OF RF EXPRESSION

A. MECHANISMS UNDERLYING RF INDUCTION

The fact that RF are a heterogeneous group of autoantibodies reactive with several epitopes localized in the Fc portion of IgG,[26] coupled with evidence that specificities of RF in various diseases may differ, such as in subacute bacterial endocarditis (SBE) and RA, suggests that alternative mechanisms likely contribute to the induction and perpetuation of RF expression in these diseases. Elucidation of such pathways should provide helpful insights concerning disease pathogenesis.

Polyclonal B cell activators have proven to be potent inducers of RF expression, both *in vitro* and *in vivo*. Several of these agents, including lipopolysaccharide (LPS),[27] pokeweed mitogen,[28] staphylococcal protein A,[29] and the Epstein-Barr virus (EBV),[30] are active in this regard. The capacity of these agents to induce RF production *in vitro* by B cells obtained from healthy individuals demonstrated that RF-programmed B cells are constituents of the normal B cell repertoire.[28,30]

Induction of RF production in animals has been accomplished using a variety of immunization techniques. Repeated immunization with several antigens elicited expression of auto-anti-IgG antibodies,[31-33] which were demonstrated to be directed against host IgG complexed to the immunizing antigen.[34,35] Secondary immunization in man is also accompanied by transient RF responses,[36,37] presumably triggered by IgG-containing immune complexes formed during the secondary immune response.

Cross-reactivities of some RF with non-IgG antigens, including DNA-histone,[38] non-histone nuclear protein,[39] denatured DNA,[40] and nitrophenyl groups,[41] have been reported and raise the possibility that these or other (as yet unidentified) antigens could contribute to RF expression in some conditions. An intriguing observation in this regard has been the similarity in binding specificity of several bacterial and viral Fc-binding proteins and some RF for the $C\gamma2$-$C\gamma3$ interface region of IgG.[42-44] It has been suggested that exposure to foreign Fc-binding proteins might induce RF through an anti-idiotypic mechanism.[43,45]

Whether polyclonal activation or antigen-driven mechanisms contribute to RF expression in human disease remains uncertain. However, RF present in autoimmune MRL/*lpr* mice exhibit patterns of variable region somatic mutations most consistent with an antigen-driven response.[46] Similar conclusions have been reached for anti-DNA antibodies also present in autoimmune MRL/*lpr* mice.[47] These data have provided compelling evidence that antigen selection plays an important role in the expansion of autoantibody-forming B cell clones in murine models of autoimmune disease. Investigations of the role of antigen selection in human autoantibody responses are in progress, but have not yet yielded conclusive results (see below).

B. POSSIBLE ROLE OF ALTERED IgG

That alterations of IgG structure might contribute to induction of RF also must be considered. Altered glycosylation of IgG in RA has indeed been demonstrated.[48-50] Normal IgG is a glycoprotein with N-linked oligosaccharides, two of which are consistently attached to asparagine residue 297 in the Fc portion of the molecule. Decreased galactose residues in the oligosaccharide moiety located at this residue with resultant termination of the oligosaccharide side-chains in *N*-acetylglucosamine has been observed in RA patients[49] and attributed to reduced levels of B cell galactosyltransferase.[51] While similar glycosylation perturbations of IgG have been observed with aging, this does not adequately explain the abnormality observed in RA.[50]

How might defective galactosylation of IgG contribute to RF expression? One possible explanation might be the unmasking of one or more epitopes, ordinarily obscured in the more completely galactosylated molecule, with consequent induction of RF production.[49] Generation of a monoclonal antibody specific for degalactosylated IgG is consistent with this notion.[52] Other evidence, however, counters this hypothesis. Deficient galactosylation of IgG is observed in Crohn's disease and ulcerative colitis,[50,53,54] diseases rarely accompanied by the appearance of serum RF. Moreover, RF present in RA sera do not bind better to IgG preparations containing abnormally elevated concentrations of degalactosylated IgG than normally galactosylated IgG.[50,55]

Alternative mechanisms leading to alteration of IgG have been identified. Ultraviolet irradiation has been shown to modify cysteine, tryptophan, tyrosine, and lysine residues of the molecule through free radical reactions,[56] leading to a characteristic autofluorescence and partial aggregation. Incubation of IgG with activated neutrophils induces similar alterations of the molecule, presumably via oxygen free radicals (e.g., superoxide anion and hydroxyl radical) released into the media. Enhanced autofluorescence and aggregation of IgG present in rheumatoid sera and synovial fluids has suggested that neutrophil-derived oxygen free radical damage to IgG occurs *in vivo*.

C. CELLULAR ORIGIN OF RF

The possibility that a discrete subpopulation of B cells might preferentially elaborate RF has been actively investigated. Particular attention has been directed to the CD5+ B cell population. Increased numbers of these B cells occur in the blood of patients with RA[57] and Sjögren's syndrome,[58] but not systemic lupus erythematosus (SLE).[59] CD5+ B cells isolated from healthy unimmunized individuals appear to preferentially elaborate several autoantibodies, including RF.[60,61] These autoantibodies characteristically exhibit low affinity and polyspecificity in that they bind to a variety of self-antigens, including the Fc portion of IgG, thyroglobulin, and denatured DNA, as well as foreign antigens such as tetanus toxoid.[62] In contrast, CD5+ B cells obtained from RA patients also produce higher-affinity monoreactive RF.[63] The precise relationship between autoantibodies elaborated by CD5+ B cells *in vitro* and those present in sera of patients with autoimmune disease has not been elucidated.

Murine CD5+ B cells appear to belong to a developmental lineage distinct from conventional B cells.[64] The propensity of these cells to elaborate IgM antibodies reactive with a host of bacterial antigens has prompted speculation that CD5+ B cells may play an important role in natural immunity.[62,65,66] In man, evidence is inconclusive as to whether CD5+ B cells constitute a distinct lineage. Indeed, CD5 may represent a B cell activation antigen in man.[67] Thus, increased circulating CD5+ B cells in RA could reflect enhanced *in vivo* B cells activation also manifested by elevated expression of other cell surface activation markers such as HLA-DR molecules.[68]

Table 2 **Cross-Reactive Idiotypes Associated with IgM Rheumatoid Factor**

	Cross-Reactive Idiotope				
	6B6.6	**17.109**	**G6**	**B6**	**LC1**
V_H/V_L	VκIIIa	VκIIIb	V_H1	V_H3	V_H4
Corresponding germline gene	Humkv328	Humkv325	V_H783	?hv3005	?

Do RF-programmed B cells subserve a physiologic role? In this regard considerable evidence suggests that RF B cells may function as antigen-presenting cells under certain circumstances. Although B cells can take up, process, and present antigen unrelated to the binding specificity of their cell surface immunoglobulin (Ig) molecules, the high concentrations of antigen required argue against this being of physiologic significance.[69] On the other hand, B cells can bind antigen recognized by their cell surface Ig and function efficiently as antigen-presenting cells,[70,71] reflecting the advantage of these cells in competing for specific antigen present in low concentrations. Expression of cell surface Ig capable of binding antigen-IgG complexes permits RF B cells to process and present antigens contained in the immune complexes to antigen-specific T helper cells as efficiently as antigen-specific B cells.[72] Thus, during the course of secondary immune responses in which IgG antibodies directed against the immunogen are elaborated and immune complexes are formed, RF B cells may serve as an increasingly important focus for antigen presentation to T cells. Alternatively, effective competition by RF B cells for antigen complexed with IgG may contribute to the negative feedback influence of antibody on specific immune responses. As previously indicated in Section III.A, antigen complexed to IgG may also lead to the appearance of RF during secondary immune responses.[26,27,73] These observations raise the possibility that RF B cells migrating into the synovium could present a variety of complexed antigens to relevant T helper cells, thereby serving to promote local immune response and enhance synovial RF production in RA patients.

D. GENETIC BASIS OF RF PRODUCTION

Advances in understanding of the molecular basis of RF expression largely derive from the study of IgM paraproteins, since approximately 10% of these monoclonal proteins exhibit RF activity.[74] Using polyclonal heteroantisera directed against variable (V) region epitopes (idiotypes) of RF paraproteins, Kunkel and colleagues defined one major and two minor idiotype families, designated Wa, Po, and Bla.[75,76] While the precise structural basis of these shared idiotypes remains uncertain, members of the Wa RF group exhibit substantial structural similarities.[77,78] The inherent difficulties in distinguishing cross-reactive RF idiotypic groups with polyclonal serologic reagents prompted efforts to generate monoclonal antibodies (mAbs) reactive with structurally defined shared idiotopes (Table 2). Two such mAbs, designated 17.109[79] and 6B6.6,[80] recognize distinct VκIII light (L) chain idiotopes expressed by approximately two thirds of IgM κ RF paraproteins.[74] The 17.109 and 6B6.6 cross-reactive idiotypes (CRI) are probably encoded by distinct germline Vκ genes, designated Humkv325[81] (renamed from Vκ RF gene[82]) and Humkv328,[83] respectively. 6B6.6 CRI (+) L chains belong to the VκIIIa sub-subgroup, whereas 17.109 CRI (+) L chains are members of the VκIIIb sub-subgroup.[74,79,80]

Efforts have also been directed toward defining CRI shared by heavy (H) chain V regions of RF paraproteins (Table 2). For example, mAb G6 recognizes a VH1 CRI

Table 3 **Restricted Pairing of V_H/V_L Gene Products Observed in RF Paraproteins**

V_L	V_H
VκIIIb (17.109)[a]	V_H1 (G6)
VκIIIa (6B6.6)	V_H4 (LC1)

[a] Designation enclosed in parentheses refers to associated CRI detected by monoclonal antibody.

encoded by the germline V_H gene 783.[84,85] Moreover, a VH3 RF-associated CRI recognized by the mAb B6 is encoded by a germline V_H gene closely related or identical to hv3005.[84,86,87] Another subgroup of RF contains H chains recognized by mAbs LC1, 5-14, and 6-10; these CRI are encoded by a V_H4 gene(s) yet to be identified.[88]

Insights concerning the origin of autoantibody genes have come from studies of the development of the human B cell repertoire. Surprisingly, of the approximately 100 V_H germline gene segments potentially available, only 12 V_H gene segments are preferentially expressed in fetal liver.[89] Of these "fetal V_H gene segments", six (20p1, 30p1, V_H6, 56p1, 51p1, and 58p2) have been shown to encode self-reactive specificities, including three (56p1, 51p1, and 58p2) that have been identified in RF.[87,90] While the significance of the apparent relationship between autoreactivity and the fetal preimmune repertoire remains unclear, Coutinho and colleagues have proposed that self-reactivity plays a critical role in shaping the early B cell repertoire in the sterile fetal environment through an interactive "network" process.[91] According to this hypothesis, inherited deletions (or other abnormalities) of these developmentally regulating germline V genes might result in subsequent aberrations of the mature B cell repertoire. Of interest in this regard is evidence of an association between deletion of the 56p1 V_H germline gene and autoimmune disease (RA and SLE).[92]

Since several conserved germline V genes are capable of encoding RF (and other self-reactive specificities), regulatory mechanisms almost certainly modulate expression of these gene products. Analysis of large panels of randomly acquired IgM paraproteins has indicated that co-expression of the 17.109 and G6 CRI or the 6B6.6 and LC1 CRI strongly correlates with RF binding activity of the paraprotein[88,93] (Table 3). Restricted V_H-V_L pairing may therefore exert an important regulatory influence on RF expression *in vivo*. Additional structural constraints may be important in determining self-reactivity. The antigen-binding site of an antibody is generated by juxtaposition of the three regions of sequence hypervariability (referred to as complementarity determining regions [CDR]) present on both H and L chains.[94] The third CDR is formed by the fusion of V, D, and J (H chain) or V and J (L chain) gene segments; the H and L chain CDR3 regions are positioned in the center of the antigen-binding site of the immunoglobulin molecule. Introduction of non-germline-encoded amino acids at these gene segment junctions, termed N region addition, can strongly influence specificity and affinity of the molecule.[94] Fetal H chain V regions characteristically exhibit limited N region addition between D and J gene segments and thus contain shorter CDR3 regions than observed in H chains appearing later in development.[95,96] N region addition in L chain V regions is unusual,[94,97] presumably reflecting transient expression of the enzyme terminal deoxynucleotidyl transferase (TdT) during B cell development. Unexpectedly, analysis of L chain sequences from nine cloned EBV-transformed B cell lines secreting RF revealed that three chains contained N region additions in their CDR3 regions.[97] It is possible that somatic modification of junctional regions which contribute to the formation of CDR3 may favor the emergence of autoantibodies exhibiting higher affinities, whereas the paucity of N region addition in the fetal repertoire may impede the generation of high-affinity self-reactive antibodies in the immature immune system. It is of interest in this regard that analysis of the κ chain repertoire expressed in the synovium of a patient with RA revealed that 5 of 17 randomly sequenced CDR3 regions exhibited N region addition.[98] It is conceivable that B cells which aberrantly regulate insertion of N region codons (as for example, through abnormal regulation of TdT expression) could be predisposed to generate potentially pathologic self-reactive antibodies.

The demonstration that a limited number of germline immunoglobulin V region genes (e.g., Humkv325 and Humkv328) encode a substantial fraction of IgM RF paraproteins suggested that these V genes might also contribute to the expression of RF occurring spontaneously in some healthy individuals and in diseases such as RA. Serologic analyses of serum RF using mAbs identifying germline-encoded RF-associated CRI (e.g., 17.109 and 6B6.6) have indicated that a substantial proportion (if not all) of RA patients synthesize some RF bearing either the 17.109 or 6B6.6 VκIII CRI.[80,99] However, only a negligible fraction (~1%) of RF in individual sera appears to express either CRI. These observations are in striking contrast to the dominance of these idiotopes among RF paraproteins and suggest either that germline genes Humkv325 and Humkv328 (or closely related genes) encode only a small proportion of RF in RA or that extensive mutation of genes encoding RF may occur in the disease. The finding of similar low proportions of 17.109 and 6B6.6 CRI (+) RF prior to disease onset[100] and minimal changes in levels of these two RF-associated CRI over time[99] is consistent with the former explanation. Germline genes Humkv325 and Humkv328 do not encode disease-specific RF, in that 17.109 and 6B6.6 CRI occur among RF in seropositive healthy adults in a pattern similar to that observed in RA.[101] Low levels of both of these VκIII CRI are also found among normal immunoglobulins.[74,80]

An alternative approach employed to investigate the V region diversity of polyclonal RF involves analysis of V region sequences of RF elaborated by cloned B cell lines obtained from healthy controls and patients with rheumatic diseases. These studies, still in their infancy, indicate that multiple V_H and V_L genes are capable of encoding RF. Both unmodified germline sequences and mutated V region sequences, consistent with antigen selection, have been observed.[87,97] It appears, therefore, that the highly restricted pattern of V gene utilization, observed among RF paraproteins, is not shared by RF-secreting B cell lines rescued from healthy individuals and patients with autoimmune diseases. However, caution must be exercised in interpreting these results, since the precise relationship between cloned B cell lines and autoantibody expression *in vivo* is far from clear.

Although serological studies have the advantage of directly analyzing RF expression *in vivo,* they are constrained by the limited number of mAbs recognizing structurally defined CRI that are currently available. Moreover, this approach is unable to distinguish between the influence of somatic mutation of a particular germline gene (with consequent loss of germline-encoded CRI) vs. utilization of alternative germline genes. Application of both serologic and cell line analyses to investigation of RF expressed in the same individual offers the best promise of ultimately elucidating the genetic origin of RF in disease. Moreover, such studies should reveal the relative importance of antigen selection vs. polyclonal activation in expression of these autoantibodies.

IV. BIOLOGIC PROPERTIES

Considerable evidence, albeit circumstantial, indicates that RF contribute to tissue injury in RA. Local production of RF has been repeatedly demonstrated at sites of tissue inflammation.[102-105] Moreover, RF are a prominent constituent of immune complexes occurring in sera and synovial fluids[106-109] and within polymorphonuclear leukocytes of patients with RA.[110] RF-IgG complexes can also be eluted from rheumatoid synovial tissue[111] and cartilage.[112] It should also be noted that disease severity and activity in RA correlate with levels of RF.[113-115]

How might RF contribute to tissue injury in RA? Both IgM-RF and IgG-RF potentiate complement activation by IgG complexes under conditions in which the target complex alone weakly fixes complement.[116-121] That local complement consumption occurs in RA is supported by the presence of depressed levels of hemolytic complement and individual complement components in rheumatoid synovial fluid.[122,123] Moreover, cleavage products of C3, C4, and Factor B are also detected in rheumatoid joints.[124] The latter observation suggests that activation of both classical and alternative complement pathways occurs in RA. Turnover rates of C4 and Factor B in patients with RA correlate with RF but not other serum antibody levels.[125] Paradoxically, complement activation by IgG complexes exhibiting strong anticomplementary activity may be attenuated by additions of IgM-RF, presumably by competing for or masking the complement-binding sites in the Fc regions of the IgG.[126-129]

Disposition of immune complexes *in vivo* appears to be strongly influenced by RF. Messner and colleagues observed that RF obtained from RA or SLE patients inhibited ingestion by human neutrophils of staphylococci opsonized with human or rabbit IgG antibody.[130] Similarly, IgM-RF inhibited phagocytosis by rabbit granulocytes of sheep red blood cells (RBCs) coated with rabbit IgG antibody[131] and immune precipitates of bovine serum albumin (BSA) and rabbit anti-BSA.[132] On the other hand, RF enhanced attachment and uptake of soluble heat-aggregated human IgG by human monocytes and mouse macrophages, although this effect declined in the presence of excess RF.[133] It was suggested that the observed biphasic effects reflected opposing influences of RF; namely, enhanced pinocytosis of small soluble immune complexes by increasing their size vs. inhibition of immune complex uptake by blocking binding of IgG to the Fc receptor of the phagocyte. The addition of RF to insoluble IgG complexes or particles opsonized with IgG exerts an inhibitory effect secondary to blockade of IgG reactivity with the Fc receptor, since no increase in size is required for phagocytosis. In the presence of complement, it is likely that RF interferes with phagocytosis of IgG complexes via complement receptors by blocking complement-binding sites in the IgG molecule. Studies in rodents have demonstrated that RF facilitates clearance of parenterally administered immune complexes.[133,134]

RF are capable of directly activating natural killer (NK) cells by cross-linking their surface Fcγ receptors (FcγRIII).[135] Indeed, lower levels of FcγRIII are found in synovial fluid compared to peripheral blood NK cells in patients with RA. Moreover, synovial fluid NK cells in RA exhibited diminished NK activity and antibody-dependent, cell-mediated cytotoxicity (ADCC) than their peripheral blood counterparts. Normal peripheral blood lymphocytes (PBL) incubated with synovial fluid containing RF or affinity-purified RF (containing IgG) from RA patients exhibited diminished FcγRIII expression, NK activity, and ADCC. Activation of synovial fluid NK cells by RF is accompanied by elaboration of interferon-γ (IFN-γ) and tumor necrosis factor-α (TNF-α). Both of these cytokines may contribute to the pathogenesis of RA.[136,137]

For the most part, studies of the role(s) of RF in RA have focused on IgM-RF and, to a lesser extent, IgG-RF. The possible contribution of IgA-RF is less clear. Polymeric IgA-RF behaves similarly to IgM-RF in its ability to enhance secretion of lysosomal enzymes (elastase and cathepsin G) from human neutrophils in the presence of heat-aggregated IgG.[138] Under the same conditions, monomeric IgA-RF was inactive. Differences in the effector functions of IgA compared to IgM and IgG would be anticipated to influence the role of IgA-RF in tissue injury. Although IgA is generally considered to be unable to fix complement by the classical pathway, it may activate the alternative pathway.[139,140] Thus, the overall contribution of RF to tissue injury in RA is likely influenced by the pattern of isotypes expressed in a particular patient or at a specific site of inflammation.

Evidence suggesting that RF has important physiological function(s) has also emerged. The frequent appearance of RF during the course of bacterial or parasitic infections[141-147] and following immunization with bacterial and viral antigens[148-152] implicated RF as being an important constituent of the host response to infectious agents. The demonstration that RF enhances complement-dependent neutralization of herpes simplex virus[153] and increases resistance to infection by trypanosomes in rats[154] supports this view.

V. CLINICAL SIGNIFICANCE OF RF

A. POPULATION STUDIES

The occurrence of RF has been studied in several populations. A longitudinal study involving approximately two thirds of the population of Tecumseh, Michigan determined that the prevalence of a positive latex fixation test for RF (>1:20 titer) was approximately 3%, with essentially identical rates observed in males and females.[155] Age significantly influenced the prevalence of RF in this population; nearly 9% of females and 14% of males over 70 years of age tested positively, a finding in agreement with several other studies. Variability in prevalences of RF among different populations also exists, as established in a study of Blackfoot and Pima Indians.[156]

Population-based studies have been helpful in elucidating the significance of a positive test for serum RF in ostensibly healthy individuals. That individuals may exhibit a positive RF test in the absence of disease is well documented. Indeed, more than two thirds of individuals with elevated serum RF in the Tecumseh study did not exhibit manifestations of RA.[155] On the other hand, strong evidence indicates that increased levels of serum RF enhance the likelihood of an individual ultimately developing RA. Ball and Lawrence observed that 7 of 19 asymptomatic individuals with elevated serum RF subsequently developed RA over a 5-year period.[157] Aho and co-workers examined sera from 30 individuals who developed RA during the course of a Finnish cardiovascular disease survey and found that 12 exhibited positive tests for RF from 4 months to 5 years prior to diagnosis of the disease.[158] More recently, del Puente et al. analyzed data obtained from a longitudinal study of 2712 Pima Indians conducted over a 19-year period.[159] A convincing correlation was observed between the incidence of RA and the RF titer (Figure 1). These results indicate that significantly elevated serum RF levels are a marker for increased susceptibility to developing RA. On the other hand, nominal concentrations of serum RF are frequently present in the sera of healthy individuals and likely reflect a physiologic role(s) of this autoantibody in normal homeostasis.[160-162] Whether RF occurring in individuals destined to develop RA differs in genetic origin,

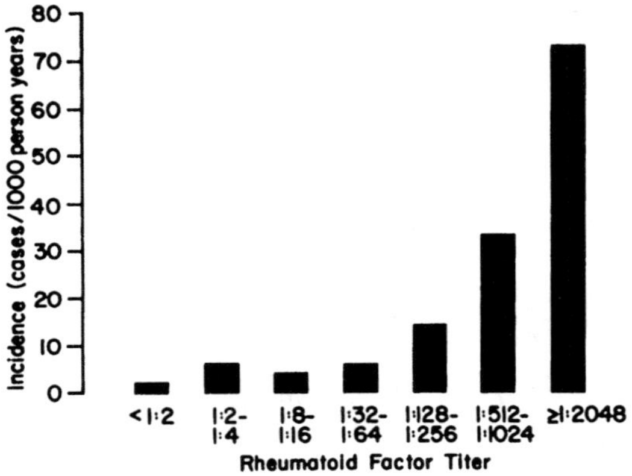

Figure 1 Association between rheumatoid factor titer and subsequent incidence of rheumatoid arthritis in the Pima Indian population ($p < .001$, controlling for age, sex, and number of clinical criteria fulfilled). (Reproduced from del Puente, A., et al., *Arthritis Rheum.*, 31, 1242, 1988. With copyright permission of the American College of Rheumatology.)

binding specificity, or affinity from RF in healthy individuals has not been resolved. A preliminary study found a similar frequency of the VκIII-associated CRI 17.109 and 6B6.6 among RF in healthy adults and those developing RA.[101]

B. RHEUMATOID ARTHRITIS

Approximately 75% of patients with RA exhibit elevated titers of serum RF when tested by conventional techniques such as the latex fixation test or the sheep cell agglutination test (SCAT). A lesser proportion of patients with other rheumatic diseases including SLE, scleroderma, polymyositis/dermatomyositis, and some types of vasculitis also manifest elevated serum RF. In contrast to RF present in non-rheumatic diseases, RF occurring in RA characteristically exhibit broad reactivity with both human and heterologous (e.g., rabbit) IgG. The broad reactivity of RF in RA reflects the occurrence of multiple subpopulations of RF in the sera of these patients.[163-165]

The precise serologic status of patients fulfilling criteria for RA, but lacking elevated serum RF by conventional testing (''seronegative'' RA), is less clear. Occasionally, ''hidden'' RF can be detected in ''seronegative'' RA patients following fractionation of their serum under conditions in which complexes of RF and autologous IgG are dissociated.[166] Approximately one half of seronegative RA patients manifest elevated levels of serum RF when measured by sensitive assays such as radioimmunoassay or enzyme-linked immunosorbent assay (ELISA), although concentrations are significantly lower than in sera from seropositive RA patients.[160] Although these observations suggest a continuum of RF levels among RA patients, the distinction between seropositive and seronegative RA (defined by conventional RF testing) has nevertheless proven to be of clinical and epidemiologic value.

Susceptibility to the development of RA is associated with inheritance of the MHC class II alleles HLA-DR4 or -DR1, while the association of DR4 with seronegative RA is generally less impressive (or absent).[167-173] While the pathogenetic mechanisms underlying the association between MHC class II genes and RA remains uncertain, molecular analysis has revealed a shared amino acid motif among the DR susceptibility alleles in the third hypervariability region of their DRβ1 chains[174] (See also Chapters 14, 15, and 16). The possibility that these MHC class II alleles support responsiveness to determinants in the Fc portion of IgG must be considered; however, DR4 does not

Table 4 **Some Diseases Associated with Elevated Serum RF**

Connective Tissue Disease
Systemic lupus erythematosus
Rheumatoid arthritis
Sjögren's syndrome
Polymyositis/dermatomyositis
Juvenile rheumatoid arthritis
Scleroderma
Chronic Bacterial Infections
Subacute bacterial endocarditis
Leprosy
Tuberculosis
Syphilis
Lyme disease
Viral Diseases
Rubella
Cytomegalovirus
Infectious mononucleosis
Influenza
Acquired immunodeficiency syndrome (AIDS)
Parasitic Diseases
Chronic Inflammatory Diseases — Etiology Uncertain
Sarcoidosis
Periodontal disease
Pulmonary interstitial disease
Liver disease
Mixed Cryoglobulinemia
Hypergammaglobulinemic Purpura

associate with increased levels of RF in the sera of healthy individuals.[175] On the other hand, DR4 was correlated with RF expression in unaffected first-degree relatives of seropositive RA patients, suggesting that DR4 may directly predispose to RF production.[176] Moreover, PBL obtained from DR4+ healthy individuals secrete higher levels of IgM RF in response to polyclonal activation than PBL from their DR4− counterparts.[177]

Despite considerable overlap, clinical distinctions between seropositive and seronegative RA clearly exist. Seropositivity is associated with more aggressive articular disease, both radiographically and functionally, and with a higher frequency of extra-articular involvement than observed in seronegative RA, including subcutaneous nodules, vasculitis, leg ulcers, and neuropathy.[178] Several studies have suggested that DR4 may also confer increased risk for more severe disease, unrelated to RF.[173,179-181]

The clinical significance of changes in RF levels has been intensively investigated, but interpretation of these studies has been frequently complicated by accompanying changes in medication. Nonsteroidal anti-inflammatory drugs (NSAIDs) were initially reported to directly suppress RF production *in vitro* and *in vivo*;[182,183] however, more recent studies indicated that decreases in serum RF following NSAID administration were correlated with improvement in disease activity.[184] A significant correlation between decreases in serum IgM-RF levels and clinical improvement was also observed in an analysis of serum samples obtained from RA patients participating in two multicenter therapeutic trials; however, methotrexate therapy per se correlated more significantly with decreases in IgM-RF levels than did changes in clinical status.[115] Abrogation of spontaneous *in vitro* RF production by PBL obtained from RA patients following initiation of methotrexate treatment is consistent with a direct effect of this agent on RF production.[185] Taken together, these studies indicate that RF levels are influenced by both clinical activity of the disease and the concomitant therapeutic regimen.

C. OTHER DISEASES

Chronic inflammatory or infectious diseases are frequently accompanied by elevated levels of serum RF, confirming that RF is not specific for RA (Table 4, see also Chapter 4, Table 3). The RF present in these diseases characteristically react preferentially with human IgG, although exceptions occur. In the case of SBE, elevated levels of RF generally disappear following treatment of the underlying infection.[144]

ACKNOWLEDGMENTS

The authors are deeply appreciative of the efforts of Ms. Evelyn Rogers in preparing this manuscript. Work alluded to in this manuscript was supported by National Institutes of Health (NIH) grants AR03555, AI18958, AI18745, AR20614, and DK40117 and a Veterans Administration Merit Award.

REFERENCES

1. **Heimer, R. and Levin, F. M.,** On the distribution of rheumatoid factors among the immunoglobulins, *Immunochemistry,* 3, 1, 1966.
2. **Dunne, J. V. et al.,** IgA rheumatoid factor in the sera and saliva of patients with rheumatoid arthritis and Sjögren's syndrome, *Ann. Rheum. Dis.,* 38, 161, 1979.
3. **Kunkel, H. G., Müller-Eberhard, H. J., Fudenberg, H. H. et al.,** Gamma globulin complexes in rheumatoid arthritis and certain other conditions, *J. Clin. Invest.,* 40, 117, 1961.
4. **Schrohenloher, R. E.,** Characterization of the γ-globulin complexes present in certain sera having high titers of anti-γ-globulin activity, *J. Clin. Invest.,* 45, 501, 1966.
5. **Zuraw, B. L., O'Hair, C. H., Vaughan, J. H. et al.,** Immunoglobulin E-rheumatoid factor in the serum of patients with rheumatoid arthritis, asthma, and other diseases, *J. Clin. Invest.,* 68, 1610, 1981.

6. **Elkon, K. B., Delacroix, D. L., Gharavi, A. E. et al.,** Immunoglobulin A and polymeric IgA rheumatoid factors in systemic sicca syndrome: partial characterization, *J. Immunol.*, 129, 576, 1982.
7. **Schrohenloher, R. E., Koopman, W. J., and Alarcón, G. S.,** Molecular forms of IgA rheumatoid factor in serum and synovial fluid of patients with rheumatoid arthritis, *Arthritis Rheum.*, 29, 1194, 1986.
8. **Pope, R. M., Teller, D. C., and Mannik, M.,** The molecular basis of self-association of antibodies to IgG (rheumatoid factors) in rheumatoid arthritis, *Proc. Natl. Acad. Sci. U.S.A.*, 71, 517, 1974.
9. **Pope, R. M., Teller, D. C., and Mannik, M.,** The molecular basis of self-association of IgG rheumatoid factors, *J. Immunol.*, 115, 365, 1975.
10. **Natvig, J. B., Gaarder, P. I., and Turner, M. W.,** IgG antigens of the Cγ2 and Cγ3 homology regions interacting with rheumatoid factors, *Clin. Exp. Immunol.*, 12, 177, 1972.
11. **Allen, J. C. and Kunkel, H. G.,** Hidden rheumatoid factors with specificity for native γ globulins, *Arthritis Rheum.*, 9, 758, 1966.
12. **Sasso, E. H. et al.,** Antigenic specificities of human monoclonal and polyclonal IgM rheumatoid factors: the Cγ2-Cγ3 interface region contains the major determinants, *J. Immunol.*, 140, 3098, 1988.
13. **Stone, G. C., Sjöbring, U., Björck, L. et al.,** The Fc binding site for streptococcal protein G is in the Cγ2-Cγ3 interface region of IgG and is related to the sites that bind staphylococcal protein A and human rheumatoid factors, *J. Immunol.*, 143, 565, 1989.
14. **Robbins, D. L., Skilling, J., Benisek, W. F. et al.,** Estimation of the relative activity of 19S IgM rheumatoid factor secreted by rheumatoid synovial cells for human IgG subclasses, *Arthritis Rheum.*, 29, 722, 1986.
15. **Robbins, D. L., Benisek, W. F., Benjamini, E. et al.,** Differential reactivity of rheumatoid synovial cells and serum rheumatoid factors to human immunoglobulin G subclasses 1 and 3 and their CH3 domains in rheumatoid arthritis, *Arthritis Rheum.*, 30, 489, 1987.
16. **Grubb, R. and Laurell, A.-B.,** Hereditary serological human serum groups, *Acta Pathol. Microbiol. Scand.*, 39, 390, 1956.
17. **Harboe, M. and Lundevall, J.,** A new type in the Gm system, anti-Gm^b, *Acta Pathol. Microbiol. Scand.*, 45, 357, 1959.
18. **Harboe, M.,** A new hemagglutinating substance in the Gm systems, anti-Gm^b, *Acta Pathol. Microbiol. Scand.*, 467, 191, 1959.
19. **Natvig, J. B.,** Gm(g) — a "new" gamma-globulin factor, *Nature*, 211, 318, 1966.
20. **Gaarder, P. I. and Natvig, J. B.,** Hidden rheumatoid factors reacting with "non a" and other antigens of native autologous IgG, *J. Immunol.*, 105, 928, 1970.
21. **Gaarder, P. I. and Natvig, J. B.,** Two new antigens of human IgG "non b^0" and "non b^1" related to the Gm system, *J. Immunol.*, 108, 617, 1972.
22. **Natvig, J. B. and Turner, M. W.,** Localization of Gm markers to different molecular regions of the FC fragment, *Clin. Exp. Immunol.*, 8, 685, 1971.
23. **Butler, V. P., Jr. and Vaughan, J. H.,** Hemagglutination by rheumatoid factor of cells coated with animal gamma globulin, *Proc. Soc. Exp. Biol. Med.*, 116, 585, 1964.
24. **Butler, V. P., Jr. and Vaughan, J. H.,** The reaction of rheumatoid factor with animal gamma-globulins: quantitative considerations, *Immunology*, 8, 144, 1965.

25. **Gaarder, P. I. and Michaelsen, T. E.,** Specificity of rheumatoid factors cross-reacting with human and rabbit IgG, *Acta Pathol. Microbiol. Scand. Sect. B,* 82, 733, 1974.
26. **Schrohenloher, R. E. and Koopman, W. J.,** Rheumatoid factor, in *Arthritis and Allied Conditions,* 12th ed., McCarty, D. J. and Koopman, W. J., Eds., Lea & Febiger, Philadelphia, 1993, 861.
27. **Dresser, D. W. and Popham, A. M.,** Induction of an IgM anti-(bovine)-IgG response in mice by bacterial lipopolysaccharide, *Nature,* 264, 552, 1976.
28. **Koopman, W. J. and Schrohenloher, R. E.,** *In vitro* synthesis of IgM rheumatoid factor by lymphocytes from healthy adults, *J. Immunol.,* 125, 934, 1980.
29. **Dalal, N. et al.,** *In vitro* secretion of human IgM rheumatoid factor. Evidence for distinct rheumatoid factor populations in health and disease, *Arthritis Rheum.,* 33, 1340, 1990.
30. **Slaughter, L. et al.,** *In vitro* effects of Epstein-Barr virus on peripheral blood mononuclear cells from patients with rheumatoid arthritis and normal subjects, *J. Exp. Med.,* 148, 1429, 1978.
31. **Abruzzo, J. L. and Christian, C. L.,** The induction of a rheumatoid factor-like substance in rabbits, *J. Exp. Med.,* 114, 791, 1961.
32. **Aho, K. and Wager, O.,** Production of anti-antibodies in rabbits. Appearance in rabbit serum of anti-antibodies reacting with autogenous and isogenous antibody following auto-stimulation with protein antigens, *Ann. Med. Exp. Biol. Fenn.,* 39, 79, 1961.
33. **Williams, R. C. and Kunkel, H. G.,** Antibodies to rabbit γ-globulin after immunizing with various preparations of autologous γ-globulin, *Proc. Soc. Exp. Med.,* 158, 529, 1983.
34. **Nemazee, D. A. and Sato, V. L.,** Induction of rheumatoid antibodies in the mouse. Regulated production of autoantibody in the secondary humoral response, *J. Exp. Med.,* 158, 529, 1983.
35. **Nemazee, D. A.,** Immune complexes can trigger specific T cell-dependent autoanti-IgG antibody production in mice, *J. Exp. Med.,* 161, 242, 1985.
36. **Welch, M. J. et al.,** Increased frequency of rheumatoid factor precursor B lymphocytes after immunization of normal adults with tetanus toxoid, *Clin. Exp. Immunol.,* 51, 299, 1983.
37. **Tarkowski, A. Czerkinsky, C., and Nilsson, L.-Å.,** Simultaneous induction of rheumatoid factor- and antigen-specific antibody-secreting cells during the secondary immune response in man, *Clin. Exp. Immunol.,* 61, 379, 1985.
38. **Aitcheson, C. T. et al.,** Characteristics of antinuclear antibodies in rheumatoid arthritis: reactivity of rheumatoid factor with a histone-dependent nuclear antigen, *Arthritis Rheum.,* 23, 528, 1980.
39. **Mason, J. C. et al.,** Characterization of non-histone nuclear proteins cross reactive with purified rheumatoid factors, *Ann. Rheum. Dis.,* 44, 287, 1985.
40. **Rubin, R. L. et al.,** Multiple autoantigen binding capabilities of mouse monoclonal antibodies selected for rheumatoid factor activity, *J. Exp. Med.,* 159, 1429, 1984.
41. **Reininger, L. et al.,** Rheumatoid factor autoantibody-binding site: a molecular analysis using monoclonal antibodies with dual anti-TNF and anti-IgG activities, *Eur. J. Immunol.,* 19, 2123, 1989.
42. **Stone, G. C. et al.,** The Fc binding site for streptococcal protein G is in the Cγ2-Cγ3 interface region of IgG and is related to the sites that bind staphylococcal protein A and human rheumatoid factors, *J. Immunol.,* 143, 565, 1989.

43. **Oppliger, I. R. et al.,** Human rheumatoid factors bear the internal image of the Fc binding region of staphylococcal protein A, *J. Exp. Med.,* 166, 702, 1987.
44. **Johansson, P. J. H. et al.,** Herpes simplex type 1-induced Fc receptor binds to the Cγ2-Cγ3 interface region of IgG in the area that binds staphylococcal protein A, *Immunology,* 66, 8, 1989.
45. **Mouritsen, S.,** Rheumatoid factors are anti-idiotypic antibodies against virus-induced anti-Fc receptor antibodies, *Scand. J. Immunol.,* 24, 485, 1988.
46. **Shlomchik, M. J. et al.,** The role of clonal selection and somatic mutation in autoimmunity, *Nature,* 328, 805, 1987.
47. **Schlomchik, M. J. et al.,** Structure and function of anti-DNA autoantibodies derived from a single autoimmune mouse, *Proc. Natl. Acad. Sci. U.S.A.,* 84, 9150, 1987.
48. **Mullinax, F. and Mullinax, G. L.,** Abnormality of IgG structure in rheumatoid arthritis and systemic lupus erythematosus (Abstract), *Arthritis Rheum.,* 18, 417, 1975.
49. **Parekh, R. B. et al.,** Association of rheumatoid arthritis and primary osteoarthritis with changes in the glycosylation pattern of total serum IgG, *Nature,* 316, 452, 1985.
50. **Tomana, M. et al.,** Abnormal glycosylation of serum IgG from patients with chronic inflammatory diseases, *Arthritis Rheum.,* 31, 333, 1988.
51. **Axford, J. S. et al.,** Reduced B-cell galactosyltransferase activity in rheumatoid arthritis, *Lancet,* ii, 1486, 1987.
52. **Rook, G. A. W., Steele, J., and Rademacher, T.,** A monoclonal antibody raised by immunizing mice with group A streptococci binds to agalactosyl IgG from rheumatoid arthritis, *Ann. Rheum. Dis.,* 47, 247, 1988.
53. **Go, M. F., Schrohenloher, R. E., and Tomana, M.,** Prevalence of IgG galactosylation deficiency in inflammatory bowel disease, *Gastroenterology,* 98 (Abstr.), A452, 1990.
54. **Dubé, R. et al.,** Agalactosyl IgG in inflammatory bowel disease: correlation with C-reactive protein, *Gut,* 31, 431, 1990.
55. **Newkirk, M. M., Lemmo, A., and Rauch, J.,** Importance of the IgG isotype, not the state of glycosylation, in determining human rheumatoid factor binding, *Arthritis Rheum.,* 33, 800, 1990.
56. **Lunec, J. et al.,** Self-perpetuating mechanisms of immunoglobulin G aggregation in rheumatoid inflammation, *J. Clin. Invest.,* 76, 2084, 1985.
57. **Plater-Zyberk, C. et al.,** A rheumatoid arthritis B-cell subset expresses a phenotype similar to that in chronic lymphocytic leukemia, *Arthritis Rheum.,* 28, 971, 1985.
58. **Sowden, J. A. et al.,** Evaluation of CD5 positive B-cells in blood and synovial fluid of patients with rheumatic diseases, *Rheumatol. Int.,* 7, 255, 1987.
59. **Casali, P. et al.,** High affinity antibodies to ssDNA are produced by $CD5^-$ B cells in systemic lupus erythematosus patients, *J. Immunol.,* 143, 3476, 1989.
60. **Casali, P. et al.,** Human lymphocytes making rheumatoid factor and antibody to ssDNA belong to $Leu\text{-}1^+$ B cells, *Science,* 236, 77, 1987.
61. **Hardy, R. R. et al.,** Rheumatoid factor secretion from human $Leu\text{-}1^+$ B cells, *Science,* 236, 81, 1987.
62. **Nakamura, M. et al.,** Human monoclonal rheumatoid factor-like antibodies from CD5 $(Leu\text{-}1)^+$ B cells are polyreactive, *J. Immunol.,* 140, 4180, 1988.
63. **Burastero, S. E. et al.,** Monoreactive high affinity and polyreactive low affinity rheumatoid factors are produced by CD5+ B cells from patients with rheumatoid arthritis, *J. Exp. Med.,* 168, 1979, 1988.

64. **Hardy, R. R. and Hayakawa, K.,** Development and physiology of LY-1 B and its human homolog, LEU-1 B, *Immunol. Rev.,* 93, 53, 1986.
65. **Mercolino, T. J. et al.,** Normal mouse peritoneum contains a large population of Ly-1$^+$ (CD5) B-cells that recognize phosphatidyl choline. Relationship to cells that secrete hemolytic antibody for autologous erythrocytes, *J. Exp. Med.,* 168, 687, 1988.
66. **Förster, I. and Rajewsky, K.,** Expansion and functional activity of Ly-1$^+$ B-cells upon transfer of peritoneal cells into allotype-congenic newborn mice, *Eur. J. Immunol.,* 17, 521, 1987.
67. **Werner-Favre, C. et al.,** Cell surface antigen CD5 is a marker for activated human B cells, *Eur. J. Immunol.,* 19, 1209, 1989.
68. **Cush, J. J. and Lipsky, P. E.,** Cellular basis for rheumatoid inflammation, *Clin. Orthop. Relat. Res.,* 265, 9, 1991.
69. **Singer, A. and Hodes, R. J.,** Mechanisms of T cell-B cell interaction, *Annu. Rev. Immunol.,* 1, 211, 1983.
70. **Chesnut, R. W. and Grey, H. M.,** Studies on the capacity of B cells to serve as antigen presenting cells, *J. Immunol.,* 126, 1075, 1981.
71. **Rock, K. L., Benacerraf, B., and Abbas, A. K.,** Antigen presentation by hapten-specific B lymphocytes, *J. Exp. Med.,* 160, 1102, 1984.
72. **Roosnek, E. and Lanzavecchia, A.,** Efficient and selective presentation of antigen-antibody complexes by rheumatoid factor B cells, *J. Exp. Med.,* 173, 487, 1991.
73. **Uhr, J. W. and Möller, G.,** Regulatory effect of antibody on the immune response, *Adv. Immunol.,* 8, 81, 1968.
74. **Crowley, J. J. et al.,** Incidence of three cross-reactive idiotypes on human rheumatoid factor paraproteins, *J. Immunol.,* 140, 3411, 1987.
75. **Kunkel, H. G. et al.,** Cross-idiotypic specificity among monoclonal IgM proteins with anti-γ-globulin activity, *J. Exp. Med.,* 137, 331, 1973.
76. **Agnello, V. et al.,** Evidence for a subset of rheumatoid factors that cross-react with DNA-histone and have a distinct cross-idiotype, *J. Exp. Med.,* 151, 1514, 1980.
77. **Andrews, D. W. and Capra, J. D.,** Amino acid sequence of the variable regions of light chains from two idiotypically cross-reactive human IgM anti-γ-globulins of the Wa group, *Biochemistry,* 20, 5816, 1981.
78. **Andrews, D. W. and Capra, J. D.,** Amino acid sequence of the variable regions of heavy chains from two idiotypically cross-reactive human IgM anti-γ-globulins of the Wa group, *Biochemistry,* 20, 5822, 1981.
79. **Carson, D. A. and Fong, S.,** A common idiotope on human rheumatoid factors identified by a hybridoma antibody, *Mol. Immunol.,* 20, 1081, 1983.
80. **Schrohenloher, R. E. et al.,** Monoclonal antibody 6B6.6 defines a cross-reactive kappa light chain idiotope on human monoclonal and polyclonal rheumatoid factors, *Arthritis Rheum.,* 33, 187, 1990.
81. **Radoux, V. et al.,** A conserved human germline Vκ gene directly encodes rheumatoid factor light chains, *J. Exp. Med.,* 164, 2119, 1986.
82. **Chen, P. P. et al.,** Isolation and characterization of human VκIII germ-line genes: implications for the molecular basis of human VκIII light chain diversity, *J. Immunol.,* 139, 1727, 1987.
83. **Chen, P. P. et al.,** Isolation and characterization of a light chain variable region gene for human rheumatoid factors, *J. Exp. Med.,* 166, 1900, 1987.

84. **Mageed, R. A. et al.,** Immunologic and antigenic epitopes of immunoglobulins. XVII. Monoclonal anti-idiotypes to the heavy chain of human rheumatoid factors, *Rheumatol. Int.*, 6, 179, 1986.
85. **Chen, P. P. et al.,** Characterization of two Ig V_H genes which are homologous to human rheumatoid factors, *Arthritis Rheum.*, 32, 72, 1989.
86. **Crowley, J. J. et al.,** The incidence of a new human cross-reactive idiotype linked to subgroup V_H III heavy chains, *Mol. Immunol.*, 27, 87, 1990.
87. **Pascual, V. et al.,** The complete nucleotide sequences of the heavy chain variable regions of six monospecific rheumatoid factors derived from Epstein-Barr virus transformed B cells isolated from the synovial tissue of patients with rheumatoid arthritis. Further evidence that some autoantibodies are unmutated copies of germline genes, *J. Clin. Invest.*, 86, 1320, 1990.
88. **Silverman, G. J. et al.,** Structural characterization of the second major cross-reactive idiotype group of human rheumatoid factors: association with the V_H4 gene family, *Arthritis Rheum.*, 33, 1347, 1990.
89. **Schroeder, H. W., Jr. and Weng, J. Y.,** Preferential utilization of conserved immunoglobulin H chain variable gene segments during human fetal life, *Proc. Natl. Acad. Sci. U.S.A.*, 87, 6146, 1990.
90. **Carson, D. A. et al.,** New roles for rheumatoid factor, *J. Clin. Invest.*, 87, 379, 1991.
91. **Coutinho, A. et al.,** Idiotypes, ballots and networks, *Ann. Inst. Pasteur Immunol.*, 139, 599, 1988.
92. **Yang, P.-M. et al.,** Possible deletion of a developmentally regulated heavy-chain variable region gene in autoimmune diseases, *Proc. Natl. Acad. Sci. U.S.A.*, 87, 7907, 1990.
93. **Silverman, G. J. et al.,** Idiotypic and subgroup analysis of human monoclonal rheumatoid factors. Implications for structural and genetic basis of autoantibodies in humans, *J. Clin. Invest.*, 82, 469, 1988.
94. **Kabat, E. A. et al.,** *Sequences of Proteins of Immunological Interest,* 4th ed., U.S. Department of Health and Human Services, Bethesda, MD, 1987.
95. **Sanz, I.,** Multiple mechanisms participate in the generation of diversity of the human H chain CDR3 regions, *J. Immunol.*, 147, 1720, 1991.
96. **Mortari, F. et al.,** The human cord blood antibody repertoire. Frequent use of the V_H7 gene family, *Eur. J. Immunol.*, 22, 241, 1992.
97. **Victor, K. D. et al.,** Rheumatoid factors isolated from patients with autoimmune disorders are derived from germline genes distinct from those encoding the Wa, Po, and Bla cross-reactive idiotypes, *J. Clin. Invest.*, 87, 1603, 1991.
98. **Lee, S. K. et al.,** The immunoglobulin kappa light chain repertoire expressed in the synovium of a patient with rheumatoid arthritis, *Arthritis Rheum.*, 35, 905, 1993.
99. **Koopman, W. J., Schrohenloher, R. E., and Carson, D. A.,** Dissociation of expression of two rheumatoid factor cross-reactive κ L chain idiotopes in rheumatoid arthritis, *J. Immunol.*, 144, 3468, 1990.
100. **Koopman, W. J. et al.,** The low proportion of 6B6.6(+) and 17.109(+) rheumatoid factor (RF) in rheumatoid arthritis is not likely related to somatic mutation (Abstract), *Arthritis Rheum.*, 33(Suppl. 5), R18, 1990.
101. **Koopman, W. J. et al.,** Rheumatoid factor (RF) VκIII idiotope expression does not distinguish benign RF(+) adults from those destined to develop rheumatoid arthritis (RA) (Abstract), *Arthritis Rheum.*, 33(Suppl. 5), R12, 1990.

102. **Smiley, J. D., Sachs, C., and Ziff, M.,** In vitro synthesis of immunoglobulin by rheumatoid synovial membrane, *J. Clin. Invest.*, 47, 624, 1968.
103. **Taylor-Upsahl, M. M., Abrahamsen, T. G., and Natvig, J. B.,** Rheumatoid factor plaque-forming cells in rheumatoid synovial tissue, *Clin. Exp. Immunol.*, 28, 197, 1977.
104. **Wernick, R. et al.,** IgG and IgM rheumatoid factor synthesis in rheumatoid synovial membrane cell cultures, *Arthritis Rheum.*, 28, 742, 1985.
105. **Koopman, W. J. et al.,** IgA rheumatoid factor: evidence for independent expression at local sites of tissue inflammation, *Ann. N.Y. Acad. Sci.*, 409, 258, 1983.
106. **Kunkel, H. G. et al.,** Gamma globulin complexes in rheumatoid arthritis and certain other conditions, *J. Clin. Invest.*, 40, 117, 1961.
107. **Schrohenloher, R. E.,** Characterization of the γ-globulin complexes present in certain sera having high titers of anti-γ-globulin activity, *J. Clin. Invest.*, 45, 501, 1966.
108. **Franklin, E. C. et al.,** An unusual protein component of high molecular weight in the serum of certain patients with rheumatoid arthritis, *J. Exp. Med.*, 105, 425, 1957.
109. **Winchester, R. J., Agnello, V., and Kunkel, H. G.,** Gamma globulin complexes in synovial fluids of patients with rheumatoid arthritis: partial characterization and relationship to lowered complement levels, *Clin. Exp. Immunol.*, 6, 689, 1970.
110. **Vaughan, J. H., Jacox, R. F., and Noell, P.,** Relation of intracytoplasmic inclusions in joint fluid leukocytes to anti-γG globulins, *Arthritis Rheum.*, 11, 135, 1968.
111. **Munthe, E. and Natvig, J. B.,** Characterization of IgG complexes in eluates from rheumatoid tissue, *Clin. Exp. Immunol.*, 8, 249, 1971.
112. **Jasin, H. E.,** Autoantibody specificities of immune complexes sequestered in articular cartilage of patients with rheumatoid arthritis and osteoarthritis, *Arthritis Rheum.*, 28, 241, 1985.
113. **Cats, A. and Hazevoet, H. M.,** Significance of positive tests for rheumatoid factor in the prognosis of rheumatoid arthritis, *Ann. Rheum. Dis.*, 29, 254, 1970.
114. **Allen, C. et al.,** IgG antiglobulins in rheumatoid arthritis and other arthritides: relationship with clinical feature and other parameters, *Ann. Rheum. Dis.*, 40, 127, 1981.
115. **Alarcón, G. S. et al.,** Suppression of rheumatoid factor production by methotrexate in patients with rheumatoid arthritis: evidence for differential influences of therapy and clinical status on IgM and IgA rheumatoid factor expression, *Arthritis Rheum.*, 33, 1156, 1990.
116. **Zvaifler, N. J. and Schur, P.,** Reactions of aggregated mercaptoethanol treated gamma globulin with rheumatoid factor-precipitin and complement fixation studies, *Arthritis Rheum.*, 11, 523, 1968.
117. **Schmid, F. R., Roitt, I. M., and Rocha, M. J.,** Complement fixation by a two-component antibody system: immunoglobulin G and immunoglobulin M anti-globulin (rheumatoid factor), *J. Exp. Med.*, 132, 673, 1970.
118. **Tesar, J. T. and Schmid, F. R.,** Conversion of soluble immune complexes into complement-fixing aggregates by IgM-rheumatoid factor, *J. Immunol.*, 105, 1206, 1970.
119. **Tanimoto, K. et al.,** Complement fixation by rheumatoid factor, *J. Clin. Invest.*, 55, 347, 1975.
120. **Brown, B. P., Nardella, F. A., and Mannik, M.,** Human complement activation by self-associated IgG rheumatoid factors, *Arthritis Rheum.*, 25, 1101, 1982.

121. **Sabharwal, U. K. et al.,** Activation of the classical pathway of complement by rheumatoid factors: assessment by radioimmunoassay for C4, *Arthritis Rheum.*, 25, 161, 1982.
122. **Pekin, T. J. and Zvaifler, N. J.,** Hemolytic complement in synovial fluid, *J. Clin. Invest.*, 43, 1372, 1964.
123. **Ruddy, S. and Austen, K. F.,** The complement system in rheumatoid synovitis. I. An analysis of complement component activities in rheumatoid synovial fluids, *Arthritis Rheum.*, 13, 713, 1970.
124. **Perrin, L. H. et al.,** Correlation between levels of breakdown products of C3, C4, and properdin factor B in synovial fluids from patients with rheumatoid arthritis, *Arthritis Rheum.*, 20, 647, 1977.
125. **Kaplan, R. A. et al.,** Metabolism of C4 and factor B in rheumatoid arthritis: relation to rheumatoid factor, *Arthritis Rheum.*, 23, 911, 1980.
126. **Zvaifler, N. J. and Bloch, K. J.,** Rheumatoid factor — an inhibitor of the complement fixation reaction, *Arthritis Rheum.*, 5, 127, 1962.
127. **Bernhard, G. C., Cheng, W., and Talmage, D. W.,** The reaction of rheumatoid factor and complement with γ-globulin-coated latex, *J. Immunol.*, 88, 750, 1962.
128. **Heimer, R., Levin, F. M., and Kahn, M. F.,** Inhibition of complement fixation by human serum. II. The activity of a γ-$_{1M}$ globulin and rheumatoid factor in complement fixation reactions, *J. Immunol.*, 91, 866, 1963.
129. **Davis, J. S. and Bollet, A. J.,** Protection of a complement-sensitive enzyme system by rheumatoid factor, *J. Immunol.*, 92, 139, 1964.
130. **Messner, R. P. et al.,** Serum opsonin, bacteria, and polymorphonuclear leukocyte interactions in subacute bacterial endocarditis: anti-γ-globulin factors and their interaction with specific opsonins, *J. Clin. Invest.*, 47, 1109, 1968.
131. **McDuffie, F. C. and Brumfield, H. W.,** Effect of rheumatoid factor on complement-mediated phagocytosis, *J. Clin. Invest.*, 51, 3007, 1972.
132. **Ward, P. A. and Zvaifler, N. J.,** Quantitative phagocytosis by neutrophils. II. Release of the C5-cleaving enzyme and inhibition of phagocytosis by rheumatoid factor, *J. Immunol.*, 111, 1777, 1973.
133. **Van Snick, J. L. et al.,** Enhancement by IgM rheumatoid factor of *in vitro* ingestion by macrophages and *in vivo* clearance of aggregated IgG or antigen-antibody complexes, *Eur. J. Immunol.*, 8, 279, 1978.
134. **Davis, J. S. and Torrigiani, G.,** Effects of rheumatoid factor on *in vivo* distribution of aggregated human IgG and antigen-antibody complexes, *Proc. Soc. Exp. Biol. Med.*, 125, 772, 1967.
135. **Hendrich, C. et al.,** Activation of CD16+ effector cells by rheumatoid factor complex, *Arthritis Rheum.*, 34, 423, 1991.
136. **Browning, J.,** Interferons and rheumatoid arthritis: insight into interferon biology, *Immunol. Today,* 8, 372, 1987.
137. **Saxne, T. et al.,** Detection of tumor necrosis factor α but not tumor necrosis factor β in rheumatoid arthritis synovial fluid and serum, *Arthritis Rheum.*, 31, 1041, 1988.
138. **Blackburn, W. D., Jr. et al.,** Induction of neutrophil enzyme release by rheumatoid factors: evidence for differences based on molecular characteristics, *Clin. Immunol. Immunopathol.*, 40, 347, 1986.
139. **Boackle, R. J., Pruitt, K. M., and Mestecky, J.,** The interactions of human complement with interfacially aggregated preparations of human secretory IgA, *Immunochemistry,* 11, 543, 1974.

140. **Pfaffenbach, G., Lamm, M. E., and Gigli, I.,** Activation of the guinea pig alternative complement pathway by mouse IgA immune complexes, *J. Exp. Med.*, 155, 231, 1982.
141. **Peltier, A. and Christian, C. L.,** The presence of the "rheumatoid factor" in sera from patients with syphilis, *Arthritis Rheum.*, 2, 1, 1959.
142. **Dresner, E. and Trombly, P.,** The latex-fixation reaction in non-rheumatoid diseases, *N. Engl. J. Med.*, 261, 981, 1959.
143. **Cathcart, E. S. et al.,** The relationship of the latex fixation test to the clinical and serologic manifestations of leprosy, *Am. J. Med.*, 31, 758, 1961.
144. **Williams, R. C. and Kunkel, H. G.,** Rheumatoid factor, complement and conglutinin aberrations in patients with subacute bacterial endocarditis, *J. Clin. Invest.*, 41, 666, 1962.
145. **Singer, J. M. et al.,** The presence of anti-gamma globulin factors in sera of patients with active pulmonary tuberculosis, *Ann. Intern. Med.*, 56, 545, 1962.
146. **Houba, V. and Allison, A. C.,** M-antiglobulins (rheumatoid factor-like globulins) and other gamma-globulins in relation to tropical parasitic infections, *Lancet,* i, 848, 1966.
147. **Carson, D. A. et al.,** IgG rheumatoid factor in subacute bacterial endocarditis: relationship to IgM rheumatoid factor and circulating immune complexes, *Clin. Exp. Immunol.*, 31, 100, 1978.
148. **Johnson, R. E. and Hall, A. P.,** Rubella arthritis: report of cases studied by latex tests, *N. Engl. J. Med.*, 258, 743, 1958.
149. **Svec, K. H. and Dingle, J. H.,** The occurrence of rheumatoid factor in association with antibody response to influenza A2 (Asian) virus, *Arthritis Rheum.*, 8, 524, 1965.
150. **Kaplan, M. E.,** Cryoglobulinemia in infectious mononucleosis: quantitation and characterization of the cryoproteins, *J. Lab. Clin. Med.*, 71, 754, 1968.
151. **Langenhuysen, M. M. A. C.,** Antibody against γ-globulin after blood transfusion and cytomegalovirus-infection, *Clin. Exp. Immunol.*, 9, 393, 1971.
152. **Levine, P. R. and Axelrod, D.,** Rheumatoid factor isotypes following immunization, *Arthritis Rheum.*, 28 (Abstr.), S100, 1985.
153. **Ashe, W. K. et al.,** Interaction of rheumatoid factor with infectious herpes simplex virus-antibody complexes, *Science,* 172, 176, 1971.
154. **Clarkson, A. B. and Mellow, G. H.,** Rheumatoid factor-like immunoglobulin M protects previously uninfected rat pups and dams from *Trypanosoma lewisi, Science,* 214, 186, 1981.
155. **Mikkelsen, W. M. et al.,** Estimates of the prevalence of rheumatic diseases in the population of Tecumseh, Michigan, 1959–60, *J. Chronic Dis.*, 20, 351, 1967.
156. **Bennett, P. H. and Burch, T. A.,** The distribution of rheumatoid factor and rheumatoid arthritis in the families of Blackfeet and Pima Indians, *Arthritis Rheum.*, 11, 546, 1968.
157. **Ball, J. and Lawrence, J. S.,** The relationship of rheumatoid serum factor and rheumatoid arthritis. A 5-year follow up of a population sample, *Ann. Rheum. Dis.*, 22, 311, 1963.
158. **Aho, K. et al.,** When does rheumatoid disease start?, *Arthritis Rheum.*, 28, 485, 1985.
159. **del Puente, A. et al.,** The incidence of rheumatoid arthritis is predicted by rheumatoid factor titer in a longitudinal population study, *Arthritis Rheum.*, 31, 1239, 1988.
160. **Koopman, W. J. and Schrohenloher, R. E.,** A sensitive radioimmunoassay for quantitation of IgM rheumatoid factor, *Arthritis Rheum.*, 23, 302, 1980.

161. **Koopman, W. J., Schrohenloher, R. E., and Solomon, A.,** A quantitative assay for IgA rheumatoid factor, *J. Immunol. Meth.,* 50, 89, 1982.
162. **Wernick, R. et al.,** Serum IgG and IgM rheumatoid factors by solid phase radioimmunoassay: a comparison between adult and juvenile rheumatoid arthritis, *Arthritis Rheum.,* 24, 1501, 1981.
163. **Butler, V. P., Jr. and Vaughan, J. H.,** The reaction of rheumatoid factor with animal gamma-globulins: quantitative considerations, *Immunology,* 8, 144, 1965.
164. **Heimer, R. et al.,** Different rheumatoid factors in the serum of one patient with rheumatic arthritis, *J. Lab. Clin. Med.,* 57, 16, 1961.
165. **Williams, R. C., Jr. and Kunkel, H. G.,** Separation of rheumatoid factors of different specificities using columns conjugated with gamma-globulin, *Arthritis Rheum.,* 6, 665, 1963.
166. **Allen, J. C. and Kunkel, H. G.,** Hidden rheumatoid factor with specificity for native γ globulin, *Arthritis Rheum.,* 9, 758, 1966.
167. **Stastny, P.,** Association of the B-cell alloantigen DRw4 with rheumatoid arthritis, *N. Engl. J. Med.,* 298, 869, 1978.
168. **Schiff, B. et al.,** Association of HLA-Aw31 and HLA-DR1 with adult rheumatoid arthritis, *Ann. Rheum. Dis.,* 41, 403, 1982.
169. **Karr, R. W. et al.,** Association of HLA-DRw4 with rheumatoid arthritis in black and white patients, *Arthritis Rheum.,* 23, 1241, 1980.
170. **Alarcón, G. S. et al.,** Sero-negative rheumatoid arthritis. A distinct immunogenetic disease?, *Arthritis Rheum.,* 25, 502, 1982.
171. **Doblough, J. H. et al.,** HLA antigens and rheumatoid arthritis, *Arthritis Rheum.,* 23, 309, 1980.
172. **Viana Queiros, M. et al.,** HLA-DR4 antigen and IgM rheumatoid factors, *J. Rheum.,* 9, 370, 1982.
173. **Olsen, N. J. et al.,** Associations of HLA-DR4 with rheumatoid factor and radiographic severity in rheumatoid arthritis, *Am. J. Med.,* 84, 257, 1988.
174. **Gregersen, P. K. et al.,** The shared epitope hypothesis: an approach to understanding the molecular genetics of susceptibility to rheumatoid arthritis, *Arthritis Rheum.,* 30, 1205, 1987.
175. **Gran, J. J. et al.,** The prevalence of HLA-DR4 and HLA-DR3 in healthy persons with rheumatoid factor, *Scand. J. Rheum.,* 14, 79, 1985.
176. **Silman, A. J. et al.,** Rheumatoid factor detection in the unaffected first degree relatives in families with multicase rheumatoid arthritis, *J. Rheum.,* 18, 512, 1991.
177. **Olsen, N. et al.,** High levels of IgM-rheumatoid factor synthesis correlate with HLA-DR4 in normal individuals, *Arthritis Rheum.,* 30, 841, 1987.
178. **Koopman, W. J. and Schrohenloher, R. E.,** Rheumatoid factor, in *Rheumatoid Arthritis. Etiology, Diagnosis, Management,* Utsinger, P. D., Zvaifler, N. J., and Ehrlich, G. E., Eds., J. B. Lippincott, Philadelphia, 1985, 217.
179. **Jaraquemada, D. et al.,** HLA and rheumatoid arthritis: susceptibility or severity, *Dis. Markers,* 4, 43, 1986.
180. **Walker, D. J. and Griffiths, I. D.,** HLA associations are with severe rheumatoid arthritis, *Dis. Markers,* 4, 131, 1986.
181. **Calin, A. et al.,** Destructive arthritis, rheumatoid factor, and HLA-DR4. Susceptibility versus severity, a case-control study, *Arthritis Rheum.,* 32, 1221, 1989.
182. **Ceuppens, J. L. et al.,** Non-steroidal anti-inflammatory agents inhibit the synthesis of IgM rheumatoid factor *in vitro, Lancet,* i, 528, 1982.

183. **Goodwin, J. S. et al.,** Administration of nonsteroidal anti-inflammatory agents in patients with rheumatoid arthritis: effects on indexes of cellular immune status and serum rheumatoid factor levels, *JAMA,* 250, 2485, 1983.
184. **Cush, J. J. et al.,** Correlation of serologic indicators of inflammation with effectiveness of nonsteroidal antiinflammatory drug therapy in rheumatoid arthritis, *Arthritis Rheum.,* 33, 19, 1990.
185. **Olsen, N. J. et al.,** Immunologic studies of rheumatoid arthritis patients treated with methotrexate, *Arthritis Rheum.,* 30, 481, 1987.

Chapter 3

Detection and Measurement of Rheumatoid Factor

Marius Teodorescu and Christopher J. Froelich

CONTENTS

I. METHODS OF DETECTION OF RHEUMATOID FACTOR

Historically rheumatoid factor (RF) activity has been measured by agglutination using either human IgG coated on latex particles or rabbit IgG bound to sheep red blood cells.[1] Although relatively sensitive, agglutination techniques are not quantitative in that a discontinuous scale or titer is used to report results and primarily IgM RF is detected (Table 1). Two widely used automated nephelometric methods, latex and turbidity, offer high throughput and quantitative results. Since IgM is an excellent agglutinator, latex nephelometry may detect primarily IgM RF. Turbidity-based nephelometry, however, has the potential to detect IgM, IgG, and IgA RF activity because all three mediate precipitation. Nevertheless, the precise contribution of each immunoglobulin class to total RF activity has not yet been determined experimentally for either method.

Enzyme-linked immunosorbent assay (ELISA), although less amenable to automation, has a distinct set of advantages: (1) specificity for RA is enhanced when rabbit IgG serves as antigen; (2) different isotypes of RF may be measured individually (IgM, IgG, IgA); (3) test sensitivity is higher than other methods; (4) the quality of the specimen (turbidity) is less likely to influence results; (5) a prozone phenomenon is not observed; and (6) relatively low instrument and reagent cost. Some commercial ELISA products use human IgG and are therefore limited to the detection of IgM RF; others use rabbit IgG, which allows for the separate detection of different Ig classes of RF.

The detection of RF by latex agglutination, sheep red cell agglutination, and nephelometry have been reviewed elsewhere.[3] Here we will focus on ELISA for the detection of IgM, IgG, and IgA RF activity toward rabbit IgG. With the help of μ and α heavy chain-specific enzyme antibody conjugates, the detection of IgM and IgA RF is relatively straightforward, based on the principle of indirect ELISA (see Chapter 1). Because IgM RF has been reported to interfere with the detection of IgG RF, techniques that measure IgG RF in the absence of IgM RF have been developed. It has been

0-8493-5974-1/94/$0.00 + $.50

Table 1 **Value and Drawbacks of Various Clinical Laboratory Methods for Detecting Rheumatoid Factor**

	Characteristics						
Method	**Precis.**	**Sensit.**	**Specific.**	**Class**	**Cost[a]**	**Prozone Effect**	**Value[b] Ranking**
ELISA with rabbit IgG	High	High	High	IgM/IgG/IgA separately	Mod.[c]	No	1
ELISA with human IgG	High	High	Low	IgM	mod.	No	2
Turbidity-based nephelometry	High	High	Low	All	High	Yes	3
Latex-based nephelometry	High	High	Low	IgM	High	Yes	4
Sheep cell agglutination	Low	Low	High	IgM	mod.	Yes	5
Latex agglutination	Low	High	Low	IgM	Low	Yes	6

[a] Reagents + labor + instrumentation. [b] 1 being the highest value and 6 the lowest. [c] mod., moderate.

proposed that IgM RF activity in the test sample may cause an overestimation of IgG RF by binding to solid-phase bound IgG while simultaneously immobilizing the patient's own IgG.[4,5] In addition, the nonspecific attachment of normal IgG to the solid-phase bound rabbit IgG, probably by Fc-Fc "aggregation", may also produce a false positive for IgG RF activity. Pepsin digestion of the test sample, a process that destroys IgM RF activity and cleaves the Fc segment of IgG, has been reported to solve these problems.[5,6] The IgG $F(ab')_2$-RF remaining after digestion binds to the solid phase and is detected with a specific antibody, anti-CH1γ,[4] or a polyclonal anti-Fab antibody conjugate. However, since Fab of monomeric IgA resists proteolysis, detection of $F(ab')_2$ fragment with a polyclonal anti-Fab (H and L chains) may also detect IgA.[7]

The significance of IgM interference with the measurement of IgG RF requires additional study. If IgM RF causes a false-positive IgG RF determination,[4,5] IgG RF levels detected in the presence of IgM RF should not correlate with the level of peptic digests — $F(ab')_2$ — of the same samples. We found, however, that the correlation between the two types of measurements on 12 randomly selected RA patients was surprisingly high ($R = 0.8$) (Figure 1) suggesting that the presence of IgM RF may not interfere with measurement of IgG RF activity and pepsin digestion may be avoided.

II. TYPE OF REACTIONS INVOLVED IN ELISA FOR RHEUMATOID FACTOR (SEE ALSO CHAPTER 1)

This is an indirect solid-phase enzyme immunoassay.[8] Alternate wells of polystyrene plate are coated with purified rabbit IgG and then all wells are saturated with bovine serum albumin (BSA) or a similar blocking reagent that does not contain IgG. Thus, each specimen, control, and standard is incubated in two wells (i.e., wells with and without antigen). To detect IgM and IgA RF, respectively, enzyme-labeled rabbit anti-human IgM (Fc5μ specific) and anti-IgA (a chain specific) are added, followed by the specific substrate. After subtracting the value for the blank, the net absorbance is calculated and related to the calibrator to determine the number of units in each sample.

To detect IgG RF two methods may be used, each with its advantages and pitfalls. First, the test is performed as for IgM and IgA RF (see above) but with an anti-Fcγ as the second antibody. This method has the advantage of simplicity but the background binding of normal IgG to the plate has to be carefully controlled to avoid false-positive reactions. Second, the serum is first incubated overnight in a pepsin solution to inactivate IgM and to remove the Fc of IgG;[4] the presence of IgG RF on the plate is detected with an anti-$F(ab')_2$ antibody conjugate. This method has the advantage of removing practically all background binding of IgG, but also may measure IgA RF.

III. SPECIMENS, SUPPLIES, REAGENTS, AND EQUIPMENT

The following are reagents that are prepared in the lab or obtained commercially (see also Chapter 1). In general, commercial reagents are stabilized for long-term storage at 4°C. Reagents manufactured "in house" also need to have supporting stability data. However, freezing some reagents, as specified below, may assure stability.

Antigen-coated microwells — Strips of 8 or 12 wells are used. A solution of 10 μg/ml of rabbit IgG is prepared in phosphate-buffered saline (PBS), pH 7.4, and incubated in the wells overnight at room temperature to assure binding. IgG binds well

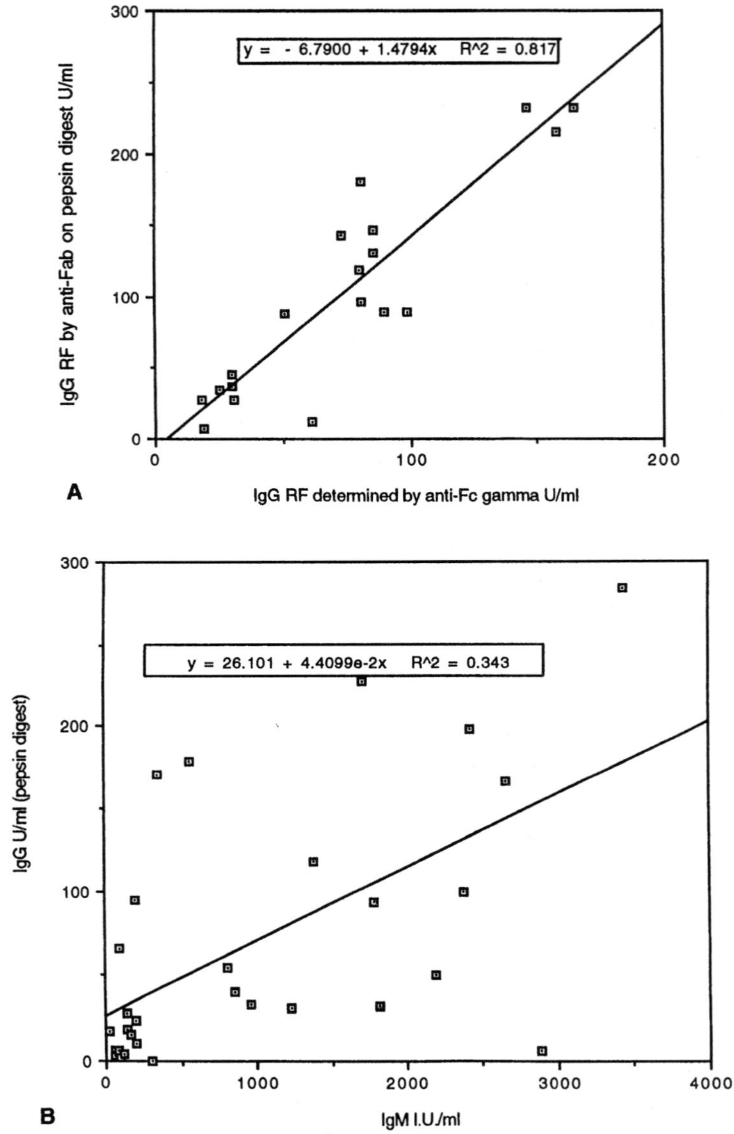

Figure 1 Relationship between various rheumatoid factor tests. (A) Correlation between IgG RF measured with and without pepsin digestion. (B) Lack of good correlation between IgM and IgG (pepsin digestion).

to a variety of ELISA-grade microtiter plates. Half of the microwells in each column or a row of wells are coated with rabbit IgG and saturated with BSA and the other half are only saturated with BSA to serve as controls (Figure 1). Plates made in house should be stored in zip-locked bags with a dessicator at −20°C.

Diluent and wash solution — The same buffer is used for both functions. PBS with 0.05% Tween 20 is prepared. It should not contain preservatives and is stored at 4°C. Water should be type 1 (tissue culture grade) or perfusion grade (USP).

Enzyme conjugate solutions — Rabbit anti-human IgM (Fc 5μ specific), IgA (α chain specific), and monoclonal anti-$(Fab')_2$ coupled with horseradish peroxidase (HRPO) are available commercially from multiple vendors (see Appendix to this volume). The optimal dilution for anti-IgM is determined as follows: patient serum (250 I.U. ± 50/ml of RF activity) and a normal donor (<25 I.U./ml) are identified. A dilution of conjugate is selected (see Chapter 1) by checkerboard arrangement that yields an absorbance value within acceptable linearity (e.g., 0.8 to 1.5) and at the same time to be very low for the normal donor (e.g., <0.15). Dilute conjugate may be stored at 4°C in commercial stabilizing buffers or frozen in aliquots.

Substrate — See Chapter 1.

Pepsin — This enzyme is used only for the detection of IgG RF by the digestion method.[6] A 100× pepsin concentrate (15 mg/ml) is prepared and stored frozen in small aliquots. It is diluted 1:100 in 0.1 *M* sodium acetate buffer, pH 4.4, immediately before use. The protease is inactivated by adding an equal volume of 0.564 *M* disodium hydrogen phosphate buffer containing Tween 20.[6] This phosphate buffer solution may be stored at 4°C (note: crystals may form in the cold).

IV. STANDARDS AND CONTROLS (SEE ALSO CHAPTER 1)

A. CALIBRATORS

IgM RF calibrator — The IgM RF international standard (1000 I.U./ml) is obtained from The Centers for Disease Control (CDC) in Atlanta, GA. An in-house calibrator is generated as follows: a standard curve is created with the CDC standard at dilutions of 1:200, 1:400, 1:800, and 1:1600. In parallel, a serum sample that will be used as the in-house calibrator is similarly diluted. The dilution of the in-house calibrator that produces an absorbance value comparable to the diluted (e.g., 1.2) CDC standard is then used to calculate the I.U./ml, (see Section V, Calculation of Results). The serum sample used to prepare the in-house calibrator should have the following specifications: at the dilution of 1:200 it produces absorbance value of 1.2 ± 0.2 and contains about 250 ± 50 I.U./ml of serum. The calibrator should be aliquoted in small tubes and may be stored at −20°C for 1 year or at −70°C for at least 5 years. This serum may be used either as a one-point standard or, to enhance precision, for generating a standard curve. If the serum contains a high level of IgM RF activity, it may be adjusted by diluting it in 6% BSA.

IgG RF calibrator — Units for the IgG RF calibrator are arbitrary. Normal range must be determined by testing a group of normals and RA patients. For testing whole sera (i.e., without pepsin digestion), the same methodology described above for the

IgM RF calibrator applies, except that the unit value for the standard is arbitrary. To establish units for pepsin-digested serum the following method is used. Pepsin digestion is performed on five normal sera and ten sera from patients with long-standing erosive RA. A concentration of anti-$(Fab')_2$ conjugate is identified: (1) that gives an absorbence of >1.0 for at least one of the patients, and (2) at which all four of the normal sera give net absorbance values of <0.15. An arbitrary number of units is assigned before validation on a large number of normal donors and on RA patients. The unit values may be adjusted to the same range as the unit value for IgM RF for the same absorbence level.

IgA RF calibrator — This calibrator is prepared based on the same principle.

B. CONTROLS

Positive control — Patient serum containing the desired RF (100 to 200 I.U./ml) is obtained and 0.1% thimerosal is added. The sample is aliquoted and stored with the calibrator.

Negative control — Human serum that contains <20 I.U./ml for IgM RF is obtained and 0.1% thimerosal is added.

Calibration and tolerance — The in-house calibrator is retested against the CDC standard at least twice a year or whenever the performance of the system is in question. The repeated measurements for the CDC standard should be ±20% of the original values. Low values tend to cause false-positive results and high values produce false-negative test results. Values for positive and negative controls should be ±25% of the original values. The value of the calibrators may be validated by testing normal donors (at least 100) and at least 30 patients with clinically confirmed rheumatoid arthritis. Normal limits are determined by excluding the highest five values (95%) of the 100 normal donors tested after repeating the test on the ten highest values at least three times.

V. ASSAY PROCEDURE, CALCULATION, AND REPORTING RESULTS

Assay procedure — If the three classes of RF activity are detected without pepsin treatment, each class may be detected separately using the principle of indirect ELISA (Chapter 1). If the pepsin treatment method is used, IgG RF can only be detected at the same time with IgM RF, due to the need to have a control for the effective digestion of IgM RF.

1. Pepsin digestion is set up 18 to 24 h prior to the performance of the test. Pepsin solution (150 μg/ml) in 100 m*M* Na acetate buffer, pH 4.4, is prepared. Serum (5 μl) (specimens, calibrator, positive and negative controls) is added to 0.5 ml of pepsin solution. The digests are incubated at 37°C for 18 to 22 h and the reaction stopped with 0.5 ml of saline containing 0.564 *M* disodium hydrogen phosphate and Tween 20.[6]
2. Dilute calibrators, controls, and specimens in PBS containing Tween 20.
3. Add each of the dilute samples and controls (100 μl/well) to parallel wells, with and without antigen (blank). Thus, for each specimen use three pairs of wells and, if the pepsin digest method is used, double the number of wells for each pepsin-digested specimen (final four pairs).

Results expressed as Units/ml

Test (ELISA method)	Patient Result	Normal Max	High Value
RF - Quant IgM	6600	55	2500
RF - Quant IgG	45	20	250
RF - Quant IgA	950	35	500

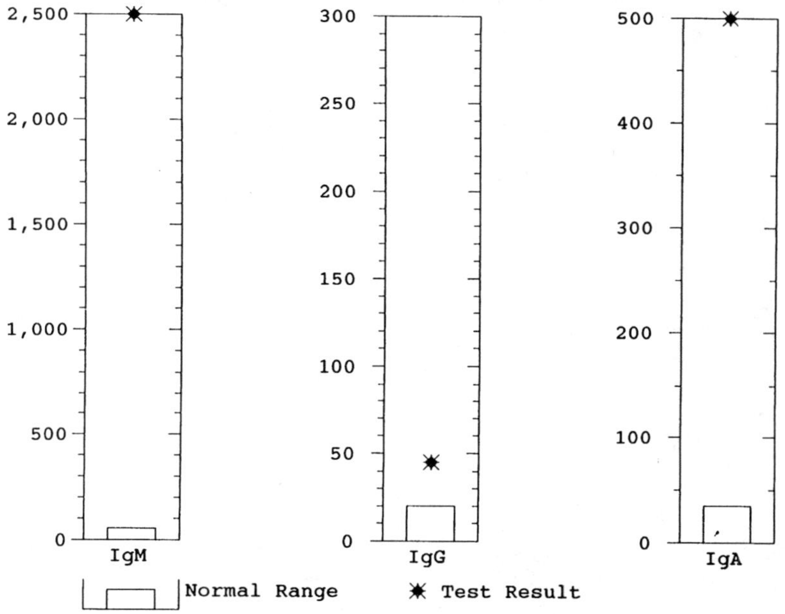

Figure 2 Graphic presentation of the results for IgM, IgG, and IgA rheumatoid factor in a patient with erosive rheumatoid arthritis.

4. Incubate the plate for 30 min at room temperature (18 to 30°C) and wash the plate three or four times with PBS/Tween 20.
5. Add the antibody conjugate specific for each Ig class. For pepsin-digested specimens add anti-Fab in one pair of wells and anti-5μ in the other to determine the effectiveness of digestion. Incubate for 30 min at room temperature.
6. Wash three or four times, add substrate, incubate for 15 min, stop the reaction with phosphoric acid (0.1 to 0.2 *M*), and read the plate.

Calculation of results (see also Chapter 1) — The specific absorbance for each specimen and control is calculated by subtracting the absorbance of the specimen blank well from the absorbance value of the specific antigen tested. Determine the net absorbance for the IgM RF calibrator, controls, and specimens. Although only a standard curve offers precision for research, one-point calibration offers sufficient precision for this assay in a clinical laboratory.

Reporting results and interpretation (see also Chapter 4) — The result is placed into perspective as follows (Figure 2) A scale of values is established to include a high value and the upper limit of normals. The high value is determined to include about

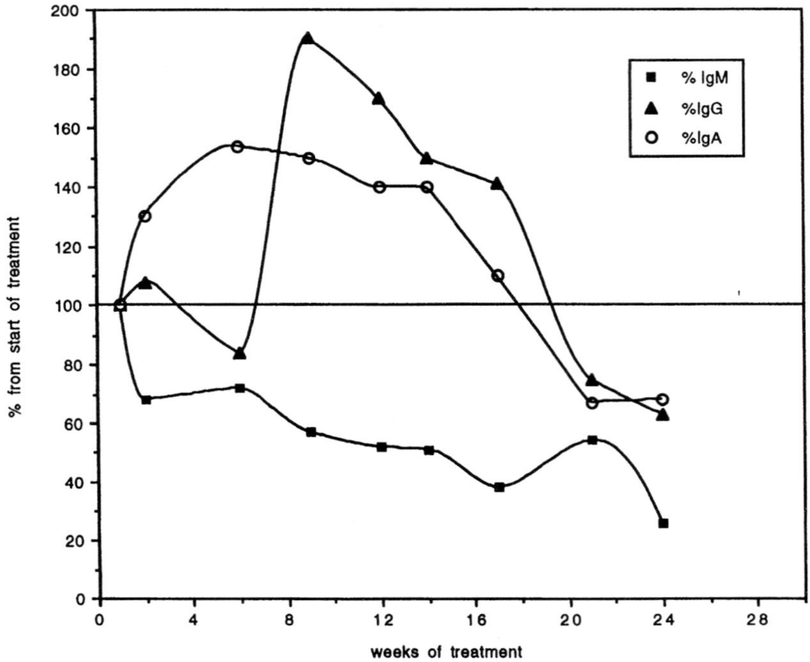

Figure 3 Changes in the level of rheumatoid factors IgM, IgG, and IgA in the serum of a rheumatoid arthritis patient treated with gold salts. The patient received 10 mg the first week, 25 mg the second week, and 50 mg per week thereafter.

95% of the patients with RF. For example, if by testing 100 patients for RF the top five values were found to be 12,000, 10,000, 6,000, 4,500, and 3,000 U/ml, the 3,000 becomes a high value for reference. It means that only about 5% of patients with this condition will exceed the high value. At the bottom of this scale is the upper limit of normal (Figure 2). Thus, reported values between these two parameters represent degrees of ''positivity''. The values may also be tracked longitudinally during treatment (Figure 3 and Table 2). With chrysotherapy it appears that IgG RF decreases most dramatically. In another published longitudinal study the most significant reduction was in IgM and IgA.[9] However, data that describe characteristic temporal change in levels under the influence of various treatments is insufficient. Commonly, for example, a transient increase in IgM RF or IgG RF occurs during early therapy with gold salts (Figure 3), which is then followed by a reduction.

Limitations of procedure — The limitations are the same as for other autoantibodies (see also Chapter 1). In addition, the level of IgM RF may be lowered by the presence of cold agglutinins. Values in units that are only up to double that of normal limits should be interpreted with caution, since RF is a normal constituent of human serum and may transiently rise as the result of relatively minor activation of the immune system.

Table 2 **Change in RF Level in Patients with Rheumatoid Arthritis Under Treatment with Gold Salts**

		% of starting level		
Patient	**Weeks of treatment**	**IgM**	**IgG**	**IgA**
MCr	18	41	28	42
YA	13	85		59
AR	13	76		34
SR	20	45	4	112
EB	26	64	5	133
AC	19	43	88	82
AG	20	58	6	66
ECh	20	108	205	94
MJ	18	55	142	44
MK	28	63	8	33
JP	18	7	4	30
RO	24	27	63	66
Median		57	18	62

Note: All patients received 10 mg at start, 25 mg the second week, and 50 mg each week thereafter.

VI. QUALITY CONTROL, IMPLEMENTATION, AND VALIDATION

Quality control (see also Chapter 1) — If the pepsin digestion method is used additional evaluations are required. To evaluate the effectiveness of digestion of IgM RF the absorbance in wells containing an IgM calibrator and positive control developed with anti-IgM conjugate should be relatively high (e.g., 1.2). This shows that the conjugate is capable of detecting IgM. At the same time the digested IgG calibrator developed with anti-IgM should have a relatively low absorbance value (e.g., <0.2) and the adjacent well treated with anti-Fab conjugate should have a relatively high value (e.g., 1.2). In the course of routine use it becomes readily apparent that the IgM is effectively destroyed, since digested patient samples with IgM RF no longer react with anti-IgM. Detection of abnormal levels of IgG RF and normal levels of IgM RF is relatively rare and suggests possible technical error.

Implementation and validation — By testing 100 normal subjects (see also Chapter 1), limits may be determined at 95 percentile by excluding the five highest values. The test is repeated for the ten highest values. Since the distribution of RF in the normal population is not gaussian, the mean plus two or three standard deviations does not offer a correct upper limit for normal subjects. Cross-validation by a different method is also desirable if the test is prepared in the lab. For example, sera from 30 normal subjects and 30 patients are examined independently by a different method (e.g., nephelometry) and correlative analysis is performed.

REFERENCES

1. **Carson, D. A.,** Rheumatoid factor, in *Textbook of Rheumatology,* 2nd ed., Kelley, W., Harris, D., Ruddy, S., and Sledge, W, Eds., 1985, 665.
2. **Goddard, D. H. and Moore, M. E.,** Common tests for rheumatoid factors: poorly standardized but ubiquitous, *Arthritis Rheum.,* 31, 432, 1988.
3. **Cook, L. and Agnello, V.,** Test for detection of rheumatoid factors, in *Manual of Clinical Laboratory Immunology,* 4th ed., Rose, N. R. et al., 1992, 762.
4. **Teitsson, I. and Valdimarsson, H.,** Use of monoclonal antibodies and $F(ab')_2$ enzyme conjugates in ELISA for IgM, IgA and IgG rheumatoid factors, *J. Immunol. Meth.,* 71, 149, 1984.
5. **Faith, A., Pontesilli, O., Unger, A., Panayi, G. S., and Johns, P.,** ELISA assays for IgM and IgG rheumatoid factor, *J. Immunol. Meth.,* 55, 169, 1982.
6. **Bampton, J. L. M., Cawson, T. E., Kyle, M. V., and Hazleman, B. L.,** Measurement of rheumatoid factors by an enzyme-linked immunosorbent assay (ELISA) and comparison with other methods, *Ann. Rheum. Dis.,* 44, 13, 1985.
7. **Rivat, C., Bourguignon, J., Fontaine, M., and Ropartz, C.,** Enzymatic fragmentation of human IgA $F(abc)'_2$: a new peptic fragment, *Immunochemistry,* 14, 69, 1977.
8. **Karsh, J., Halbert, S. P., Klima, E., and Steinberg, A. D.,** Quantitative determination of rheumatoid factor by an enzyme-labeled immunoassay, *J. Immunol. Meth.,* 32, 115, 1980.
9. **Hanly, J. G., Hassan, J., Whelan, A., Feighery, C., and Bresnihan, B.,** Effects of gold therapy on the synthesis and quantity of serum and synovial fluid IgM, IgG and IgA rheumatoid factors in rheumatoid arthritis patients, *Arthritis Rheum.,* 29, 480, 1986.

Chapter 4

Clinical Value of Rheumatoid Factor Measurement

James S. Grober and Christopher J. Froelich

CONTENTS

I. INTRODUCTION

Over 50 years ago, Waaler[1] and Rose et al.[2] showed that certain human sera were able to agglutinate sheep erythrocytes. Since the phenomenon was found to be mediated by agglutinating antibodies identified primarily in the sera of patients with rheumatoid arthritis (RA), the name rheumatoid factor (RF) was adopted. RFs can be defined as autoantibodies that bind antigenic determinants in the CH_2 and CH_3 domains (Fc fragment) of IgG molecule. Although early laboratory studies demonstrated the existence of IgM RF antibodies, more recent work has shown that the immune system produces IgG, IgA, and IgE RFs. Whether RF plays a dominant role in the immunopathogenesis of RA or merely is a consequence of polyclonal B cell activation during the chronic inflammatory process remains unclear. Insights have been provided by sequencing studies which showed that RFs exist either in a germline (e.g., monoclonal RFs of gammopathies) or somatically mutated configuration (e.g., RF in the synovium, see Chapter 2). Nevertheless, epidemiologic studies also may offer clues to the role of RF in the disease process (see below).

RF activity is detected by a variety of methods. The most widespread technique measures agglutination using either sheep erythrocytes, IgG-coated latex, or bentonite beads as the indicator. Newer, sensitive and quantitative methods include radioimmunoassay (RIA), enzyme-linked immunosorbent assay (ELISA), and nephelometric techniques (see Chapters 2 and 3 for details).

II. DEFINITION OF SENSITIVITY, SPECIFICITY, AND PREDICTIVE VALUE

Although RF is primarily associated with RA, RF activity also has been identified in the sera of patients with other rheumatic disorders (e.g., Sjögren's syndrome), with nonrheumatic infectious and inflammatory diseases (e.g., sarcoidosis, subacute bacterial

0-8493-5974-1/94/$0.00+$.50

endocarditis), and with aging. The widespread availability of RF testing and the high prevalence of musculoskeletal complaints in the general population conspire to make "RF assay" the most commonly ordered immunologic test in clinical medicine. These circumstances have led to the overutilization of RF testing and have resulted in the inadvertent misdiagnosis and mismanagement of patients with vague musculoskeletal complaints.

Consequently, in order to use RF test results in a cost-effective and rational manner, one should have a thorough understanding of the test's diagnostic sensitivity, specificity, and predictive value for RA and other diseases, as well as be cognizant of the prognostic value of RF positivity in RA patients and asymptomatic individuals. Based on the principles of sensitivity, specificity, and predictive value (see introduction), a serological test used for screening groups of normal subjects should be very sensitive but have moderate specificity and predictive value. When the test is used for diagnosis, however, both specificity and predictive value must be high, while a somewhat lower sensitivity may be acceptable. Because the more sophisticated immunoassays possess high test sensitivity (and hence disease sensitivity), they may have lower disease specificity, which results in reduced predictive value. This problem, however, may be partially circumvented by broadening the range of normal values and by insuring that age-matched controls are used.

III. PREVALENCE OF RF IN RANDOM POPULATION

Differences in the diagnostic sensitivity and specificity of RF testing can be attributed to the following interrelated factors: (1) the failure to perform standardized testing, (2) the frequency of RF in the normal population from which the test sample is derived, (3) the effect of aging on prevalence of RF positivity, and (4) the test method chosen to measure RF activity. The clinical goals of RF testing are to screen and "quantify" the serum level of RF activity. The most common screening practice is to perform a semiquantitative agglutination assay in which the result is reported as positive or negative at a defined cut-off value (titer). Thereafter, endpoint dilution is performed to determine the level of RF activity (usually titer). Reporting test results of the RF assay as titers is archaic. This unit of measure reduces test precision, compromising the value of the agglutination assay as a screening test. As described for anti-nuclear antibody testing, the conversion of titers to units based on an external standard would significantly improve test precision and hence the value of the RF test for screening. If the goal of testing is to determine the level of RF activity, then external standardization is mandatory and a more precise assay (e.g., ELISA, nephelometry) should be considered a substitute for the agglutination method. A standard reference serum, with RF activity designated in international units, is provided by the Centers for Disease Control.[3] In addition, organizations that administer proficiency testing programs (e.g., the College of American Pathologists) allow clinical laboratories to evaluate the precision of their methods[3] by testing samples that contain various levels of RF.

The revised 1987 American College of Rheumatology (ACR) criteria for RA suggest that less than 5% of normal subjects should be positive for RF.[4] The issues of converting titers to unit values for agglutination assays and the utilization of an international standard irrespective of the assay method performed are not addressed in the ACR criteria. Given the pitfalls of RF testing, it is not surprising that some investigators have chosen a cut-off for the presence of RF as low as 1:20, while others use values of 1:80, 1:128, or (rarely) higher. Since the current problems in RF testing result in reduced precision and concordance, the reported values obtained from population-based prevalence analyses will vary widely and consequently should be interpreted with caution.

Using the latex fixation test to detect RF in 5461 normal subjects, Waller et al.[5] reported RF positivity in 3 to 5% of individuals younger than age 60, whereas 28% of those older than age 60 were seropositive. However, by sheep cell agglutination test, 2% of the older and less than 1% of the younger individuals were positive. In Tecumseh, Michigan, testing 6590 persons by latex agglutination demonstrated an overall prevalence of 3% which increased to 11% for individuals over age 70.[6] A population survey of 7200 Finns showed that RF positivity (by sheep cell agglutination) existed in 1 to 2% of subjects between ages 30 and 70 and in only 3% of subjects older than 70.[7] While only 6% of 902 normal Eskimos younger than 55 years had positive RF tests, 14% of the older age group were seropositive by bentonite flocculation.[8] Thus, irrespective of the agglutination methods, the prevalence of RF positivity in younger individuals (age less than 55 to 60) is less than 5%, whereas upwards of 25% of persons older than 60 may be RF-positive, particularly if latex fixation is used to detect RF activity. If approximately 1 to 3% of the population has RA and approximately 80% are RF-positive (see below), it becomes apparent that the reported frequencies of RF positivity in these random population studies exceeds the values that can be accounted for by the inadvertent inclusion of RA patients in the tested groups. The relatively high prevalence of RF in a young normal population is most readily attributed to the imprecision of agglutination testing and the reporting of results as titers.

As noted above, upwards of 25% of persons greater than age 60 in random populations may be RF-positive by agglutination techniques. Although RF titers in these individuals are usually low, a substantial percentage (as high as 20%) have titers higher than 1:160. The increased frequency of RF positivity in the elderly is likely due to the enhanced production of autoantibodies (see Chapter 2). This observation indicates that age-adjusted normal values are necessary for evaluating the results of RF tests in the elderly. Measurement of RF isotypes may help to clarify this issue. Teittson[9] reported that IgM RF but not IgA RF levels increase with age in patients with RA. In contrast, it should be noted that Wolfe et al.[10] found no significant correlation of RF *positivity* (defined as titer ⩾1:80) with age in 8287 rheumatic disease clinic patients using a commercial latex kit. However, RF *titer* did increase with age in 1362 RA patients but not in the 6925 patients with other rheumatic diseases.

Are asymptomatic RF-positive individuals at increased risk of developing RA? Ball and Lawrence reported that 7 of 19 asymptomatic RF-positive subjects developed RA over a 5-year period.[11] A survey of 2712 Pima Indians over 19 years by del Puente et al.[12] found a positive correlation between the development of RA (i.e., person years of risk) and RF titer elevation. Nevertheless, all individuals with high RF titers did not develop RA. The fact that the study involved a genetically homogenous group which has an increased incidence of RA limits the generalizability of the data. This is because the high incidence of risk exaggerates the risk associated with a positive RF test. In 1985, Aho et al. retrospectively analyzed sera from 30 patients with new-onset RA identified during a Finnish longitudinal cardiovascular study and detected RF in 12 sera obtained 4 to 60 months before the diagnosis of RA.[7] The results of their more recent work are consistent with earlier findings.[13] Both these reports confirm the potentially long latent period between RF production and RA presentation. The prevalence of RF in the original groups of healthy individuals was not stated and there were no data on

Table 1 **ACR Diagnostic Criteria for Rheumatoid Arthritis (1987)**

Criterion	Definition
1. Morning stiffness	Morning stiffness lasting at least 1 h
2. Symmetrical joint involvement	
3. Arthritis of 3 or more joints	Observed soft tissue swelling or fluid of at least three joints; 14 possible areas: PIP, MCP, wrist, elbow, knee, ankle, and MTP joints
4. Arthritis of hand joints	One swollen area in wrist, MCP, or PIP joint
5. Rheumatoid nodules	Subcutaneous nodules, over bony prominences, or extensor surfaces, or in juxta-articular regions
6. Serum rheumatoid factor	
7. Radiographic changes	

comparative disease outcomes in the original healthy seronegative and seropositive groups. Despite their shortcomings, the studies illustrate important features of RF as a predictor of RA. The presence of RF in an otherwise healthy individual is clearly associated with increased risk of RA. As many as 50% of all patients with RA have antecedent history of positive RF. Nevertheless, at the population level, *RF is a poor predictor* of disease. Although these data are intriguing, routine screening of asymptomatic individuals does not appear to be useful to identify those at high risk for RA until new therapeutic modalities become available.

IV. DIAGNOSTIC SENSITIVITY, SPECIFICITY, AND PREDICTIVE VALUE OF RF TESTING IN RHEUMATOID ARTHRITIS

Rheumatoid arthritis affects an estimated 1 to 3% of the general population, with peak onset at ages 35 to 45. Women are three times more likely than men to develop the disease, and a positive family history may confer additional risk. The presence of serum RF is one of the ACR diagnostic criteria for the classification of RA (Table 1). According to this scheme, individuals meeting at least four of the seven criteria can be diagnosed with RA. Primarily designed to facilitate the standardization of patients enrolled in various research protocols, the ACR criteria have enabled investigators to assess the sensitivity and specificity of RF testing for the diagnosis of RA.

Standard rheumatology texts state that the prevalence of IgM RF positivity among RA patients is between 70 and 90%. These figures are based primarily on clinical studies that employed less sensitive agglutination techniques.[6] Using the sensitive ELISA technique with rabbit IgG as antigen, we observed that 57 of 61 patients with RA at the University of Illinois Arthritis Center (93%) were positive for RF. Along similar lines, very little information exists that describes the prevalence of IgG RF and IgA RF in RA. When IgG and IgA RF reactivity of the above-mentioned patients was determined by ELISA, the distribution by class showed that about 70% had all three isotypes (IgM, IgG, and IgA), 20% had IgM and IgA, and 3% had only IgM RF. Isolated IgG RF without IgM or IgM and IgG without IgA are very rare (<1%).

In several older population-based cross-sectional studies, RF diagnostic sensitivity was low. These studies applied the 1958 American College of Rheumatology criteria and reported RA prevalence of 2.4 to 6.1%. Although the specificity of RF testing in these studies was 92 to 98%, the prevalence of RF seropositivity in these RA patients (i.e., the sensitivity of RF testing) ranged from only 19 to 33%. Possible explanations for the reported low sensitivities include: (1) a higher prevalence of milder, self-limited seronegative RA existing in the general population compared to cohorts in clinical studies (e.g., only 28% of Tecumseh RA patients had evidence of RA 3 to 5 years later); (2) the absence of a precise, sensitive, and standardized method for RF detection in population studies (e.g., 44% of RF-positive Tecumseh patients were negative on repeat testing); and (3) population studies likely include patients with early seronegative disease. In the study used to develop the 1987 ACR criteria for the classification of RA, 80.4% of RA patients were positive for RF.[4] Similarly, RF positivity was noted in 87% of 200 RA patients followed at a university-based rheumatology clinic.[14] The study by Wolfe et al.[10] of 8287 consecutive new outpatient arthritis clinic patients revealed a sensitivity of 78% at a titer of 1:80 (latex fixation).

The discrepancies in diagnostic sensitivity of RF testing for clinical and population studies described above raise questions about the positive and negative predictive value of RF testing. According to probability theory, the pretest probability of RA influences the likelihood that RA is present given a positive result and, conversely, the likelihood that it is absent given a negative result. Pretest probability is determined by: (1) the prevalence of RA in the "normal" population from which the patient comes and (2) the physician's estimate of disease likelihood as based on clinical experience and relevant published data. Since the pretest probability of RA is significantly greater for the rheumatologist than for the generalist, the predictive value of a positive RF test should be lower for the generalist.

Fortunately, these issues have been critically addressed by Wolfe et al. in a 14-year study of outpatient arthritis clinic patients, in whom the prevalence of RA (according to either 1958 or 1987 ACR criteria) was 16.4%.[10] The non-RA patients were divided into groups that had either inflammatory rheumatic disease (IRD) (e.g., systemic lupus erythematosus [SLE], Sjögren's syndrome) or noninflammatory rheumatic disease (NIRD) (e.g., osteoarthritis, gout). Among the combined IRD and NIRD patients, RF was positive in 3.2%. The authors calculated that the respective post-test probabilities of RA in a seropositive and a seronegative patient were greater than 0.80 and less than 0.05. The generation of curves for physician operating characteristic that describe the true-positive and false-positive rates for the RA, IRD, and NIRD groups then allows the assessment of post-test probabilities in other clinical settings. For example, if community and general practice patients are considered to be roughly comparable to the NIRD patients in this study, and assuming a prevalence of 1% for RA in the community, a positive RF would indicate a 10% likelihood of RA. It should be noted, however, that 92.8% of the patients in this study were Caucasian. Whether these data are valid for clinic populations of different racial and ethnic makeup remains to be determined. Nonetheless, they offer the clearest guidelines to date for clinicians trying to assess post-test probabilities of RA.

Despite the attempts to develop criteria that would delineate clinically homogeneous groups of RA patients, not all RA patients have elevated serum levels of RF. Several explanations of RF seronegativity in RA have been offered. Foremost, the prevalence of RF among RA patients will be influenced by the sensitivity of the assay procedure.

Also, widely used agglutination techniques measure IgM RF but rarely detect RFs of other isotypes (see cases 1, 2, 3). So-called "hidden IgM RFs" have also been implicated.[15] Hidden IgM RFs do not react in standard tests of sera, perhaps because they have higher avidity for human IgG than do classical RFs. They can be detected by ELISA or if standard tests are performed using the IgM fraction of sera. Nevertheless, recent evidence suggests that hidden IgM RFs are found in 65 to 75% of juvenile RA sera but only rarely in seronegative adult RA sera.[15] Of course, some patients may be seronegative because of testing early in the disease course. Jacoby et al.[16] found that the prevalence of seropositivity in RA patients after 3 months of disease was only 33%; the prevalence rose to 55% after 6 months and, ultimately, to 88% in 100 patients followed for 11 years.

V. PROGNOSTIC VALUE IN RHEUMATOID ARTHRITIS

The presence of RF in patients with RA has been widely accepted as a poor prognostic factor. In comparison to their seronegative counterparts, seropositive RA patients have been reported to develop more severe joint erosions and extra-articular complications.[17-23] Several recent studies have expanded this conventional view. By ELISA, elevation of IgG RF is associated with more severe RA; patients with vasculitis and nodules have high serum levels of IgG RF.[24] As measured by RIA, Jones and Jacoby[25] found that the frequency of erosive disease correlated with serum levels of IgM RF (and, to a lesser degree, IgA and IgG RF). IgA RF levels have been associated with increased disease severity, as assessed by standard clinical parameters and by erythrocyle sedimentation rate (ESR).[9] In a prospective study of 58 RA patients, Mottinen et al.[26] found that patients with elevated levels of IgA RF levels were more likely to develop joint erosions within the first 2 years of disease onset. IgA RF and IgG RF levels within the first year of RA have also been correlated with the time of first appearance of joint erosions, as well as with the severity of erosive changes and the functional grade in 119 patients after a mean follow-up period of 10 years.[27] Additional studies are warranted to determine the associations of the different RF isotypes with disease manifestations.

Kinoshita et al. have investigated the clinical utility of measuring the binding specificity of RF for substances other than the Fc region of IgG.[28] They found that levels of RFs that cross-react with ssDNA (CRRF), present in a variety of rheumatic diseases, are increased in RA patients with extra-articular disease manifestations. Whether CRRF levels are elevated before the development of extra-articular disease, and might therefore offer prognostic information, remains to be determined.

Noritake et al.[29] developed a double-binding ELISA to measure RFs that bind and cross-link human IgG and sheep IgG. Seropositivity identified by this method was highly specific (99%) for RA but only 36% sensitive in the entire group of 108 patients. However, the test was 88% sensitive for moderately severe RA (40 patients) and was positive primarily in those with active disease.

Several studies have evaluated the effects of treatment on RF levels. Compared with pretreatment values, Cush et al. reported decreases in IgM RF levels in RA patients who responded to either flurbiprofen or ibuprofen.[30] Patients who did not respond to treatment showed no significant change in RF level, as assessed by either rate nephelometry or ELISA. Goodwin et al.[31] noted significant decreases in mean serum RF titers associated with clinical improvement in patients who received piroxicam for 10 weeks. In our experience as well as that of others,[24] immunosuppressive therapy that resulted in clinical improvement was also associated with a reduction in IgM RF levels.

Table 2 **Rheumatoid Factor in Rheumatic Disease**

Disease	Frequency (%)
Rheumatoid arthritis	50–90
Sjögren's syndrome	55–95
Cryoglobulinemia[47]	40–100
Mixed connective tissue disease	15–60
Systemic lupus erythematosus	15–35
Systemic sclerosis	10–30
Polymyositis/dermatomyositis	5–10
Juvenile polyarticular RA	60–75
Polymyalgia rheumatica	5–10
Lyme disease	5–10

Table 3 **Rheumatoid Factor in Nonrheumatic Diseases**

Primary biliary cirrhosis	30–70%
Parasitic infection[49]	10–70%
Viral infection[50-52]	15–65%
Leprosy	5–60%
Subacute bacterial endocarditis	25–50%
Silicosis	30–50%
Interstitial pulmonary fibrosis	10–50%
Hepatitis	15–40%
Sarcoidosis	3–33%
Asbestosis	30%
Syphilis	0–15%

Data from Reference 48.

VI. DIAGNOSTIC UTILITY IN OTHER DISORDERS

RFs have been reported to be elevated in the serum of patients with a wide variety of rheumatic and nonrheumatic disorders (Tables 2 and 3). The diagnosis of these varied diseases, however, does not require and usually is not assisted by RF testing. Thus, the significance of RF positivity in these diseases lies in their potential confusion with rheumatoid arthritis — that is, the problem of false positivity. Fortunately, the clinical features of these disorders permit distinction from RA, especially as patients are followed over time. Nevertheless, it may be difficult to differentiate the patient with incidental IgM RF from the patient destined to develop RA. Under these circumstances the measurement of RF isotypes may be helpful. As mentioned above, we have observed that upwards of 70% of RA patients at the University of Illinois Arthritis Center (unpublished observations) had all three RF isotypes (IgM, IgG, and IgA), 20% had IgM and IgA, and 3% had only IgM RF. We have preliminary evidence that suggests RF reactivity without evidence of RA is due only to IgM RF activity. Thus, measurement of RF isotypes may differentiate the patient with early RA from the patient without RA but who has an elevated IgM RF level (see Case 4, below).

Some authors have advocated a role for RF testing in other diseases to provide information about prognosis and disease activity. Davis and Bollett were the first to suggest that RF played a protective role against nephritis in SLE patients.[32] The most commonly postulated mechanism is more efficient reticuloendothelial clearance of larger, less soluble immune complexes formed by RF interaction with circulating immune complexes. Several subsequent studies that used either agglutination techniques or ELISA to detect RF support this view.[33-35] A recent retrospective analysis of 102 lupus clinic patients found a significant negative association between detectable RF (by latex agglutination) at any time during a patient's course and clinically significant renal disease as defined by either persistent proteinuria greater than 0.5 g/day or the presence of cellular casts in the urinary sediment.[36] This association was unrelated to the presence or absence of anti-ds DNA antibodies (by *Crithidia luciliae* indirect immunofluorescence). On the other hand, Turner-Stokes and co-workers[37] found only a trend toward a protective role for RF by latex slide test and no protective effect when analyzed by RIA, an observation consistent with several previous studies using different test methods. The studies (both positive and negative) vary according to RF test method, cut-off for RF positivity, and definition of renal disease. Thus, the issue of whether RF protects SLE patients from developing nephritis remains controversial.

The utility of RF testing in another renal disease, minimal change nephrotic syndrome (MCNS), has also been explored. Because previous work demonstrated elevated serum IgE levels and spontaneous *in vitro* Ig production in patients with MCNS, Endoh et al. measured RF by a solid-phase fluorescence immunoassay in 20 affected patients.[38] Serum IgG and IgM RFs were significantly increased during nephrotic stages and normalized during complete remission. The authors therefore suggest that periodic RF measurement in MCNS patients may assist with the evaluation of disease activity and response to treatment in this setting.

Serial RF testing may offer important prognostic information in Sjögren's syndrome. As noted in Table 2, the prevalence of RF in Sjögren's syndrome (primary or secondary) is high, presumably reflecting chronic polyclonal B cell hyperactivity. It is well established that patients with Sjögren's syndrome occasionally evolve a clinical picture termed "pseudolymphoma" and carry a 44-fold increased risk of ultimately developing non-Hodgkin's lymphoma. Such patients may exhibit a decrease in RF titer or even "convert" from RF-positive to RF-negative, due to suppression of previously polyclonal Ig production by the malignant clone.[39] Serologic conversion of this type may therefore help to alert the clinician to the possibility of neoplastic transformation in the Sjögren's patient with a changing clinical picture (e.g., weight loss, increased lymphadenopathy, new pulmonary infiltrates).

Because of the multitude of central nervous system abnormalities reported in Sjögren's syndrome, Olsen et al.[40] measured RF (along with anti-nuclear antibody [ANA] and lupus anticoagulant) in 100 patients consecutively admitted to an in-patient neurology service and hospitalized on that service longer than 72 h. While only two patients had a known rheumatic disease (SLE and RA) on admission, three of ten other patients in whom rheumatic disease was felt to be responsible for the neurologic symptoms were recognized as having Sjögren's syndrome. Of these three patients, one was RF-positive (titer >1:80); of the remaining seven RF-positive patients, two had chronic infections, one had RA, and four had unexplained titers of 1:160, 1:320, 1:1280, and 1:2560. The authors advocate randomized prospective studies of systematic screening of neurology patients for rheumatic disease by measuring RF, ANA, and lupus anticoagulant and assessing salivary and lacrimal gland function in order to determine whether such an approach can uncover more patients with treatable causes of neurologic disease.

RF testing has long been advocated as part of the evaluation of patients with fever of undetermined origin (FUO).[41,42] However, a sustained or significant fever secondary to RA is extremely unusual. The exceptions are patients with concomitant rheumatoid vasculitis,[43] in whom RA is usually chronic and clinically apparent. Prolonged, daily fever is a hallmark of a related disorder, Still's disease, but affected patients are almost always RF-negative.[44] One series of FUO patients found no clinical utility in measuring RF in this setting.[45] In a more recent study, fever was attributed to RA in 2 of 199 FUO patients.[46]

V. CASE REPORTS

Case #1 — A 41-year-old male of Iranian descent presented with asymmetric polyarthritis that involved, in an additive fashion over 4 months, his right wrist followed by his left knee and then the right ankle. He had otherwise been well except for a recent history of partial resection of the penis for squamous cell carcinoma. At the time of the visit he was experiencing 2 hours of morning stiffness and significant swelling of his left knee. There were no rash, nodules, pleural pain, oropharyngeal or urogenital ulceration. Review of systems was negative for symptoms consistent with seronegative spondyloarthropathies. Physical exam demonstrated a healthy male with significant synovitis of the aforementioned joints without enthosopathic changes (e.g., Achilles' tendonitis). Laboratory testing revealed Westergren ESR85, normochromic normocytic anemia, and polyclonal hypergammaglobulinemia; RF (nephelometry) <30 I.U./ml. Except for soft tissue swelling and effusions, joint X-rays were normal. By ELISA (Figure 1A) IgA RF was 150 U/ml (Nl <35 U/ml), and IgM RF and IgG RF were normal. Over the next 2 months, the patient was unsuccessfully treated with various nonsteroidal anti-inflammatory drugs (NSAIDs). The decision was made to begin methotrexate (25 mg IM). At that time IgA RF and IgM RF were elevated (324 I.U./ml) (Figure 1B); the IgG RF was still negative. The patient responded well to the methotrexate therapy.

Discussion: Clinically the patient appeared to have a seronegative spondyloarthropathy, but the initial elevation of IgA RF suggested RA.

Case #2 — A 22-year-old white female presented with a 6-month history of episodic bilateral pain and stiffness in her groin areas. A usual "attack", the most recent being her sixth, lasted 2 weeks. Treatment with various NSAIDs produced modest benefits. No other joints have been involved and family history was positive for RA (maternal aunt). Studies performed by a consulting orthopedist showed a normal complete blood count (CBC), ESR, ANA, and RF. Magnetic resonance imaging (MRI) of the hips during a painful episode was normal except for mild effusions bilaterally. An exam at the time of an attack showed painful reduction in bilaterally hip range of motion. IgM RF (nephelometry) was <30 I.U./ml; by ELISA (Figure 1C), IgA RF was 110 U (NL <35) while IgM and IgA RF were normal. Patient had prompt resolution of her attack with diclofenac (75 mg BID) and remained well after cessation of the NSAID. However, 3 months later she returned with symmetric stiffness and swelling of her 2nd, 3rd, and 4th metacarpophalangeal (MCP) joints, wrists, and elbows. The hip pain was also present. At this time laboratory tests showed Westergren ESR55 and IgM RF (nephelometry) 66 I.U./ml. By ELISA the IgM RF, IgG RF, and IgARF were now elevated: IgM RF, 420 (Nl <55) and IgG RF, 104 (Figure 1D).

Discussion: Clinically it appeared that this young woman had palindromic rheumatism. The detection of IgG RF as the first antibody suggested the diagnosis of rheumatoid arthritis.

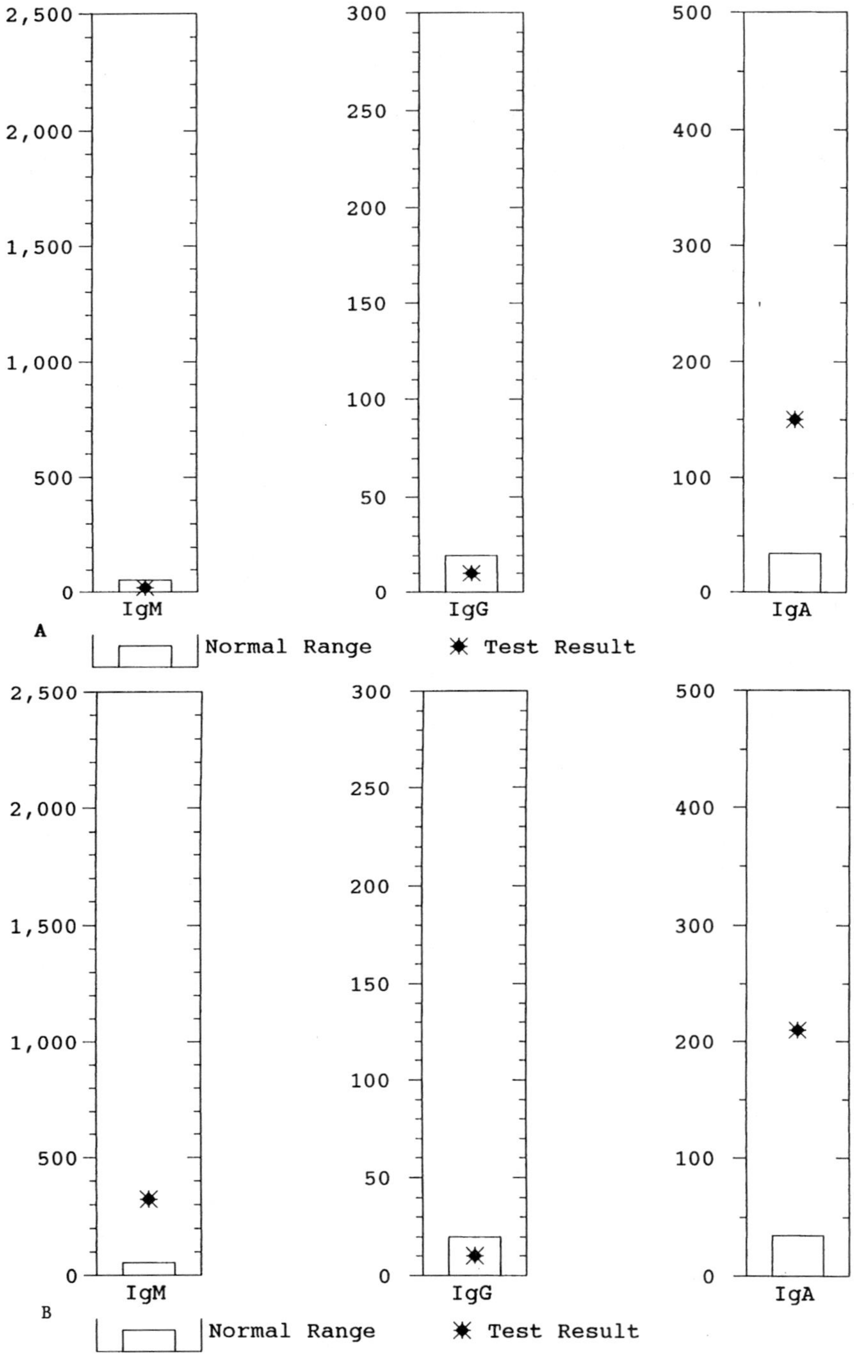

Figure 1 Rheumatoid factor profile of four patients with rheumatoid arthritis (see case reports). A and B: case #1; C and D: case #2; E: case #3; F: case #4.

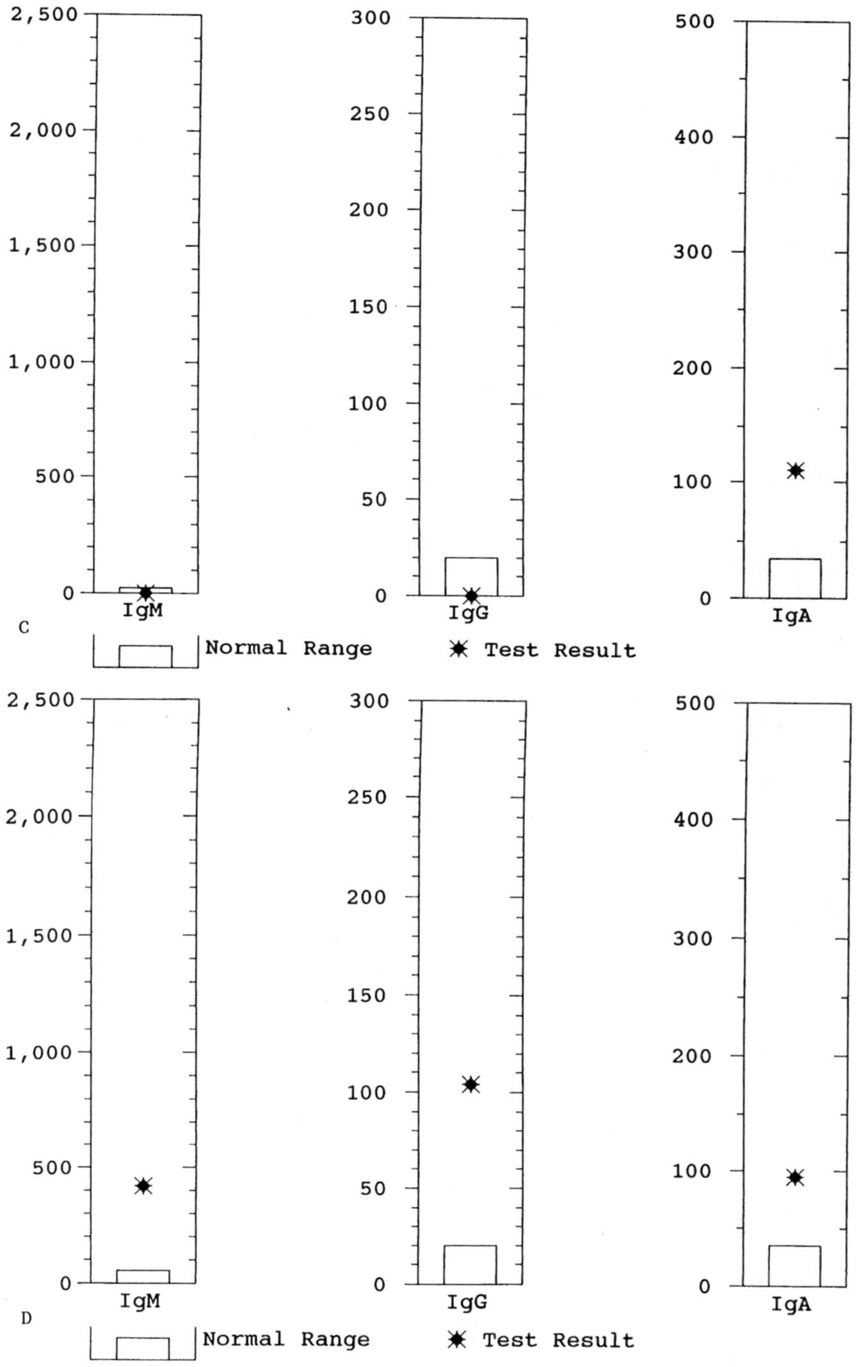

Figure 1 (continued).

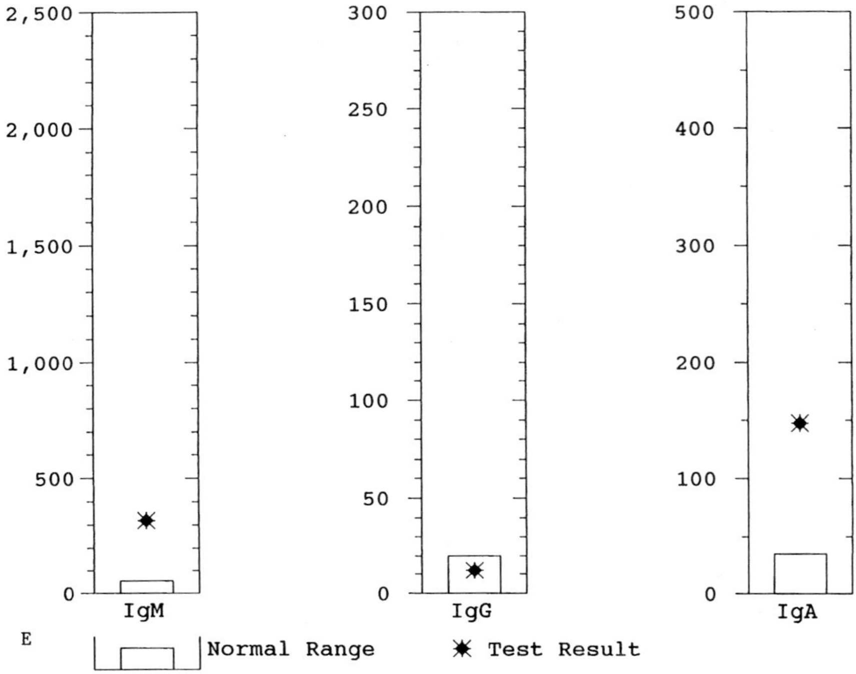

E

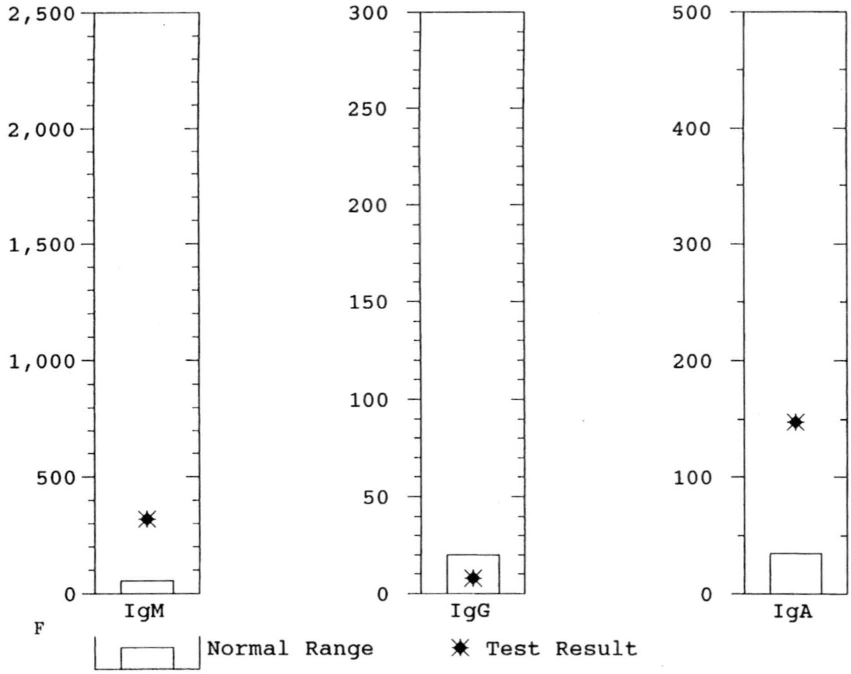

F

Figure 1 (continued).

Case #3 — A 35-year-old white female of Irish descent had a 4-month history of symmetric morning stiffness involving her MCPs, proximal interphalangeal (PIPs), wrists, elbows, and knees. No swelling was observed by the consulting rheumatologist at that time. Laboratory tests showed ESR65, mild normochromic normocytic anemia, negative RF, and an ANA-1:80 speckled. Based on the data, a diagnosis of SLE was made and the patient was treated with NSAIDs and hydroxychloroquine. However, because of a lack of response the patient obtained a second opinion. At the time of the visit, the patient had 2 hours of morning stiffness and complained of swelling of her wrist and 2nd/3rd PIP joints. Exam revealed pain and mild synovial thickening of the aforementioned joints. Laboratory testing showed ESR51, RF negative (nephelometry), and ANA-1:160 speckled. By ELISA IgM RF was 544 I.U. (Figure 1E); IgA, RF, and IgG RF negative; anti-ssDNA, -dsDNA, -Sm, -RNP, -SSA, -SSB, -histone, -Scl70, were normal.

Discussion: The case demonstrates the increased sensitivity of the ELISA method for the detection of IgM RF and suggests that the combined measurements of all three classes of RF may have enhanced diagnostic specificity compared to IgM RF alone.

Case #4 — A 75-year-old white female presented with a left knee monoarthritis. The process resolved after 1 year. At the time of her evaluation, the patient complained of 1 hour of morning stiffness in the left knee. Clinical exam showed warmth, swelling, and erythema. Laboratory tests showed ESR45 and IgM RF (nephelometry) 95 I.U./ml. X-ray showed joint space narrowing and chondrocalcinosis of the medial compartment. Arthrocentesis showed calcium pyrophosphate crystals. RF by ELISA showed IgM RF 320 I.U./ml and IgA RF 147 U/ml (Figure 1F). IgG RF was normal. The patient was treated with NSAID for presumptive diagnosis of pseudogout. On return visit 1 month later, she had symmetric synovitis of both knees and wrists, consistent with the diagnosis of rheumatoid arthritis.

Discussion: This case demonstrates the utility of measuring all three classes of RF in elderly individuals who may be IgM RF-positive as a consequence of polyclonal B cell activation. In this instance the diagnostic specificity of all three RF classes exceeded that for IgM RF alone.

REFERENCES

1. **Waaler, E.,** On the occurrence of a factor in human sera activating the specific agglutination of sheep blood corpuscles, *Acta Pathol. Microbiol. Scand.*, 17, 172, 1940.
2. **Rose, H. M., Ragan, C., Pearce, E., and Lipman, M. O.,** Differential agglutination of normal and sensitized sheep erythrocytes by sera of patients with rheumatoid arthritis, *Proc. Soc. Exp. Biol. Med.*, 68, 1, 1948.
3. **Goddard, D. and Moore, M.,** Common tests for rheumatoid factors: poorly standardized by ubiquitous, *Arthritis Rheum.*, 31, 432, 1988.
4. **Arnett, F. C., Edworthy, S. M., Bloch, D. A. et al.,** The American Rheumatism Association 1987 revised criteria for the classification of rheumatoid arthritis, *Arthritis Rheum.*, 31, 315, 1988.
5. **Waller, M., Toone, E. C., and Vaughan, E.,** Study of rheumatoid factors in a normal population, *Arthritis Rheum.*, 7, 513, 1964.
6. **Mikkelsen, W. M., Dodge, H. J., Duff, I. F., and Kato, H.,** Estimates of the prevalence of rheumatic diseases in the population of Tecumseh, Michigan, 1959–60, *J. Chronic Dis.*, 20, 351, 1967.

7. **Aho, K., Palosuo, T., Raunio, V., Puska, P., Aromaa, A., and Salonen, J. T.,** When does rheumatoid disease start?, *Arthritis Rheum.*, 28, 485, 1985.
8. **Beasley, R. P., Retailliau, H., and Healey, L. A.,** Prevalence of rheumatoid arthritis in Alaskan Eskimos, *Arthritis Rheum.*, 16, 737, 1973.
9. **Teitsson, I.,** IgA rheumatoid factor as predictor of disease activity, *Scand. J. Rheumatol.*, S-75, 233, 1988.
10. **Wolfe, F., Cathey, M., and Roberts, F. K.,** The latex test revisited: rheumatoid factor testing in 8,287 rheumatic disease patients, *Arthritis Rheum.*, 34, 951, 1991.
11. **Ball, J. and Lawrence, J. S.,** The relationship of rheumatoid serum factor to rheumatoid arthritis: a 5-year follow-up of a population sample, *Ann. Rheum. Dis.*, 22, 311, 1963.
12. **del Puente, A., Knowler, W. C., Pettitt, D. J., and Bennett, P. H.,** The incidence of rheumatoid arthritis is predicted by rheumatoid factor titer in a longitudinal population study, *Arthritis Rheum.*, 31, 1239, 1988.
13. **Aho, K., Heliovaara, M., Maatela, J., Tuomi, T., and Palosuo, T.,** RF antedating clinical RA, *J. Rheumatol.*, 18, 1282, 1991.
14. **Fuchs, H. A., Kaye, J. J., Callahan, L. F., Nance, E. P., and Pincus, T.,** Evidence of significant radiographic damage in rheumatoid arthritis within the first 2 years of disease, *J. Rheumatol.*, 16, 585, 1989.
15. **Moore, T., Dorner, R., Osborn, T., and Zuckner, J.,** Hidden 19S IgM rheumatoid factors, *Semin. Arthritis Rheum.*, 18, 72, 1988.
16. **Jacoby, R. K., Jayson, M. I. V., and Cosh, J. A.,** Onset, early stages, and prognosis of rheumatoid arthritis: a clinical study of 100 patients with 11-year follow-up, *Br. Med. J.*, 2, 96, 1973.
17. **Cats, A. and Hazevoet, H. M.,** Significance of positive tests for rheumatoid factor in the prognosis of rheumatoid arthritis: a follow-up study, *Ann. Rheum. Dis.*, 29, 254, 1970.
18. **Feigenbaum, S. L., Masi, A. T., and Kaplan, S. B.,** Prognosis in rheumatoid arthritis — a longitudinal study of newly diagnosed younger patients, *Am. J. Med.*, 66, 377, 1979.
19. **Alarcon, G. S., Koopman, W. J., Acton, R. T., and Barger, B. O.,** Seronegative rheumatoid arthritis: a distinct immunogenetic disease?, *Arthritis Rheum.*, 25, 502, 1982.
20. **van der Heijde, D. M., van Riel, P. L., van Rijswijk, M. H., and van de Putte, L. B.,** Influence of prognostic features on the final outcome in rheumatoid arthritis: a review of the literature, *Semin. Arthritis Rheum.*, 17, 284, 1988.
21. **Schneider, H. A., Yonker, R. A., Katz, P., Longley, S., and Panush, R. S.,** Rheumatoid vasculitis: experience with 13 patients and review of the literature, *Semin. Arthritis Rheum.*, 14, 280, 1985.
22. **Geirsson, A. J., Sturfelt, G., and Truedsson, L.,** Clinical and serological features of severe vasculitis in rheumatoid arthritis: prognostic implications, *Ann. Rheum. Dis.*, 46, 727, 1987.
23. **Gordon, D. A., Stein, J. L., and Broder, I.,** The extra-articular features of rheumatoid arthritis: a systematic analysis of 127 cases, *Am. J. Med.*, 54, 445, 1973.
24. **Scott, D., Bacon, P., Allen, C., Elson, C., and Wallington, T.,** IgG rheumatoid factor, complement and immune complexes in rheumatoid synovitis and vasculitis: comparative and serial studies of cytotoxic therapies, *Clin. Exp. Immunol.*, 43, 53, 1981.

25. **Jones, V. E. and Jacoby, R. K.,** Rheumatoid arthritis: rheumatoid factors, immune complexes, and C-reactive protein are raised shortly after the onset of symptoms [letter], *Arthritis Rheum.*, 32, 117, 1989.
26. **Mottonen, T., Hannonen, P., Jokinen, I., Arvilommi, M., and Oka, M.,** Relation between bone erosions and rheumatoid factor IgA and IgM isotypes in recent onset rheumatoid arthritis, *Scand. J. Rheumatol.*, S-75, 244, 1988.
27. **Wiloch, H., Thompson, K., Young, A., Corbett, M., Shipley, M., and Hay, F.,** IgA and IgM rheumatoid factors as markers of later erosive changes in rheumatoid arthritis, *Scand. J. Rheumatol.*, S-75, 238, 1988.
28. **Kinoshita, M., Aotsuka, S., and Yokohari, R.,** Cross-reactive rheumatoid factors in rheumatoid arthritis with extra-articular disease, *Clin. Exp. Immunol.*, 79, 72, 1990.
29. **Noritake, D., Colburn, K., and Weisbart, R.,** Rheumatoid factor specific for active rheumatoid arthritis, *Ann. Rheum. Dis.*, 49, 910, 1990.
30. **Cush, J. J., Lipsky, P. E., Postlethwaite, A. E., Schrohenloher, R. E., Saway, A., and Koopman, W. J.,** Correlation of serologic indicators of inflammation with effectiveness of nonsteroidal antiinflammatory drug therapy in rheumatoid arthritis, *Arthritis Rheum.*, 33, 19, 1990.
31. **Goodwin, J. S., Cueppens, J. L., and Rodriguez, M. A.,** Administration of nonsteroidal anti-inflammatory agents in patients with rheumatoid arthritis: effects on indices of cellular immune status and serum rheumatoid factor levels, *JAMA*, 250, 2485, 1983.
32. **Davis, J. S. and Bollet, A. J.,** Complement levels, rheumatoid factor and renal disease in systemic lupus erythematosus, *Arthritis Rheum.*, 9, 499, 1966.
33. **Tarkowski, A. and Westberg, G.,** Rheumatoid factor isotypes and renal disease in systemic lupus erythematosus, *Scand. J. Rheumatol.*, 16, 309, 1987.
34. **Hill, G. S., Hinglais, N., Tron, F., and Bach, J. F.,** SLE morphologic correlations with immunologic and clinical data at the time of biopsy, *Am. J. Med.*, 64, 61, 1978.
35. **Helin, H., Lorpela, M., Mustonen, J., and Pasternack, A.,** Rheumatoid factor in rheumatoid arthritis-associated renal disease and in lupus nephritis, *Ann. Rheum. Dis.*, 45, 508, 1986.
36. **Howard, T., Iannini, M., Burge, J., and Davis, J., IV,** Rheumatoid factor, cryoglobulinemia, anti-DNA, and renal disease in patients with systemic lupus erythematosus, *J. Rheumatol.*, 18, 826, 1991.
37. **Turner-Sokes, L., Jones, M., Addison, I., Mansell, M., and Isenberg, D.,** Does rheumatoid factor protect lupus patients from the development of nephritis?, *Ann. Rheum. Dis.*, 48, 14, 1989.
38. **Endoh, M., Miyazaki, M., Suga, T., Miura, M., Nomoto, Y., and Sakai, H.,** Rheumatoid factors in patients with minimal change nephrotic syndrome, *Clin. Nephrol.*, 35, 93, 1991.
39. **Anderson, L. G. and Talal, N.,** The spectrum of benign to malignant lymphoproliferation in Sjogren's syndrome, *Clin. Exp. Immunol.*, 10, 199, 1972.
40. **Olsen, M., O'Connor, S., Arnett, F., Rosenbaum, D., Grotta, J., and Warner, N.,** Autoantibodies and rheumatic disorders in a neurology inpatient population: a prospective study, *Am. J. Med.*, 90, 479, 1991.
41. **Esposito, A. L. and Gleckman, R. A.,** A diagnostic approach to the adult with fever of unknown origin, *Arch. Intern. Med.*, 139, 575, 1979.
42. **Jacoby, J. A. and Swartz, M. N.,** Fever of undetermined origin, *N. Engl. J. Med.*, 289, 1407, 1973.

43. **Scott, D. G., Bacon, P. A., and Tribe, C. R.,** Systemic rheumatoid vasculitis: a clinical and laboratory study of 50 cases, *Medicine,* 60, 288, 1992.
44. **Ohta, A., Yamaguchi, M., Kaneoka, H., Nagayoshi, T., and Hilda, M.,** Adult Still's disease: review of 228 cases from the literature, *J. Rheumatol.,* 14, 1139, 1987.
45. **Larson, E. B., Featherstone, H. J., and Petersdorf, R. G.,** Fever of undetermined origin: diagnosis and follow-up of 105 cases, 1970–1980, *Medicine,* 61, 269, 1982.
46. **Knockaert, D. C., Vanneste, L. J., Vanneste, S. B., and Bobbaers, H. J.,** Fever of unknown origin in the 1980s: an update of the diagnostic spectrum, *Arch. Intern. Med.,* 152, 51, 1992.
47. **Meltzer, M., Franklin, E., Elias, K., McCluskey, R., and Cooper, N.,** Cryoglobulinemia — a clinical and laboratory study. II. Cryoglobulins with rheumatoid factor activity, *Am. J. Med.,* 40, 837, 1966.
48. **Dresner, E. and Trombly, P.,** The latex fixation reaction in nonrheumatic diseases, *N. Engl. J. Med.,* 261, 981, 1959.
49. **Houba, V. and Allison, A.,** M-Antiglobulins (rheumatoid factor-like globulins) and other gamma globulins in relation to tropical parasitic infections, *Lancet,* 1, 848, 1966.
50. **Naides, S. and Field, E.,** Transient rheumatoid factor positivity in acute human parvovirus B19 infection, *Arch. Intern. Med.,* 148, 2587, 1988.
51. **Johnson, R. and Hall, A.,** Rubella arthritis, *N. Engl. J. Med.,* 258, 743, 1958.
52. **Kaplan, M.,** Cryoglobulinemia in infectious mononucleosis: quantitation and characterization of cryoproteins, *J. Lab. Clin. Med.,* 71, 754, 1968.

III. Antinuclear and Anticytoplasmic Antibodies

Chapter 5

Nuclear and Cytoplasmic Antigens and Induction of Autoantibodies

Christopher J. Froelich and Robert G. Lahita

CONTENTS

I. INTRODUCTION

Systemic lupus erythematosus (SLE) is the prototypic systemic autoimmune disease in which greater than 95% of patients have positive anti-nuclear antibodies (ANAs). Specific ANAs appear to have phlogistic properties that may be necessary for the expression of certain clinical manifestations. Investigators have posited numerous theories to explain the formation of anti-nuclear autoantibodies in SLE. Mechanistically, ANA production is secondary either to polyclonal B cell activation or to antigen-induced B cell activation with coexistent T cell help. An analysis of autoantibody specificities in SLE sera supports a primary role for antigen-driven immune response against a limited number of autoantigens (Table 1). The potential antibody repertoire exceeds 10^7. If autoantibody production was due primarily to polyclonal B cell activation, then lupus sera should bind hundreds of intracellular proteins. However, using immunoblotted lysates of HeLa cells, a recent study showed that SLE sera reacted with less than 100 intracellular proteins.[1] The results, therefore, indicate that relatively few intracellular proteins (e.g., Sm, RNP, Ro, La, Ku, among others) are targets for SLE autoantibodies (see Table 1).

0-8493-5974-1/94/$0.00+$.50

Table 1 **Frequency of Various Autoantibodies in SLE**

Autoantibody Specificity	**Frequency (%)**
Native (double stranded) DNA	40–75
Denatured (single stranded) DNA	60–90
Sm	15–55
RNP (nuclear RNP)	30–80
SSA	35–60
SSB	15–50
Histone (total)	70–90
Ribosomal P	10
Ku	10

Note: Values compiled from various sources in the References.

The purpose of this chapter is not to describe the expanding list of anti-nuclear antibody specificities. Rather the intent is to synthesize recent advances in our understanding of the more common SLE antibodies (Table 1), particularly when asked in the context of the question — what are the physiochemical and antigenic attributes that enable the nuclear antigens to provoke the tolerant immune system to produce these potentially phlogistic antibodies? In this framework, the following will be reviewed:

1. The biochemical structure of the autoantigen complex
2. The binding specificities of the antibodies (i.e., epitope analysis)
3. Description of recent advances in the structural analysis of the autoantibodies
4. Description of idiotype interactions
5. An overview on recent thoughts about ANA autoantibody induction

II. ANTI-DNA ANTIBODIES

A. Antigenic Determinants of DNA

The most specific serologic indicator of SLE is the presence of anti-double stranded (ds) DNA antibodies. dsDNA is an elongated double helical polymer in which base-paired purines and pyrimidines orient toward the center of the helix and two spirally wound polydeoxyribose-phosphate backbones form the outer aspect of the helix. dsDNA may exist as a supercoiled closed circular structure, a relaxed circular form, or a long flexible linear structure. The major antigenic determinants reside on the pentose-phosphate backbone of the dsDNA molecule. However, due to subtle conformational changes induced by variation in base composition, in the sidechains expressed, and in the sequence of the double-chain backbone, a dsDNA molecule may have considerable antigenic polymorphism (see Reference 2 for review). Supporting the notion that dsDNA indeed expresses antigenic heterogeneity, studies by Pisetsky et al. have provided evidence that sufficient differences exist between bacterial and mammalian DNA to allow the recognition of bacterial DNA as foreign by the immune system.[3-5] Single-stranded DNA (ssDNA) clearly manifests many different epitopes. Determinants may be contributed by: (1) the sequences of bases, nucleosides, nucleotides, and oligonucleotides;

(2) the conformational arrangement of a single chain; or (3) the double-chain backbone of a short helical structure. What remains obscure is whether the complexing of polynucleotides with structural and/or regulatory proteins enhances their autoantigenic potential.

B. Polyreactivity of Anti-DNA Antibodies

Murine and human monoclonal anti-ssDNA antibodies possess various degrees of polyspecificity. While some antibodies primarily bind repetitive base or nucleotide sequences, others react preferentially with dsDNA.[6] Nevertheless, the majority of the monoclonal antibodies, which are primarily IgM, react with several nucleic acids, with ssDNA, and with synthetic polynucleotides. Perhaps more remarkable was the observation that many monoclonal anti-DNA antibodies also cross react with cytoskeletal proteins (e.g., vimentin), phospholipids (e.g., cardiolipin), and glycolipids. In related studies, monoclonal anti-DNA antibodies also bound to platelets, Raji cell membrane,[7] the Fc portion of IgG, and nucleosomes.[8] Recent work has shown, however, that the apparent polyspecificity of a monoclonal anti-DNA antibody is less diverse than initially appreciated. In this regard, the DNA in an anti-DNA/DNA complex may directly contribute to the binding reaction or the DNA may complex with a nonantibody protein that then acts as the binding protein. For example, histone in anti-DNA-DNA complexes mediates the binding to cell membranes.[9] While the formation of DNA-anti-DNA complexes may explain cross reactions with protein structures, such immune complexes cannot account for the binding of anti-DNA antibodies to biochemically distinct phospholipids and glycolipids.[10,11] Hence, the reported cross reaction between platelets and anti-DNA antibodies, is due to an epitope that is possessed both by DNA and by a glycolipid structure on the platelet.[12]

In summary, the apparent polyspecificity of anti-DNA may not be as manifold as previously suspected. Nevertheless, anti-DNA antibodies specific for polynucleotides do cross react with phospholipids. The polyreactivity of a monoclonal anti-DNA antibody may be due to its ability to bind with variable affinity to related conformational epitopes present on seemingly diverse structures. X-ray crystallographic studies that employ a monoclonal antibody that binds two or more epitopes on biochemically distinct molecules will be necessary to document this phenomenon of conformational polyspecificity.

C. Anti-DNA Idiotypes

Idiotypes represent serologically defined antigenic determinants on the Fab regions of the antibody molecule. Anti-idiotypes may be private, identifying a single antibody clone, or cross-reactive (CRI), manifesting multiple specificities toward either distinct or disparate molecules. The epitope identified by the anti-idiotype antibody may be linear (i.e., amino acid sequences on the H or L chains) or conformational. In some instances, the tertiary structure of the anti-idiotype resembles the antigen determinant and hence describes the internal image of the antigen. An additional type of anti-idiotype reacts with both the idiotype of the antibody and the antigen recognized by the antibody (epibody).

Before the advent of molecular biology, anti-DNA idiotype antibodies were developed in an attempt to identify variable region gene expression of anti-DNA antibodies (e.g., anti-DNA idiotypes). Investigators have identified approximately 20 different anti-DNA-associated idiotypes in man.[13] The diversity of materials that serve as the immunogen, the nature of the anti-idiotype reagents, and at a more fundamental level, the validity of using a serological tool to accurately identify a unique idiotype, have complicated the analysis of the immunological and clinical relevance of anti-DNA idiotype antibodies. Anti-DNA antibodies, isolated either from SLE patients, normal individuals, or fetal tissue, have served as the immunogens. The anti-idiotype reagents generated have been similarly diverse and have included both monoclonal and polyclonal antibodies.

The immunizing idiotype may potentially represent a constant, variable, and/or hypervariable regions of the heavy and/or light chains of the antibody. A recent three-dimensional analysis of an idiotype-anti-idiotype interaction demonstrated that the epitope can be conformationally dependent.[14] Employing X-ray diffraction analysis, the data showed that the idiotype of an anti-lysozyme Fab, as defined by anti-monoclonal anti-idiotype, comprised 13 amino acid residues that resided on the complementary determining region of *both* the V_H and V_L framework residues. Based on this observation, the potential does exist for cross reactions between biochemically distinct but conformationally related idiotypes.

If the epitope recognized by an anti-DNA idiotype is conformational, different anti-DNA antibodies that possess this idiotype should have dissimilar amino acid sequences in the variable portions of their H and L chains. Asking this question, Young and colleagues[15] sequenced the V_H regions of human monoclonal anti-DNA antibodies (16/6 idiotype). They found dissimilar amino acid compositions for the V_H regions, providing indirect evidence that idiotypic determinants are conformational. In a related study, Manheimer-Lory et al.[16] generated a panel of idiotype-bearing antibodies to assess patterns of heavy and light chain usage. The amino acid sequence analysis of IgM and IgG anti-DNA monoclonal antibodies obtained from Epstein-Barr Virus (EBV)-transformed B cells of a SLE patient showed that idiotype markers do not correspond directly to a heavy or light chain sequence or family.[16] Demonstrating the extent of cross-reactive idiotypy, Grayzel et al. emphasized that anti-DNA idiotype antibodies occur in normal subjects without circulating anti-DNA antibodies.[17] Following the immunization of patients with a pneumococcal vaccine, all 10 individuals showed a rise in the titer of anti-pneumococcal antibodies bearing the anti-DNA-associated idiotype (31 idiotype). No anti-DNA antibodies were present in post-vaccination sera.[17]

Overall, these studies warrant the following comments. The evidence indicates that comparable conformational determinants on antibodies with disparate specificities may result in cross-reactive anti-idiotype antibodies. Why should anti-bacterial antibodies display a DNA idiotype? An appealing likelihood is that CRIs represent idiotype-anti-idiotype interactions that provide the economic dual purpose of suppressing anti-DNA production while simultaneously modulating an effective antibacterial response. Since the attributes of pathogenic DNA antibodies remain unclear, anti-idiotype reagents capable of discriminating between pathologic and benign anti-DNA antibodies will remain unidentified. Despite the limitations of idiotypic analysis, certainly, one may conclude that a unique set of variable genes, exclusively expressed in SLE patients, cannot be responsible for pathogenic anti-DNA idiotypes. Also, idiotype analyses suggest that anti-DNA antibodies are not constrained by unique idiotype-anti-idiotype interactions. Despite the rather limited utility of anti-DNA idiotype antibodies, however, these reagents may serve to correlate levels of an idiotype with disease activity. In a collaborative study, an analysis of 18 different idiotypes in 180 SLE sera showed that although no anti-idiotype marker was disease specific, many of the reagents correlated with total IgM and anti-ssDNA levels.[13]

D. STRUCTURAL ANALYSIS OF ANTI-DNA ANTIBODIES

With the availability of molecular biologic techniques, investigators have determined the degree of clonality and extent of genomic diversity among IgG anti-DNA antibodies.[18,19] Using ten monoclonal IgG anti-DNA antibodies from one NZB/NZW mouse, Marion et al. partially sequenced the variable regions and observed four patterns overall, including one group with six members.[18] Interestingly, the antibodies were oligoclonal and somatically mutated, suggesting that the hybridomas represented mutationally divergent members from a limited number of clones. Other investigators who employed similar techniques showed that antibodies from a single NZB/NZW mouse came from several different V_H families.[20] Finally, analysis of mRNA sequences from the variable, diversity, and joining regions of IgG anti-DNA hybridomas (MRL mice) revealed that many of the hybridoma clones had a common progenitor, that underwent *clonal expansion, sequential somatic mutation, and antigenic selection* to yield multiple variants with different fine specificities.[19] Although these results clearly demonstrate that an anti-DNA antibody response is antigen driven, the data do not resolve whether DNA acts as the stimulating immunogen.

On the basis of gene usage, two general classes of anti-DNA antibodies exist: antibodies containing germline gene segments and antibodies with variable gene segments that have undergone somatic mutation. The former category likely includes natural polyreactive IgM antibodies,[21,22] whereas the latter are primarily IgG antibodies that bind dsDNA and ssDNA with high affinity. An analysis that lends support to the concept that high-affinity IgG antibodies arise from natural IgM antibodies showed that the V_H gene that encoded an NZB/NZW IgG anti-DNA antibody was a mutation of a gene closely related to the germline VH130 gene for MRL IgM anti-DNA antibody.[23] Van Es and co-workers[24] analyzed the gene elements that encoded a high-affinity IgG anti-dsDNA antibody secreted by EBV-transformed B cells from an active SLE patient. This group also cloned and sequenced the germline counterparts of the V_H and V_L genes expressed for this autoantibody. The comparison of both sets of gene elements showed that the autoantibody V_H and V_L regions contained numerous somatic mutations. The light chain expressed in this autoantibody was a somatically mutated variant of the kv 325 germline gene that frequently exists in paraproteins. Furthermore, investigators have identified this utilized D_H segment repeatedly in multireactive, low-affinity IgM anti-DNA autoantibodies from healthy individuals and SLE patients.[24]

Does the substitution of certain amino acids in the complementary binding site enhance the affinity of anti-DNA antibodies? Various proteins rich in arginine and asparaginine residues bind DNA either electrostatically or by hydrogen bonds. In this context, two high-affinity anti-DNA monoclonal antibodies from separate mice (J885 and S107 VH families) were found to contain arginine and tyrosine residues among the amino acids lining the walls and the base of the antigen-binding cleft. The data imply that these residues may contribute significantly to the avidity of DNA binding by the antibody. Shlomchik et al.[19] also have found that DNA binding capacity of murine hybridomas Ig heavy chains increased with arginine and asparaginine substitutions in the third framework region and the complementary-determining region of the heavy chain. In related work Radic and co-workers[25] examined the influence of Ig light chain on heavy chain binding affinity. They reported that the 3H9 heavy chain, derived from a high-affinity anti-dsDNA antibody, could interact with all of six tested k light chains to yield antibodies that bound ssDNA. Moreover, the light chain dictated the binding avidity of the heavy chain for ssDNA, dsDNA, RNA, and cardiolipin. Strikingly, the pairing of different light chains with the 3H9 heavy chain resulted in anti-DNA antibodies with different nuclear and, in some instances, cytoplasmic and cell membrane immunofluorescence staining patterns. These intriguing observations suggest that some anti-DNA antibodies may recognize complex epitopes produced by the interaction of DNA or RNA with cellular proteins. Thus, the asparagine-containing heavy chains of the Ig heterodimer could stabilize the interaction with the nucleic acid, thereby facilitating the remainder of the Ig binding site to interact with nucleic acid-protein complex.

E. CHARACTERISTICS OF PATHOGENIC ANTI-DNA ANTIBODIES

Polyreactivity is considered a characteristic of natural IgM antibodies, whereas pathogenic IgG anti-DNA antibodies minimally express this attribute. The issue of polyreactivity, however, may be more quantitative than qualitative. Sabbaga et al.[26] have reported that anti-DNA antibodies isolated from normal sera had the most restricted specificity (polynucleotide of deoxythymidine and ssDNA), while anti-DNA antibodies in the lupus serum possessed more polyspecificity by binding several different polynucleotides, including ssDNA and dsDNA. Antibodies with the broadest cross-reactivity (multiple polynucleotides and phospholipids) were eluted from kidney tissue of the SLE patients.[26] Overall, the data suggest that a positive correlation may exist between the level of polyspecificity and pathogenicity of IgG anti-DNA antibody. Nevertheless, polyspecificity cannot, in isolation, serve as a marker for pathogenic antibodies.

Analysis of the available data suggests that natural anti-DNA antibodies are IgM isotype, circulate in both normal subjects and patients, have germline coding, and, as manifested by their relatively low binding affinity with multiple epitopes, polyreactivity. On the other hand, pathogenic anti-dsDNA antibodies have the following characteristics: (1) IgG class, (2) T cell dependent, (3) high affinity for dsDNA, (4) derived from multiple V_H and V_L genes, (5) cross-reactive idiotypes manifested by conformational epitopes, and (6) polyreactivity.

Available studies support the likelihood that deposition of DNA/anti-DNA immune complexes mediate significant tissue damage. However, it is unclear if the physical properties of the complexes or the DNA (or DNA-histone aggregates) in the anti-DNA/DNA complexes dictate the site of deposition (glomerular tissue).[27,28] The nature of the DNA and its ability to bind to different basement membrane molecules require further study. Furthermore, do anti-DNA antibodies *directly* mediate tissue damage by a cross-reactive mechanism? Raz et al. showed that human IgG anti-DNA antibodies, when injected into the renal artery of rats, bound to antigenic determinants in the rat kidney and subsequently induced renal dysfunction.[29] Other investigators have provided additional evidence that anti-DNA antibodies bind to glomerular membrane constituents by showing that high-affinity anti-dsDNA antibodies bind to laminin in the glomerular basement membrane.[30] Additional studies are needed to clarify the direct role of anti-DNA vs. anti-DNA/DNA complexes in the pathogenesis of tissue injury.

III. ANTI-snRNP PARTICLE (Sm AND RNP) AUTOANTIBODIES

Anti-Sm and anti-snRNP antibodies are distinct sets of antibody specificities that share partial identity in Ouchterloney immunodiffusion. Both autoantibodies or, rather, sets of autoantibody specificities bind to components of the splicesome apparatus, an RNA-protein complex that excises introns from the heteronuclear RNA, and then splices the remaining exons together. Splicesomes are RNA-protein particles (U snRNP) which consist of subsets of peptides bound to various small U RNAs (i.e., U1, U2, U4, U5, and U6 small RNAs). A number of minor cellular snRNPs also exists in eukaryote (U7, U8, U9, and U10) and in viral systems (herpes virus saimiri — HSUR 1 through 4). The core protein particle for all described U snRNPs consists of a common group of peptides that bear Sm antigenic determinants *and* additional peptides that are unique to the particular U snRNP. The common peptides that react with anti-Sm autoantibodies (i.e., possess Sm antigenicity) are B (28 kDa), B′ (29 kDa), D (16 kDa), E (13 kDa), F (9 kDa), and G (8 kDa). For the U1 snRNP, the unique proteins are A (33 kDa), C (22 kDa), and a 68-kDa nuclear matrix associated protein. The 68-kDa protein reacts with the vast majority of "anti-RNP antibodies". The U2 snRNP contains the peptides A′ (27 kDa) and B″ (21 kDa). The proteins unique to other U snRNPs (U4, U5, U6) have not been thoroughly characterized.

Virtually all the cDNAs for the common and known unique proteins of the snRNPs have been cloned and sequenced. Sequencing of the cDNAs for B and B′ showed that these two proteins are nearly identical and differ only at the carboxy terminus. Because of alternative splicing of a single RNA transcript, the proline-rich sequence PPPPGMR repeats twice in B′.[31-33] The N protein displayed 92% amino acid sequence homology with B′.[33] The D protein has minimal sequence homology with the B/B′ proteins, and it binds relatively few lupus sera.[32] Significant homologies between B/B″, A, and C also exist, particularly for proline-rich repeats.[33]

A number of investigators have performed epitope mapping studies to determine if each snRNP possesses unique immunodominant epitopes and/or if cross reactivity exists between the proteins. Immunoblotting studies with fusion protein fragments for B and B′ peptides showed that SLE sera bound different fusion proteins with variable frequency, suggesting that these peptides contained multiple epitopes.[34] However, analysis of binding frequencies designated the proline-rich carboxyl terminus as a major autoepitope.[34] Whether those sera that bound these peptides also cross react with the proline-rich sequence of other snRNPs was not explored. Addressing this issue, Habets et al. isolated human autoantibodies by affinity chromatography with a proline-rich U1 snRNP A protein fragment.[35] They obtained selective enrichment of antibodies that cross reacted with the B, B′, C, and N proteins. Furthermore, this group identified additional subsets of antibodies to this A fragment that can be characterized as follows: one set of antibodies reacted only with an "epitope" on the A protein, a second cross reacted with an epitope on B and B′, and a third set of antibodies cross reacted with B″. Other investigators have shown that the A protein contains multiple epitopes.[36] In related work, even though B, B′, and N sequences showed minimal similarity to the D protein, Habets et al. showed that the four proteins shared a common epitope.[35]

Mapping studies for epitopes on the 68-kDa protein have revealed three to six binding regions.[37-39] Using immunoblotted fusion protein fragments and a panel of connective tissue disease sera, Cram et al. observed that all sera that reacted with native 68-kDa protein did not bind the fusion proteins.[39] They concluded that additional antibody specificities may exist either toward epitopes that span the border of two contiguous fusion products or toward conformationally dependent epitopes.

This observation exemplifies a limitation of immunoblotted fusion proteins, a methodology that preferentially identifies linear epitopes, to perform epitope mapping. Unlike linear epitopes, conformational epitopes may have greater biologic relevance for antibody-mediated autoimmunity.[40] Hence, reports that describe linear autoepitopes should be interpreted with caution. Visualization of the spatial arrangement of oligopeptide fusion fragment in the snRNP protein complex by computer modeling analysis will be necessary to verify the autoimmunogenic relevance of an identified epitope. Methodologically, both immunoblotting and enzyme-linked immunosorbent assay (ELISA) have been used for mapping studies. Although antigen-coating procedures are more disruptive, both methods may variably affect the tertiary structure of protein fragments bound to the solid phase. If the tertiary structure of a fusion protein provides a conformationally dependent autoantigenic determinant, the blotting or coating process may sufficiently disrupt its tertiary structure to prevent recognition by the complementary autoantibody. Additional studies will be necessary to clarify this methodologic problem.

Although preliminary investigations suggest that the anti-snRNP response is antigen driven,[39,41] available data do not resolve whether the antibody response is stimulated by autoantigenic RNA-protein complexes or by molecular mimicry. As noted, various investigations have demonstrated that autoimmune sera contain a diversity of autoantibodies that cross react with several snRNP proteins. The apparent polyclonality of the antibody response to these proteins suggests, but not proves, that snRNPs may be the autoantigens of SLE and mixed connective tissue disease (MCTD).

Anti-snRNP autoantibodies may be induced by molecular mimicry. In this regard, sequence homology *and* immunological cross reactivity have been identified between the 68-kDa protein and both a retroviral gag protein and the M1 matrix protein of the influenza B virus.[38,42] Thus, these viral proteins could initiate the anti-68-kDa response, which is subsequently perpetuated by a cross-reactive immune reaction toward snRNPs. In another study, the 4B4 murine anti-Sm monoclonal antibody was found to bind a C-terminus proline-rich epitope of B/B′.[43] The 4B4 antibody cross reacted with the p24 gag protein of HIV-1 and with other polypeptides rich in proline residues, including collagen. These data suggest that the Sm B/B′ antigen contains a poly-proline epitope that is shared by several autoantigens and retroviral proteins. If molecular mimicry is indeed operative, antibodies directed primarily toward these viral protein epitopes should be present early in the clinical course, before the more diverse polyclonal anti-snRNP response.

Although additional work is necessary to determine how and which epitopes identified on the snRNPs contribute to the initiation and perpetuation of autoimmunity, the recombinant proteins offer an attractive source of material for the performance of diagnostic testing. Do recombinant proteins require conformationally intact epitopes for an assay to have diagnostic utility? Since most SLE sera react with epitopes on the B and B′ peptides,[44] Shields et al.[45] have determined if a recombinant B protein was suitable for the detection of anti-Sm reactive sera. Using an ELISA, a method that facilitates denaturation of native proteins, the investigators found that only 90% of sera positive by counterimmunoelectrophoresis were also positive by ELISA.[46] The inability of ELISA to detect anti-Sm antibodies in 10% of the SLE patients may be due to the fact that the recombinant B protein lacked native conformational epitopes. Alternately, the recombinant protein may contain all the autoepitopes, but some determinants are lost during the coating process. Similar issues may be relevant when assessing the specificity and sensitivity of other recombinant snRNP antibodies for the diagnosis and management of connective tissue disorders.[47-51]

IV. ANTI-RO (SSA) AUTOANTIBODIES

Anti-Ro (SSA) autoantibodies bind particles that contain at least a 60-kDa peptide plus one of four RNAs termed hY RNAs (for human cYtoplasmic). Ro RNP particles can be segregated into three discrete subpopulations with characteristic physicochemical properties: one containing hY4 RNA (Ro^{hY4}), another only hY5 RNA, RohY5, and the third with hY1, hY3, and hY4 RNAs ($Ro^{hY1\text{-}hY4}$).[52] The hY RNAs consist of 84 to 112 unmodified bases, are uridine rich, and are products of RNA polymerase III. The sequences for the 60-kDa protein[53,54] and the hY RNAs have been described. The 60-kDa protein contains a RNA binding motif and a zinc finger. The 60-kDa protein does not have substantial homology with amino acid sequences of other known proteins (see below). Each of the four hY RNAs has two highly homologous 11 base regions found close to the 3′ and 5′ ends; these are predicted to interact via hydrogen bonding.[53] The 5′ end has a polyuridine tail that could potentially bind the La protein.

At least three other antigenically distinct Ro proteins have been identified (46, 52, and 54 kDa).[55-58] The antigenic and physiochemical relationships of these peptides to the aformentioned 60-kDa Ro protein require further analysis. The 46-kDa protein, assigned by amino acid sequencing, migrated on sodium dodecyl sulfate polyacrylamide gel electrophoresis (SDS-PAGE) at an apparent molecular weight of approximately 60 kDa. This 46-kDa protein has sequence homology with the N-terminus of the rabbit calregulin gene product and contains a hydrophobic leader sequence, an endoplasmic reticulum retention sequence, and a possible calcium-binding domain.[56,59] Rabbit antibodies raised against the 6-19 amino acid sequence of the 46-kDa protein immunoprecipitated small RNAs from cell extracts with mobilities similar to the hY 1-5 RNA particles. However, it is unknown if this 46-kDa (apparent mol wt 60 kDa) binds hY RNA particles *in vivo.* Since this protein has characteristics of cell membrane proteins, an interaction between the 46-kDa peptide and hY RNA particles seems unlikely. Rather, this calregulin-like nature protein may contain a cross-reactive epitope that binds the anti- 60-kDa ''Ro'' protein. Such antigenic cross reactivity may explain why ultraviolet light induces cell membranes to express structures with anti-Ro reactivity.[60]

The 54-kDa ''Ro'' protein exists primarily in cells of erythroid lineage; its limited cellular distribution may also reflect a restricted hY RNA binding capacity.[60] The contribution of the 54-kDa ''Ro'' protein to the genesis of an anti-Ro antibody response is unknown. The recently cloned 52-kDa ''Ro'' protein shares no homology with the 60-kDa protein.[61] As determined by ELISA and immunoblotting, human sera with anti-Ro specificities, defined by counterimmunoelectrophoresis (CIE), bound the expressed 52-kDa ''Ro'' protein. The protein contains zinc finger domains, therefore it may play a role in RNA processing. Nevertheless, further studies are needed to determine if the protein binds hYRNAs and the RNA-protein aggregate elicits an ''Ro'' antibody response.

The source of Ro antigen, for clinical testing, is either bovine[62] or human spleen.[63] Although certain antigenic determinants on human SSA may be absent on bovine SSA, only a minor percentage of patients react with human and not bovine SSA. This observation implies that anti-Ro antibody activity is against both highly conserved epitopes and epitopes unique to the human species.[64] As mentioned, conformational epitopes may have greater biologic relevance than linear epitopes.[40] Also, the techniques commonly used to perform epitope mapping — ELISA and, to a lesser degree, immunoblotting — may favor the detection of determinants on denatured proteins. Considering these caveats, Scofield et al.[119] have identified a carboxy-terminal 13-kDa fragment (120 amino acids) that bound 62% of tested anti-Ro-positive sera. Overlapping octapeptides of the 120 amino acid sequence were synthesized and tested for binding of these sera. Three binding regions were identified. One major antigenic region in the 13-kDa fragment appeared to contain amino acid residues 477 to 492 (AIALREYRKKMDIPA). Using three-dimensional computer modeling, it was predicted that this sequence was an α-helix structure that resided on the surface of the 60-kDa Ro molecule. In addition, the binding of a reference serum to the most reactive octapeptide (EYRKKMDI, 477 to 492) was inhibited by the free peptide and by affinity-purified Ro antigen. Besides showing binding specificity, the results also indicated that the octapeptide was a "linear" as well as a conformational epitope for this serum sample. Thus, this may be an example of a linear epitope which, upon exposure to the isotonic solvent, acquires the necessary confirmational attributes.

Other anti-Ro antibody specificities also may be conformationally dependent.[65] Boire and co-workers identified an epitope present on the 60-kDa protein that would only bind anti-Ro antibody when the protein was complexed with hY5 RNA.[66] A Ro fusion protein (60-kDa) facilitated identification of the majority of, but not all, serum anti-Ro antibodies when studied by immunoblotting.[67] The results suggest that the "immunoblot negative" anti-Ro-positive sera contained antibodies directed only toward conformational epitopes.

V. ANTI-LA (SSB) AUTOANTIBODIES

Anti-La antibodies bind a particle composed of a 46- to 48-kDa peptide. This peptide binds 5′ terminal polyuridine sequences, especially if they are triuridine or longer.[68] A group of RNA polymerase III transcripts exists (e.g., 7s-RNA, pre-5SRNA) that the La particle probably bind through this mechanism. In addition, the leader sequence of the RNA of vesicular stomatitis virus, Epstein-Barr virus, and certain adenoviruses bind the La peptide.[69,70] Bachman et al. demonstrated that La, mechanistically, is a nucleic acid-dependent ATPase/dATPase that participates in transcription termination.[71] Work by Gottleib and Steitz supports this notion by showing that the La protein influenced both the accuracy and the efficiency of RNA polymerase III transcription.[72] Although uncorroborated, another study indicated that the La protein may participate in the repair of DNA.[73]

When anti-La antibody is present in the serum of an SLE patient, anti-Ro antibody almost always coexists. Anti-Ro antibodies, however, may exist in isolation.[74,75] Recent work may clarify why anti-Ro and anti-La frequently but not always coexist.[52,76] Ro RNP particles segregate into three discrete subpopulations with characteristic physicochemical properties: one containing hY4 RNA (Ro^{hY4}), another only hY5 RNA RohY5, and the third with hY1, hY3, and hY4 RNAs, ($Ro^{hY1\text{-}hY4}$).[52] Apparently the La protein associates with hY5 RNA (Ro^{hY5}) and not the other Ro snRNPs. Hence, one may postulate that whereas Ro^{hY5} may stimulate an immune response in which both anti-Ro and anti-La antibodies occur, other autoimmunogenic Ro RNP particles may induce primarily an anti-Ro antibody response.

As for Ro, multiple epitopes, primarily linear, have been identified for La.[77-82] One particular epitope consists of an amino acid sequence (88 to 101) that is similar to the feline sarcoma virus gag protein.[83] In an important study, it was asked if the fine specificity of human anti-La autoantibodies, identified by immunodiffusion, differed from antibodies deliberately generated by immunization of mice with recombinant La protein.[84] The binding specificities of the human and the generated murine anti-La antibodies were compared by ELISA using synthetic peptides for several portions of the recombinant La protein. The data demonstrated that only murine anti-La reactive sera reacted with the solid-phase-bound oligopeptides. The differences in binding specificities between the murine and human antibodies can be explained by the following possibilities. The human sera likely contained antibodies toward epitopes present on the native La protein. Due either to lack of glycosylation or as a consequence of purification, the recombinant La protein is probably denatured and would preferentially stimulate antibodies toward epitopes on "denatured" La protein. Since the ELISA detection system preferably identifies antibodies directed toward denatured protein fragments, it was not surprising that human anti-La sera failed to react in the ELISA assay. The data, thus, suggest that conformational epitopes are relevant for the study of fine specificity of the La autoantibody response.

As for other nuclear antigens, data support an antigen-driven autoantibody response against La. The anti-La specificities of patient sera that were collected longitudinally were tested by ELISA using four fusion proteins from different regions of the La molecule. Antibody levels against the different specificities varied independently in individual patients.[77]

VI. ANTI-KU AUTOANTIBODIES

The structure and function of the Ku antigen has not been as thoroughly studied as other autoantigens. Ku is a DNA-protein complex consisting of two proteins (approximately 70 and 80 kDa) that interact noncovalently with the ends of dsDNA.[85,86] A recent report has shown that Ku may be similar or identical to a cellular DNA-binding protein, NFIV, that binds to dsDNA termini at the adenovirus DNA replication origin and translocates along the DNA, resulting in the formation of a multimeric protein complex.[87,88] Sequencing of the 70-kDa cDNA revealed a structure comparable to certain transcription activation factors.[89-91] The sequence of 80 kDa has no homology with the 70-kDa protein.[90,91] One autoepitope has been identified on the C terminus of the 70-kDa protein. Autoantibodies that were immunoaffinity purified with 70-kDa fusion proteins had no cross reactivity with the 80-kDa protein, and vice versa.[87] Therefore, these two structures are both structurally and immunologically distinct.

What remains unanswered is why autoantibodies to the 70- and 80-kDa proteins tend to coexist in patient sera. Epitope mapping studies with fusion proteins generated from fragments of cDNAs for both have identified three major determinants on each protein.[92] The presence of conformational epitopes was determined by an antigen capture ELISA. Both proteins displayed confirmational epitopes in the carboxy terminus region. Longitudinal autoantibody studies of SLE showed that anti-70-kDa and anti-80-kDa antibodies can be produced in tandem independently of other autoantibodies, indicating that the antibody responses to these antigens also are antigen driven.[93]

VII. ANTI-RIBOSOMAL P AUTOANTIBODIES

Anti-ribosomal autoantibodies consist of an expanding group of antibodies that identify the following highly conserved ribosomal proteins: P_0, P_1, P_2, S10, L5, and L12 molecules (38, 19, 17, 6, and 20 kDa).[94-96] All apparently associate with the 60S ribosomal subunit in eukaryote cells, participating in the elongation of ribosomal protein synthesis. Epitope mapping studies, although preliminary, have revealed an immunodominant determinant on P_0, P_1, and P_2 that resides within the 22 amino acid sequence of the C terminus.

Twelve to 16% of sera from SLE patients have been reported to contain anti-P.[97,98] Immunoblotting techniques, however, have revealed that anti-P, anti-S10, and anti-L12 occur in 41, 31, and 2% of 89 randomly selected SLE patients without sacrificing specificity.[99] These results suggest that anti-ribosomal antibodies may be more specific for SLE than anti-Sm. Further, anti-ribosomal P antibodies have been associated with the neuropsychiatric manifestations of SLE.[97,98] Using the 22 amino acid peptide for immunoaffinity purification of anti-P, Koren et al. have reported that the purified antibodies cross react with a 38-kDa cell membrane structure.[100] This molecule has been identified on the surface of hepatoma and neuroblastoma cells. Although the biological significance is unclear, the observation suggests that anti-P antibodies may cross react with similar structures on neuronal cells of the central nervous system (CNS) and thereby contribute to the manifestations of diffuse CNS dysfunction (e.g., psychosis).

VIII. ANTI-HISTONE AUTOANTIBODIES

Histones occur in the nucleus in a highly organized nucleosomal structure that consists of three subunits, two H2A-H2B dimers flanking a H3-H4 tetramer, surrounded by approximately two helical turns of DNA. The nucleosomes are connected by varying lengths of linker DNA that associates with H1 histone. Within the chromatin strands of the nucleus, conditions promote further conformational alterations in the polynucleosomal complex that results in additional levels of organized condensation.[101]

Antibodies to all classes of mammalian histones, H1, H2A, H2B, H3, and H4 are observed in SLE and other connective tissue diseases. Furthermore, additional specificities are directed toward DNA-histone complexes. They represent the most prevalent group of antibodies in SLE (50 to 70%) of unselected patients. Nevertheless, each connective tissue disorder likely has its own pattern of restricted antihistone antibody specificities.[102-104] This relationship is illustrated by the different antibody specificities observed in drug-induced and idiopathic SLE. In idiopathic SLE, perhaps as a consequence of methodologic differences, specificities toward all histones been described. However, H1 and H2B appear to be the most common. For procainamide-induced lupus, patients have elevated levels of IgG antibodies to the H2A-H2B dimer. Interestingly, a recent report has demonstrated that the anti-dimer antibodies are more reactive if DNA is associated with H2A-H2B.[105] This observation lends credence to the notion that antibodies are generated to released nucleosomes and not free histones.

Evidence suggests that anti-histone antibodies react with a number of distinct epitopes, which reside either on the N-terminal (H2B,H4), C-terminal, or the core regions of the histone proteins (H1).[106,107] Using proteolytic digest of histone and synthetic peptides, investigators have tentatively shown that N-terminal determinants may be pathologically relevant. When the core histones are associated to form the nucleosome octamer, only the N-terminal region is accessible and susceptible to trypsin digestion. Trypsin markedly decreases the binding of anti-histone antibodies, suggesting that many of the antibody specificities are located in the N-terminal region, perhaps toward confirmational epitopes. This observation has been partially validated by using synthetic N-terminal petides to block binding of the anti-histone antibodies.[108]

IX. ANTI-NEUTROPHIL CYTOPLASMIC AUTOANTIBODIES (ANCA)

Anti-neutrophil cytoplasmic antibodies directed toward proteins in the primary granules of neutrophils and lysosomes of monocytes have been reported to assist in the diagnosis and management of various forms of vasculitis.[109] The most frequently reported technique to detect ANCA-positive serum is a variant of the F-ANA test. When alcohol-fixed neutrophils are used as substrate, two dominant patterns are observed: (1) Cytoplasmic-ANCA (cANCA) and (2) perinuclear ANCA (pANCA). The cANCA pattern has been associated with antibodies that bind proteinase 3 while the pANCA pattern defines antibodies to myeloperoxidase (MPO) and less frequently to elastase.[110,111]

Using either immunoprecipitation or immunoelectrophoresis (IEF) and capillary immunoblotting, recent work from Bini and colleagues[112] indicates the cANCA-positive sera recognize conformational epitope(s) on proteinase 3. Reduction, acidification, or SDS treatment of proteinase 3 markedly reduced reactivity. This data may explain why the techniques of sandwich ELISA or western blotting with purified proteinase 3 yield lower frequencies of detection for the antibody with known cANCA-positive sera. Further, they point out the necessity of Ag capture ELISA to identify this particular autoantibody. Although less rigorously proven, it is likely that epitopes recognized by anti-myeloperoxidase are also conformationally dependent.[113]

X. INDUCTION OF AUTOANTIBODIES

The immune system is endowed with a high and apparently complex level of connectivity, an attribute dependent upon the processes of self-recognition and self-reaction. Secondary to cognitive pressures engendered by this process of connectivity, the immune system maintains a vigilant posture that readily allows discrimination between self and non-self. For example, through the connectivity of idiotype/anti-idiotype interactions, dominant Ig idiotypic motifs for normal serum immunoglobulins are compelled to emerge. Maintenance of these motifs insures tolerance at the B cell level.[114] Although unproved, it is likely that these dominant patterns of immunoglobulin interactions also influence the selection of regulatory T cells that, in turn, contribute an additional level of control. These regulatory T cells likely interconnect with a parallel T cell receptor (TCR) idiotypic network that has its own hierarchy. Effective regulation of autoreactive B and T cells occurs through the existence of favorable Ig and TCR idiotypic patternings manifested by anti-idiotype antibodies and by anti-idiotype regulatory T cells.

Within this controlled immune network, Ig and TCR idiotypic motifs that mimic the images of particular self-antigens are likely to be abundant. Manifested as self-tolerance, the dominance of these images blinds the system to many other similar but not identical self-antigens. Consequently, when an injurious event causes release of self-antigens capable of stimulating an autoimmune response, the extant regulatory processes that maintain these dominant Ig and TCR idiotypic patterns favor dampening and "elimination" of the autoantibody and auto-effector cell responses.[115] When the immune system encounters a pathogen, the organism essentially presents two broad categories of antigenic epitopes: (1) non-self epitopes and (2) by molecular mimicry, autoepitopes. In this context, non-self or foreign epitopes quickly stimulate an aggressive immune reaction. However, the autoepitopes (self-antigens) displayed by the organism also stimulate an immune response. Fortuitiously, the B and T cell idiotypic networks that control this autoreactivity automatically restrain the anti-self response. As a consequence, exposure to the pathogens that display self-epitopes reinforces the visibility of the dominant idiotypic patterns and hence the maintenance of tolerance to self.

The levels of certain idiotypes for normal immunoglobulins fluctuate on a regular basis, implying the existence of reactive homeostatic regulation. For unexplained reasons, this pattern of control is altered in autoimmunity.[116] Since perpetuation of the autoimmune response requires T cell help, similar perturbations may exist at the level of TCR idiotypes. Although unable to initiate an autoimmune reaction, circumstances that shift the pattern of idiotype dominance toward T cell autoreactivity would certainly provide the environment for its inception when the immune system is provoked with the proper precipitant.

A. PERTURBATIONS OF THE IDIOTYPIC NETWORK

Although we have considered the role of a perturbed idiotypic network as a necessary prerequisite for the development of an autoimmune response, changes in this network theoretically could contribute directly to its inception. As discussed, cross-reactive idiotypes represent an attribute of the controlled connectivity of the immune system. Perturbations in the idiotype/anti-idiotype network of anti-DNA idiotypes may lead to the generation of pathogenic anti-DNA antibodies. Mendlovic et al.[117] demonstrated that immunization of normal mice with monoclonal anti-DNA antibody bearing the cross-reactive 16/6 idiotype developed a lupus-like illness. The corresponding anti-idiotype antibody also induced the disorder. These provocative observations suggest that alteration in connectivity by either a ''pathogenic'' idiotype or anti-idiotype can initiate an autoimmune diathesis. What remains unclear is the mechanisms through which the idiotypes become pathogenic.

Using a light chain Ig that reacted with snRNP, Puccetti et al. immunized normal mice and showed that they developed not only anti-snRNP antibodies but also anti-dsDNA and anti-ssDNA antibodies. The light chain immunogen displayed two unusual characteristics. The third hypervariable region of the light chain contained the idiotype of anti-DNA and anti-snRNP network for MRL-lpr/lpr mice and the amino acid sequence showed significant homology with 68-kDa RNP antigen. While the generation of an anti-RNP response seems obvious, the origin of the anti-DNA response is problematic. When the aforementioned data are coupled with observations by Radic et al.,[25] one plausible explanation would be as follows. During an immune reaction against a pathogen, somatic mutation from an anti-non-self to anti-self antibody response occurs. Normally, the anti-self response is attenuated by idiotypic connectivity. However, in the genetically susceptible individual, the transition from the anti-non-self to anti-self antibody response may provide L or H chains that alter the idiotypic network to facilitate an anti-self response or the mutated L or H chains may directly serve as an autoantigen. Irrespective of the mechanism, the results of this extraordinary study further implicate aberrant idiotype interactions in the development of autoimmunity.

B. MOLECULAR MIMICRY AND COGNATE T-B CELL RECOGNITION

Although the autoantibody response in SLE appears to be antigen driven, the events that cause certain self-antigens to become the focus of an autoreactive response necessitate further investigation. Viral infections have long been associated with the development of autoimmune disease. With the availability of data bases that contain known amino acid sequences, the list of homologies between viral and human proteins is growing rapidly.[118] Thus, it comes as no surprise that investigators have identified nuclear autoantigens that contain amino acid sequences homologous with sequences for various viral proteins. Presumably, a portion of these homologies may represent potential autoepitopes recognized by anti-nuclear antibodies. In this context, an autoepitope on the carboxy terminus of the Ro antigen was highly homologous with a sequence for the vesicular stomatitis virus nucleocapsid protein.[119] Sequence homology and immunological cross reactivity also have been reported between the 68-kDa protein of U1 snRNP and both a retroviral gag protein and the M1 matrix protein of the infleunza B virus.[38,42] Data also suggest that the Sm B/B′ antigen contains a poly-proline epitope that is shared by several retroviral proteins.[43] As amino acid sequences in the data bases accrue, investigators will certainly identify additional examples of biochemical cross reactivity. For most of these homologies, immunologic cross reactivity has not been demonstrated. Furthermore, it will be important to demonstrate that antigen processing of a viral protein, containing a sequence homology with a self-protein, will produce an antigenic determinant that contains a sequence homologous to the self protein determinants. The viral antigenic determinant then could focus a cognate T cell-assisted B cell anti-self antibody response.

While mammalian DNA is virtually nonimmunogenic, other DNA, particularly bacterial DNA, can induce pathogenic anti-DNA antibodies.[4,5,120] However, while prokaryotic DNA may stimulate autoreactive anti-DNA B cells, this loss of B cell tolerance is not sufficient to generate a sustained autoimmune response. A breakdown of T cell tolerance (T helper cell level) is an obligatory prerequisite for an autoantibody response to occur. In a novel study, when B cells were stimulated with foreign antigen to make antibody that cross reacted with a self protein, the activated autoreactive B cells were able to present the self protein in immunogenic form to T cells, producing T cell autoreactivity.[121] Hence, molecular mimicry, coupled with robust antigen-presenting B cells, offers the potential not only to induce autoantibody production, but also to stimulate autoreactive T cells that drive the antibody response. Along these lines, Zinkernagel et al.[122] have reported experiments in which transgenic mice expressing the cell membrane-associated glycoprotein of the vesicular stomatitis virus (VSV-G) were generated and found to be tolerant to this protein. The investigators then found that mice did not produce IgG anti-VSV-G antibodies when immunized either by VSV-G in adjuvant or by recombinant vaccinia virus expressing VSV-G. However, when infected with wild-type VSV, the mice produced anti-VSG "autoantibodies". The data showed that helper T cell tolerance is crucial in the maintenance of B cell nonreactivity, that cognate T-B recognition is necessary to break tolerance of self-reactive B cells, and that infectious agents, with proteins homologous to the host, could disrupt the tolerance of self-reactive B cells.

XI. CONCLUSION

The above information provides new fragments about the structure of autoantibodies and their autoantigens and reviews recent data that offer insights to the mechanisms that contribute to the genesis of autoimmune disease. It is unlikely that a single "mechanism" will lead to the development of autoimmune disease. Nevertheless, a picture that describes a final common pathway is emerging.

ACKNOWLEDGMENTS

C.J.F. would like to thank E. S. Kurtides, M.D. for his support. He also appreciates the assistance of the Rice Foundation and the Illinois Chapter of the Arthritis Foundation.

REFERENCES

1. **Gharavi, A. E., Chu, J.-L., and Elkon, K.,** Autoantibodies to intracellular proteins in human systemic lupus erythematosus are not due to random polyclonal B cell activation, *Arthritis Rheum.*, 31, 1337, 1988.
2. **Stollar, B. D.,** Anti-DNA antibodies, *Crit. Rev. Biochem.*, 20, 1, 1986.
3. **Messina, J. P., Gilkeson, G. S., and Pisetsky, D. S.,** Stimulation of in vitro murine lymphocyte proliferation by bacterial DNA, *J. Immunol.*, 147, 1759, 1991.
4. **Pisetsky, D. S., Grudier, J. P., and Gilekson, G. S.,** A role for immunogenic DNA in the pathogenesis of SLE, *Arthritis Rheum.*, 33, 153, 1990.
5. **Wu, D. P., Gilkeson, G. S., Armitage, J., Reich, C. F., and Pisetsky, D. S.,** Selective recognition of DNA antigenic determinants by murine monoclonal antibodies, *Clin. Exp. Immunol.*, 82, 33, 1990.
6. **Shoenfeld, Y., Rauch, J., Massicotte, H., and Stollar, B.,** Polyspecificity of monoclonal lupus autoantibodies, *N. Engl. J. Med.*, 308, 414, 1983.
7. **Jacob, L., Tron, F., Bach, J., and Louvard, D.,** Binding of a monoclonal anti-DNA autoantibody to identical proteins present at the surface of several human cell types involved in lupus pathogenesis, *J. Clin. Invest.*, 75, 315, 1985.
8. **Hannested, R., Rekvig, O., and Husebekk, A.,** Cross reacting rheumatoid factors and lupus (LE) factors, *Springer Semin. Immunopathol.*, 4, 133, 1981.
9. **Jacob, L., Viard, J., Allenet, B., Anin, M., Slama, F., Vandekerckhove, J., Primo, J., Markovits, J., Jacob, F., Bach, J. F., Lepecq, J., and Louvard, D.,** A monoclonal anti-dsDNA autoantibody binds to a 94kD cell surface structure protein on various cells via nucleosomes or a DNA-histone, *Proc. Natl. Acad. Sci. U.S.A.*, 86, 4669, 1989.
10. **Brinkman, K., Termant, R., de Jong, J., Van den Brink, H., Berden, J., and Smeenk, R. J. T.,** Crossreactive binding patterns of monoclonal antibodies to DNA are often caused by DNA/anti-DNA complexes, *Res. Immunol.*, 140, 595, 1989.
11. **Subiza, J., Caturla, A., Pascual-Salcedo, D., Chamorro, M., Gazapo, E., Figueredo, M., and De la Concha, E.,** DNA-anti-DNA complexes account for part of the anti-histone activity found in patients with SLE, *Arthritis Rheum.*, 32, 406, 1989.
12. **Lampman, G., Furie, B., Schwartz, R., and Stollar, B.,** Amino acid sequence of a human lupus monoclonal autoantibody, IgM HF2-2/17, that binds ssDNA and platelets, *Blood,* 74, 262, .
13. **Isenberg, D., Williams, W., Axford, J., et al.,** Comparison of DNA antibody idiotypes in human sera: an international collaborative study of 19 idiotypes from 11 different laboratories, *J. Autoimmun.*, 3, 393, 1990.
14. **Bentley, G., Boulot, G., Riottot, M., and Poljak, R.,** Three-dimensional structure of an idiotype-anti-idiotype complex, *Nature,* 348, 254, 1990.
15. **Young, F., Tucker, L., Rubinstein, D., Guillaume, T., Andre-Schwartz, J., Barret, K., Schwartz, R. S., and Logtenberg, T.,** Molecular analysis of a germ line-encoded idiotypic marker of pathogenic human lupus autoantibodies, *J. Immunol.*, 145, 2545, 1990.

16. **Manheimer-Lory, A., Davidson, A., Watkins, D., Hannigan, N., and Diamond, B.,** Generation and analysis of clonal IgM- and IgG-producing human B cell lines expressing an anti-DNA idiotype, *J. Clin. Invest.*, 87, 1519, 1991.
17. **Grayzel, A., Solomon, A., Aranow, C., and Diamond, B.,** Antibodies elicited by pneumococcal antigens bear an anti-DNA-associated idiotype, *J. Clin. Invest.*, 87, 842, 1991.
18. **Marion, T., Bothwell, A., Briles, D., and Janeway, C. A., Jr.,** IgG anti-DNA antibodies within an individual autoimmune mouse are the products of clonal selection, *J. Immunol.*, 142, 4269, 1989.
19. **Shlomchik, M., Mascelli, M., Shan, H., Radic, M., Pisetsky, D., and Weigert, M.,** Anti-DNA antibodies from autoimmune mice arise from clonal expression and somatic mutation, *J. Exp. Med.*, 171, 265, 1990.
20. **Panosian-Sahakian, N., Klotz, J., Ebling, F., Kronenberg, M., and Hahn, B.,** Diversity of Ig V gene segments found in anti-DNA autoantibodies from a single (NZB/NZW) F1 mouse, *J. Immunol.*, 142, 4500, 1989.
21. **Cairns, E., Kwong, P., Misener, V., Ip, P., Bell, D., and Siminovitch, K.,** Analysis of variable region genes encoding a human anti-DNA antibody of normal origin. Implications for the molecular basis of autoimmune responses, *J. Immunol.*, 143, 685, 1989.
22. **Baccala, R., Quang, T., Gilbert, M., Ternynck, T., and Avrameas, S.,** Two murine natural polyreactive autoantibodies are encoded by nonmutated germ-line genes, *Proc. Natl. Acad. Sci. U.S.A.*, 86, 4624, 1989.
23. **Eilat, D., Webster, D., and Rees, A.,** V region sequences of anti-DNA and anti-RNA autoantibodies from NZB/NZW F1 mice, *J. Immunol.*, 141, 1745, 1988.
24. **Van Es, J. H., Meyling, H. J. G., van de Akker, R. M., Aanstoot, H., Derksen, R. H. W. M., and Logtenberg, T.,** Somatic mutations in the variable regions of a human IgG anti double stranded DNA autoantibody suggest a role for antigen in the induction of SLE, *J. Exp. Med.*, 173, 461, 1991.
25. **Radic, M., Mascelli, M., Erikson, J., Shan, H., and Weigert, M.,** Ig H and L chain contributions to autoimmune specificities, *J. Immunol.*, 146, 176, 1991.
26. **Sabbaga, J., Pankewycz, O. G., Lufft, V., Schwartz, R. S., and Madaio, M. P.,** Cross-reactivity distinguishes serum and nephritogenic anti-DNA antibodies in human lupus from their natural counterparts in normal serum, *J. Autoimmun.*, 3, 215, 1990.
27. **Termaat, R. M., Brinkman, K., Nossent, J. C., Swaak, A. J. G., Smeenk, R. J. T., and Berden, J. H. M.,** Anti-heparan sulphate reactivity in sera from patients with systemic lupus erythematosus with renal or non-renal manifestations, *Clin. Exp. Immunol.*, 82, 268, 1990.
28. **Smeenk, R., Brinkman, K., van den Brink, H. G., Termaat, R. M., Berden, J., Nossent, J. C., and Swaak, A. J. G.,** Antibodies to DNA in patients with SLE: their role in the diagnosis, the follow-up, and the pathogenesis of the disease, *Clin. Rheumatol.*, 9, 100, 1990.
29. **Raz, E., Brezis, M., Rosenmann, E., and Eilat, D.,** Anti-DNA antibodies bind directly to renal antigens and induce kidney dysfunction in the isolated perfused rat kidney, *J. Immunol.*, 192, 3076, 1989.
30. **Sabbaga, J., Line, S., Potocnjak, P., and Madaio, M.,** A murine nephritogenic monoclonal anti-DNA autoantibody binds directly to mouse laminin, the major non-collagenous protein of the glomerular basement membrane, *Eur. J. Immunol.*, 19, 137, 1989.

31. **Rokeach, L. A., Jannatipour, M., Haselby, J. A., and Hoch, S. O.,** Primary structure of a human small nuclear ribonucleoprotein polypeptide as deduced by cDNA analysis, *J. Biol. Chem.*, 264, 5024, 1989.
32. **Ohosone, Y., Mimori, T., Griffith, A., Akizuki, M., Homma, M., Craft, J., and Hardin, J. A.,** Molecular cloning of cDNA encoding Sm autoantigen: derivation of a cDNA for a B polypeptide of the U series of small nuclear ribonucleoprotein particles, *Proc. Natl. Acad. Sci. U.S.A.*, 86, 4249, 1989.
33. **Van Dam, A., Winkel, I., Zijlstra-Baalbergen, J., Smeenk, R., and Cuypers, H. T.,** Cloned human snRNP proteins B and B″ differ only in their carboxyl-terminal part, *EMBOJ.*, 8, 3853, 1989.
34. **Elkon, K. B., Hines, J. J., Chu, J. L., and Parnassa, A.,** Epitope mapping of recombinant Hela Sm B and B′ peptides obtained by polymerase chain reaction, *J. Immunol.*, 145, 636, 1990.
35. **Habets, W. J., Sillekens, P. T. G., Hoet, M. H., McAllister, G., Lerner, M. R., and van Venrooij, W. J.,** Small nuclear RNA-associated proteins are immunologically related as revealed by mapping of autoimmune reactive B-epitopes, *Proc. Natl. Acad. Sci. U.S.A.*, 86, 4674, 1989.
36. **Barakat, S., Briand, J. P., Abuaf, N., Van Regenmortel, M. H. V., and Muller, S.,** Mapping of epitopes on U1 snRNP polypeptide A with synthetic peptides and autoimmune sera, *Clin. Exp. Immunol.*, 86, 71, 1991.
37. **Guldner, H., Nettler, H., Szostecki, C., Lahomek, H., and Will, H.,** Epitope mapping with a recombinant human 68kD(u1) ribonucleoprotein antigen reveals heterogeneous autoantibody profiles in human autoimmune disease, *J. Immunol.*, 141, 469, 1988.
38. **Query, C. and Keene, J.,** A human autoimmune protein associated with U1 RNA contains a region of homology that is cross-reactive with retroviral p30 gag antigen, *Cell*, 51, 211, 1987.
39. **Cram, D. S., Fisicaro, N., Coppel, R. L., Whittingham, S., and Harrison, L. C.,** Mapping of multiple B cell epitopes on the 70kd autoantigen of the U1 ribonucleoprotein complex, *J. Immunol.*, 145, 630, 1990.
40. **Laver, W. G., Air, G., Webster, R., and Smith-Gill, S.,** Epitopes on protein antigens: misconceptions and realities, *Cell*, 61, 553, 1990.
41. **Habets, W. J., Hoet, M. H., and van Venrooij, W. J.,** Epitope patterns of anti-RNP antibodies in the rheumatic diseases: evidence for antigen driven autoimmune response, *Arthritis Rheum.*, 33, 834, 1990.
42. **Guldner, H. H., Netter, H. J., Szostecki, C., Jaeger, E., and Will, H.,** Human anti-p68 autoantibodies recognize a common epitope of U1 RNA containing small nuclear ribonucleoprotein and influenza B virus, *J. Exp. Med.*, 171, 819, 1990.
43. **De Keyser, F., Hoch, S. O., Takei, M., Dang, H., De Keyser, H., Rokeach, L. A., and Talal, N.,** Cross-reactivity of the B/B′ subunit of the Sm ribonucleoprotein autoantigen with proline-rich polypeptides, *Clin. Immunol. Immunopathol.*, 62, 285, 1992.
44. **Habets, W., de Rooij, D., Hoet, M., van der Putte, L., and van Ventooij, W.,** Quantitation of anti-RNP and anti-Sm antibodies in MCTD and SLE patients by immunoblotting, *Clin. Exp. Immunol.*, 59, 457, 1985.

45. **Shields, M. J., Siegel, J. N., Clark, C. R., Hines, K. K., Potempa, L. A., Gewurz, H., and Anderson, B.,** An appraisal of polystyrene-(ELISA) and nitrocellulose-based (ELIFA) enzyme immunoassay systems using monoclonal antibodies reactive toward antigenically distinct forms of human C-reactive protein, *J. Immunol. Meth.*, 141, 253, 1991.
46. **Hines, J. J., Danho, W., and Elkon, K. B.,** Detection and quantification of human anti-Sm antibodies using synthetic peptide and recombinant SmB antigens, *Arthritis Rheum.*, 34, 572, 1991.
47. **Takeda, Y., Wang, G. S., Wang, R. J., Anderson, S. K., Pettersson, I., Amaki, S., and Sharp, G.,** ELISA using isolated (U) small nuclear ribonucleoprotein polypeptides as antigens to investigate the clinical significance of autoantibodies to these polypeptides, *Clin. Immunol. Immunopathol.*, 50, 213, 1989.
48. **Habets, W. J. A., Hoet, M. H., Sillkens, P. T. G., de Rooij, D. J. M., van de Putte, L. B. A., and van Venrooij, W. J.,** Detection of autoantibodies in a quantitative ELISA using recombinant ribonucleoprotein antigens, *Clin. Exp. Immunol.*, 76, 172, 1989.
49. **ter Borg, E., Horst, G., Limburg, P., van Venrooij, W., and Kallenberg, C. G. M.,** Changes in levels of antibodies against the 70kDa and A polypeptides of the U1RNP complex in relation to exacerbations of systemic lupus erythematosus, *J. Rheumatol.*, 18, 363, 1991.
50. **Seelig, H. P., Ehrfeld, H., Schroeter, H., Heim, C., and Renz, M.,** A recombinant 70K protein ELISA. Screening for antibodies against U1snRNP proteins in human sera, *J. Immunol. Meth.*, 143, 11, 1991.
51. **St. Clair, E. W., Query, C. C., Bentley, R., Keene, J. D., Polisson, R. P., Allen, N. B., Caldwell, D. S., Rice, J. R., Cox, C., and Pisetsky, D. S.,** Expression of autoantibodies to recombinant (U1) RNP-associated 70K antigen in systemic lupus erythematosus, *Clin. Immunol. Immunopathol.*, 54, 266, 1990.
52. **Boire, G. and Craft, J.,** Human Ro ribonucleoprotein particles: characterization of native structure and stable association with the La polypeptide, *J. Clin. Invest.*, 85, 1182, 1990.
53. **Deutscher, S., Harley, J. B., and Keene, J. D.,** Molecular analysis of the 60kD human Ro ribonucleoprotein, *Proc. Natl. Acad. Sci. U.S.A.*, 85, 9479, 1988.
54. **Ben-Chetrit, E., Gandy, B., Tan, E., and Sullivan, K.,** Isolation and characterization of cDNA encoding the 60kD component of the human SSA/Ro ribonucleoprotein, *J. Clin. Invest.*, 83, 1284, 1989.
55. **Ben-Chetrit, E., Fox, R., and Tan, E.,** Dissociation of immune responses to the SSA 52 kD and 60 kD polypeptides in SLE and Sjogren's syndrome, *Arthritis Rheum.*, 33, 349, 1990.
56. **McCauliffe, D. P., Lux, F. A., Lieu, T. S., Sanz, I., Hanke, J., Newkirk, M. M., Bachinski, L. I., Itoh, Y., Siciliano, M. J., Reichlin, M., Sontheimer, R. D., and Capra, J. D.,** Molecular cloning, expression, and chromosome localization of a human Ro/SSA autoantigen, *J. Clin. Invest.*, 85, 1379, 1990.
57. **Ben-Chetrit, E., Chan, E., Sullivan, K., and Tan, E.,** The 52kD protein is a novel component of the SSA/Ro antigenic particle, *J. Exp. Med.*, 167, 1560, 1988.
58. **Rader, M., O'Brien, C., Liu, Y., Harley, J., and Reichlein, M.,** Heterogeneity of the Ro/SSA antigen. Different molecular forms in lymphocytes and in red blood cells, *J. Clin. Invest.*, 83, 1293, 1989.

59. **McCauliffe, D., Zappi, E., Lieu, T., Michalak, M., Sontheimer, R., and Capra, J.,** A human Ro/SSA autoantigen is the homologue of calreticulin and highly homologous with onchocercal RAL-1 antigen and an aplysia "memory molecule", *J. Clin. Invest.*, 86, 332, 1990.
60. **Furukawa, F., Kashihara-Sawami, M., Lyons, M. B., and Norris, D. A.,** Binding of autoantibodies to the extractable nuclear antigens SSA and SSB is induced on the surface of human keratinocytes by UV light: implications for the pathogenesis of photosensitive cutaneous lupus, *J. Invest. Dermatol.*, 94, 77, 1990.
61. **Chan, E. K. L., Hamel, J. C., Buyon, J. P., and Tan, E. M.,** Molecular definition and sequence motifs of the 52-kD component of human SS-A/Ro autoantigen, *J. Clin. Invest.*, 87, 68, 1991.
62. **Fields, R. A., Toubbeh, H., Searles, R. P., and Bankhurst, A. D.,** The prevalence of anticardiolipin antibodies in a healthy elderly population and its association with antinuclear antibodies, *J. Rheumatol.*, 16, 623, 1989.
63. **Hollingsworth, P. N., Bonifacio, E., and Dawkins, R. I.,** Use of standard curve improves precision and concordance of ANA measurement, *J. Clin. Lab. Immunol.*, 22, 197, 1987.
64. **Reichlin, M. and Reichlin, M. W.,** Autoantibodies to the Ro/SSA particle react preferentially with the human antigen, in *Sjögren's Syndrome: A Model for Understanding Autoimmunity,* Talal, N., Ed., Academic Press, New York, 1989, 51.
65. **Boire, G., Lopez-Longo, F.-J., Lapointe, S., and Ménard, H.-A.,** Sera from patients with autoimmune disease recognize conformational determinants on the 60-kd Ro/SS-A protein, *Arthritis Rheum.*, 34, 722, 1991.
66. **Boire, G. and Craft, J.,** Biochemical and immunological heterogeneity of the Ro ribonucleoprotein particles, *J. Clin. Invest.*, 84, 270, 1989.
67. **James, J., Dickey, W., Fujisaku, A., O'Brien, C., Deutscher, S., Keene, J., and Harley, J.,** Antigenicity of a recombinant Ro (SSA) fusion protein, *Arthritis Rheum.*, 33, 102, 1990.
68. **Stephano, J. E.,** Purified lupus antigen La recognizes an oligo uridylate stretch common to the 3′termini of RNA polymerase II transcripts, *Cell,* 36, 145, 1984.
69. **Kurilla, M. and Keene, J.,** The leader RNA of vesicular stomatitis virus is bound by a cellular protein reactive with anti-La antibodies, *Cell,* 34, 837, 1983.
70. **Lerner, M., Andrews, N., Miller, G., and Steitz, J.,** Two small RNAs encoded by EBV and complexed with proteins are precipitated by antibodies from patients with SLE, *Proc. Natl. Acad. Sci. U.S.A.*, 78, 805, 1981.
71. **Bachman, M., Pfeifer, K., Schroder, H. C., and Muller, E. G.,** Characterization of the autoantigen La (SSB) as a nucleic acid-dependent ATPase/dATPase with melting properties, *Cell,* 60, 85, 1990.
72. **Gottleib, E. and Steitz, J.,** The RNA binding protein La influences both the accuracy and the efficiency of RNA polymerase III transcription *in vitro, EMBO J.*, 8, 841, 1989.
73. **Coverley, D., Kenney, M. K., Munn, M., Rupp, W. D., Lane, D. P., and Wood, R. D.,** Requirement for the replication protein SSB in human DNA excision repair, *Nature,* 349, 538, 1991.
74. **Maddison, P. J., Isenberg, D. A., Goulding, N. J., Leddy, J., and Skinner, R. P.,** Anti-SSB identifies a distinctive subgroup of systemic lupus erythematosus, *Br. J. Rheumatol.*, 27, 27, 1988.

75. **Harley, J., Yamagata, H., and Reichlin, M.,** Anti-La(SSB) antibody is present in some normal sera and is coincident with Ro(SSA) precipitins in SLE, *J. Rheumatol.*, 11, 309, 1984.
76. **Mamula, M., Siverman, E., Laxer, R., Bentur, L., Isacovics, B., and Hardin, J.,** Human monoclonal anti-La antibodies: the La protein resides on a subset of Ro particles, *J. Immunol.*, 143, 2923, 1989.
77. **St. Clair, E. W., Burch, J. A., Jr., Ward, M. W., Keene, J. D., and Pisetsky, D. S.,** Temporal correlation of antibody responses to different epitopes of the human La autoantigen, *J. Clin. Invest.*, 85, 515, 1990.
78. **Bini, P., Chu, J. L., and Elkon, K.,** Analysis of autoantibodies to recombinant La (SSB) peptides in systemic lupus erythematosus and Sjogrens syndrome, *J. Clin. Invest.*, 85, 325, 1990.
79. **Chan, E. K., Sullivan, K. F., Fox, R. I., and Tan, E.,** Sjogren's syndrome nuclear antigen (SSB): cDNA cloning, structural domains, and autoepitopes, *J. Autoimmun.*, 2, 321, 1989.
80. **St. Clair, E. W., Talal, N., Moutsopoulos, H. M., Ballester, A., Zerva, L., Keene, J. D., and Pisetsky, D. S.,** Epitope specificity of anti-LA (SSB) antibodies from patients with Sjogren's syndrome, *J. Autoimmun.*, 2, 335, 1989.
81. **Rauh, J., Hornig, H., and Luhrmann, R.,** At least three distinct B cell epitopes reside in the C-terminal half of the La protein as determined by recombinant DNA approach, *Eur. J. Immunol.*, 18, 2049, 1988.
82. **Sturgess, A., Peterson, M., McNeilage, L., Whittingham, S., and Coppel, R.,** Characteristics and epitope mapping of cloned autoantigen, La, *J. Immunol.*, 140, 3212, 1988.
83. **Koshaka, H., Yamamoto, K., Fujii, H., Miura, H., Miyasaaka, N., Nishioka, K., and Miyamoyo, T.,** Fine epitope mapping of the human SS-B/La protein: identification of a distinct autoepitope homologous to the viral gag polyprotein, *J. Clin. Invest.*, 85, 1566, 1990.
84. **St. Clair, E., Kenan, D., Burch, J., Keene, J., and Pisetsky, D.,** The fine specificity of anti-La antibodies induced in mice by immunization with recombinant human La autoantigen, *J. Immunol.*, 144, 3868, 1990.
85. **Reeves, J.,** Use of monoclonal antibodies for the characterization of novel DNA-binding proteins recognized by human autoimmune sera, *J. Exp. Med.*, 161, 18, 1985.
86. **Mimori, J.,** Mechanism of interaction between Ku and DNA, *J. Biol. Chem.*, 261, 10375, 1986.
87. **De Vries, E., Van Driel, W., Bergsma, W. G., Arnberg, A. C., and Van Der Vliet, P. C.,** Hela nuclear protein recognizing DNA termini and translocating on DNA forming a regular DNA-multimeric protein complex, *J. Mol. Biol.*, 208, 65, 1989.
88. **Stuiver, M., Coenjaerts, F., and Vandervliet, P.,** The autoantigen Ku is indistinguishable from NF IV, a protein forming multimeric protein-DNA complexes, *J. Exp. Med.*, 172, 1049, 1990.
89. **Reeves, W. H. and Sthoeger, Z.,** Molecular cloning of cDNA encoding the p70 (Ku) lupus autoantigen, *J. Biol. Chem.*, 264, 5047, 1989.
90. **Yaneva, M., Wen, J., Ayala, A., and Cook, R.,** cDNA derived amino acid sequence of the 80kD subunit of the Ku autoantigen, *J. Biol. Chem.*, 264, 13407, 1989.

91. **Mimori, T., Ohosone, Y., Hama, N., Suwa, A., Akizuki, M., Homma, M., Griffith, A., and Hardin, J.,** Isolation and characterization of cDNA encoding the 80kD subunit protein for the human autoantigen Ku (p70/p80) recognized by autoantibodies from patients with scleroderma-polymyositis overlap syndrome, *Proc. Natl. Acad. Sci. U.S.A.*, 87, 1777, 1990.
92. **O'Brien, R. M., Cram, D. S., Coppel, R. L., and Harrison, L. C.,** T-cell epitopes on the 70-kDa protein of the (U1RNP) complex in autoimmune rheumatologic disorders, *J. Autoimmun.*, 3, 747, 1990.
93. **Reeves, W., Sthoeger, Z., and Lahita, R.,** Role of antigen selection in autoimmune responses to the Ku antigen, *J. Clin. Invest.*, 85, 562, 1989.
94. **Elkon, K., Parnassa, A., and Foster, C.,** Lupus autoantibodies target ribosomal P proteins, *J. Exp. Med.*, 162, 459, 1985.
95. **Saito, T., Uchiumi, T., Kominami, R., and Arakava, M.,** Autoantibodies specific for the 20-kd ribosomal large subunit protein L12, *Biochem. Biophys. Res. Commun.*, 172, 496, 1990.
96. **Bonfa, E., Parnassa, A., Rhoades, A., Roufa, D., Wool, I., and Elkon, K.,** Antiribosomal S10 antibodies in humans and MRL mice with SLE, *Arthritis Rheum.*, 32, 1252, 1989.
97. **Bonfa, E., Golombeck, S., Kaufman, L., Skelly, S., Weissback, H., Brot, N., and Elkon, K.,** Association between lupus psychosis and anti-ribosomal P protein antibodies, *N. Engl. J. Med.*, 317, 265, 1987.
98. **Schneebaum, A. B., Singleton, J. D., West, S. G., Blodgett, J. K., Allen, L. G., Cheronis, J. C., and Kotzin, B. L.,** Association of psychiatric manifestations with antibodies to ribosomal P proteins in systemic lupus erythematosus, *Am. J. Med.*, 90, 54, 1991.
99. **Saito, T., Uchiumi, T., Ozawa, T., Kikuchi, M., Nakano, M., Kominami, R., and Arakawa, M.,** Autoantibodies against ribosomal proteins found with high frequency in patients with systemic lupus erythematosus with active disease, *J. Rheumatol.*, 18, 1681, 1991.
100. **Koren, E., Reichlin, M. W., Koscec, M., Fugate, R. D., and Reichlin, M.,** Autoantibodies to the ribosomal P proteins react with a plasma membrane-related target on human cells, *J. Clin. Invest.*, 89, 1236, 1992.
101. **Fritzler, M. J. and Tan, E.,** Antibodies to histone in drug-induced and idiopathic lupus erythematosus, *J. Clin. Invest.*, 62, 550, 1978.
102. **Totoriis, M., Tan, E., McNally, E., and Rubin, R.,** Association of anti-Histone (H2A-H2B) complex antibody with symptomatic procainamide-induced lupus erythematosus, *N. Engl. J. Med.*, 318, 1431, 1988.
103. **Gioud, M., Aitkaci, M., and Monier, J. C.,** Histone antibodies in systemic lupus erythematosus, *Arthritis Rheum.*, 35, 407, 1982.
104. **Monestier, M., Losman, J. A., Fasy, T. M., Debbas, M. E., Massa, M., Albani, S., Bohm, L., and Martini, A.,** Antihistone antibodies in antinuclear antibody-positive juvenile arthritis, *Arthritis Rheum.*, 33, 1836, 1990.
105. **Burlingame, R. W. and Rubin, R. L.,** Subnucleosome structures as substrates in enzyme-linked immunosorbent assays, *J. Immunol. Meth.*, 134, 187, 1990.
106. **Goohill, J., Cary, P., Couppez, M., and Fritzler, M.,** Antibodies from patients with drug-induced and idiopathic SLE react with epitopes restricted to the amino and carboxyl termini of histone, *J. Immunol.*, 135, 3116, 1985.

107. **Portnova, J., Arndt, R., Tan, E., and Kotzin, B. L.,** Antihistone antibodies in idiopathic and drug-induced lupus recognize distinct intra-histone regions, *J. Immunol.,* 138, 446, 1987.
108. **Portanova, J., Cheronis, J., Blodget, J., and Kotzin, B.,** Histone autoantigens in murine lupus. Definition of a major epitope within the accessible region of chromatin, *J. Immunol.,* 144, 4633, 1990.
109. **Venning, M. C., Quinn, A., Broomhead, V., and Bird, A. G.,** Antibodies directed against neutrophils (C-ANCA and P-ANCA) are of distinct diagnostic value in systemic vasculitis, *Q. J. Med.,* 77, 1287, 1990.
110. **Savige, J. A., Gallicchio, M., Georgiou, T., and Davies, D. J.,** Diverse target antigens recognized by circulating antibodies in anti-neutrophil cytoplasm antibody-associated renal vasculitides, *Clin. Exp. Immunol.,* 82, 238, 1990.
111. **Savage, C. O. S., Pottinger, B. E., Gaskin, G., Pusey, C. D., and Pearson, J. D.,** Autoantibodies developing to myeloperoxidase and proteinase 3 in systemic vasculitis stimulate neutrophil cytotoxicity toward cultured endothelial cells, *Am. J. Pathol.,* 141, 335, 1992.
112. **Bini, P., Gabay, J. E., Teitel, A., Melchior, M., Zhou, J.-L., and Elkon, K. B.,** Antineutrophil cytoplasmic autoantibodies in Wegener's granulomatosis recognize conformational epitope(s) on proteinase 3, *J. Immunol.,* 149, 1409, 1992.
113. **Falk, R. J., Terrell, R., Becker, M., and Jennette, J. C.,** Anti-myeloperoxidase autoantibodies are specific for the native but not denatured MPO and do not abrogate peroxidase activity, *J. Am. Soc. Nephrol.,* 1, 521, 1990.
114. **Freitas, A., Viale, A., Sunblad, A., Heuser, C., and Coutinho, A.,** Normal serum immunoglobulins participate in the selection of the peripheral B cell repertoire, *Proc. Natl. Acad. Sci. U.S.A.,* 88, 5640, 1991.
115. **Cohen, I. and Young, D.,** Autoimmunity, microbial immunity, and the immunological homunculus, *Immunol. Today,* 12, 105, 1991.
116. **Varela, F., Anderson, A., Dietrich, G., Sunblad, A., Holmberg, D., Kazatchkine, M., and Coutinho, A.,** The population of antibodies in normal and autoimmune individuals, *Proc. Natl. Acad. Sci. U.S.A.,* 88, 5917, 1991.
117. **Mendlovic, S., Segal, R., Shoenfeld, Y., and Mozes, E.,** Anti-DNA idiotype- and anti-idiotype-specific T cell responses in patients with systemic lupus erythematosus and their first-degree relatives, *Clin. Exp. Immunol.,* 82, 504, 1990.
118. **Barnett, L. and Fujinami, R.,** Molecular mimicry: a mechanism for autoimmune injury, *FASEB J.,* 6, 840, 1992.
119. **Scofield, R. H., Dickey, W. D., Jackson, K. W., James, J. A., and Harley, J. B.,** A common autoepitope near the carboxyl terminus of the 60-kD Ro ribonucleoprotein: sequence similarity with a viral protein, *J. Clin. Immunol.,* 11, 378, 1991.
120. **Gilkeson, G. S., Grudier, J. P., Karounos, D. G., and Pisetsky, D. S.,** Induction of anti-dsDNa antibodies in normal mice by immunization with bacterial DNA, *J. Immunol.,* 142, 1482, 1989.
121. **Lin, R.-H., Mamula, M., Hardin, J., and Janeway, C. A., Jr.,** Induction of autoreactive B cells allows priming of autoreactive T cells, *J. Exp. Med.,* 173, 1433, 1991.
122. **Zinkernagel, R., Cooper, S., Chambers, J., Lazzarini, R., Hengartner, H., and Arnheiter, H.,** Virus-induced autoantibody response to a transgene viral antigen, *Nature,* 345, 68, 1990.

Chapter 6

Detection and Measurement of Anti-Nuclear and Anti-Cytoplasmic Antibodies

Marius Teodorescu and Christopher J. Froelich

CONTENTS

0-8493-5974-1/94/$0.00 + $.50

I. INTRODUCTION

Intended to maximize the detection of antibodies toward a vast array of antigens, the screening anti-nuclear antibody (ANA) techniques include fluorescence microscopy (F-ANA), brightfield microscopy (e.g., peroxidase-ANA), and, recently, enzyme-linked immunosorbent assay (ELISA).[1,2] To determine if a specimen is abnormal, most laboratories serially dilute the sample (e.g., 1:40, 1:80, 1:160, etc.) and report the highest positive dilution. The relatively low precision and reproducibility of this procedure may be partially obviated by using an international standard (see below Section II.C.1).

Because F-ANA staining patterns (speckled, homogeneous, etc.) have been reported to increase the likelihood that a sample contains certain specific autoantibodies, laboratories often append such information to their results. Most specialists, however, do not rely on this data since, overall, the predictive value of this information is low and methods that directly detect specific ANAs are now widely available. Two caveats still warrant notice: (1) the pattern of fluorescence for proliferating HEp-2 cells identifies anti-centromere antibodies, and (2) anti-neutrophil cytoplasmic antibodies (ANCA) are reported as either cytoplasmic ANCA (C-ANCA) or perinuclear ANCA (P-ANCA). As reliable assays that measure ANCA specificities enter the clinical workplace, a description of centromere and ANCA patterns will also become unnecessary *(vide infra).*

The indirect ELISA is commonly used to screen or to test for a specific ANA (see Chapter 1). The ''antigen'' for ANA screening incorporates either whole or sonified HEp-2 nuclei, cellular extracts, or a combination of purified antigens (see Appendix to this volume for resources). Neutrophil salt extracts serve this function for ANCA.[3] Studies that use the international ANA standard[4] will determine if the sensitivity, specificity, and predictive value of the ELISA ANA compares favorably to F-ANA.[2,5] ELISA ANA and ANCA testing will soon supplant microscopic assays.

The testing of sera for ANAs is basically a two-step process. First, the clinical lab screens multiple specimens at a predetermined dilution for positive reaction by microscopy or ELISA. Subsequently, the positive specimen undergoes evaluation for specific autoantibodies if the screening test suggests an abnormality (see also Chapter 7). A variety of techniques are employed to measure individual or various combinations of autoantibodies (see Chapter 1). If the patient's symptoms suggest a connective tissue disease (systemic lupus erythematosus [SLE] Sjögren's syndrome, mixed connective tissue disease [MCTD], scleroderma, or overlap syndrome), then anti-ssDNA (denatured), -dsDNA, -Sm, -RNP, -SSA, -SSB, -histone, and -Scl-70 should be measured, either singly or in combination. For patients likely to have scleroderma, anti-centromere enhances diagnostic specificity for CREST (calcinosis, Raynaud's phenomenon, esophageal dysmotility, sclerodactyl, and telangiectasia). Most commonly, however, the clinical data are sufficiently ambiguous to warrant the simultaneous measurement of all these antibodies (see Chapter 7).

In order to enhance throughput and process control, the clinical lab may choose to implement reflex testing. The performance of reflex testing avoids: (1) the processing of multiple specimens that different specialists may choose to order on the same patient; (2) delayed diagnosis, and (3) inaccurate patient perception. For example, a patient with ''fibrositis'', a benign nonautoimmune syndrome, may inadvertently be given the diagnosis of SLE if their F-ANA test is ''positive''. Thereafter, the patient proffers the ''positive ANA'' to validate the seriousness of their illness. However, by completely evaluating the patient's ANA status as a reflex, the laboratory provides specific and reliable data. Reflex testing would have shifted the focus from the initial positive ANA to results that failed to demonstrate clinically relevant autoantibodies. This analysis becomes even more valuable when a patient has SLE and fibrositis or SLE and an infection (see Chapter 7).

II. CONSTRUCTION OF ELISA TESTS FOR ANA/ANCA

A. PREPARATION OF ANTIGENS FOR ELISA

1. ANA Screen Antigen Mixture

To ensure that ANA and ANCA screening tests have maximal sensitivity, the "antigenic material" should be as complex as possible. Hep2 cell nuclear suspension,[5] neutrophil extracts,[6] or a combination of purified antigens[2] may fulfill this purpose. Cultured mammalian cells are detached from the growth surface, washed, counted, and the plasma membrane is solubilized with a nonionic detergent (e.g., 0.5% NP 40). After 10 min at 37°C, nuclei are washed and resuspended. The nuclei may be coated to a solid phase[5] or converted to a homogeneous mixture by ultrasound treatment. Efficiency of sonication is monitored microscopically.

2. DNA (Single- and Double-Stranded)

Calf thymus, bacteriophage lambda, and circular plasmid DNA are available commercially (see Appendix). Bacteriophage and circular plasmid DNA are highly stable. Because calf thymus dsDNA is labile, ssDNA segments frequently appear after the coating process; this phenomenon increases the risk that the assay will inadvertently detect anti-ssDNA antibodies. Not all vendors offer products with sufficient purity for ELISA testing. ssDNA may be readily obtained from calf thymus DNA by boiling the solution for 5 min followed by rapid cooling on ice.[7] The solution should be sufficiently diluted during boiling and cooling to avoid the formation of "clots" of DNA.

3. Histone

The laboratory may obtain histone complexes as well as separated fractions (e.g., H2a-H2b) commercially (Appendix) or choose to prepare the antigens "in house".[8] To detect antibodies in symptomatic patients with drug-induced lupus, H2A-H2B-DNA complexes may be purified by the lab[9] or obtained from commercial suppliers.

4. Sm and RNP

Anti-SM and anti-RNP antibodies are distinct sets of antibody specificities that share partial identity by Ouchterlony immunodiffusion. Anti-Sm and anti-RNP react with components of the splicesome apparatus, an RNA-protein particle (U snRNP). The splicesome consists of various peptides bound to a family of small U RNAs (i.e., U1, U2, U4, U5, and U6 small RNAs) (see Chapter 5). All described U snRNPs contain a common group of polypeptides that bear Sm antigenic determinants plus additional proteins unique to a particular U snRNP. The common proteins that react with anti-Sm autoantibodies are B (28 kDa), B′ (29 kDa), D (16 kDa), E (130 kDa), F (9 kDa), and G (8 kDa). For the U1 snRNP, the unique proteins are A (33 kDa), C (22 kDa), and a 68-kDa protein (nuclear matrix-associated protein). "anti-RNP antibodies" primarily react with the 68-kDa protein. The U2 snRNP contains the peptides A′ (27 kDa) and B″ (21 kDa). The unique proteins in the remaining U snRNPs have not been completely characterized. ELISA grade Sm and RNP as well as the other non-histone nuclear antigens are isolated from various tissues[10] or as fusion proteins from recombinant DNA expression systems (see Chapter 7). Purification schemes for some polypeptides can be used to isolate Sm and RNP as a Sm/RNP complex from tissue sources. While RNP epitopes can be destroyed to yield free Sm, ''natural'' RNP maintains antigenicity only when complexed with Sm.

Calf thymus acetone powder is the usual source for Sm and RNP/Sm complex.[10] The powder is prepared from fresh (or freshly frozen at −70°C) calf thymus by high-speed grinding in cold acetone. The acetone precipitate is washed in a Buchner funnel and dried overnight at −20°C. The powder is hydrated overnight with phosphate-buffered saline (PBS) at 4°C and then centrifuged at 4000 *g* (30 min) to remove particulates. The supernatant undergoes a 30% saturated ammonium sulfate salt cut and the precipitate is discarded after centrifugation at 4000 *g*. The supernatant is increased to 60% ammonium sulfate saturation and the resultant precipitate is collected and dissolved in PBS. After dialysis against PBS, the solution should produce a line of precipitation in Ouchterlony double diffusion when tested with anti-Sm and anti-RNP antibody containing sera. To assure clarity the solution is centrifuged at 100,000 × *g*. To isolate Sm, the crude antigen preparation is applied to an anti-Sm antibody (IgG) immunoaffinity column. The column is prepared as follows: IgG from sera containing high anti-Sm reactivity is isolated with protein G column (Pharmacia LKB, Piscataway, NJ) and subsequently coupled through the Fc portion to affi-Prep HZ support gel (Biorad, Richmond, CA). Mouse monoclonal antibodies specific for desired Sm proteins are also effective.[10] The eluate is heat-inactivated for 60 min at 56°C to destroy the RNP component.

The presence of all antigenic components of Sm and RNP/Sm is identified by western blotting. However, western blotting does not guarantee that all the Sm polypeptides have been effectively coated to the solid phase. Thus, unless monoclonal antibodies specific to each polypeptide are available, binding is indirectly verified by testing the reactivity of a large battery of Sm-positive SLE sera ($n = 20$ by double diffusion).

The RNP/Sm complex also is isolated from calf thymus acetone powder by sequential ammonium sulfate salt precipitation (see above). Thereafter, the clarified supernatant is applied to an affinity column coupled with anti-RNP antibodies obtained from patients with MCTD. After coating to the solid phase, the antigen should react with at least 10 random anti-RNP sera from patients with MCTD. Since the 68-kDa protein and the A protein appear to be sufficient to identify most anti-RNP-positive sera,[11] these polypeptides may be substituted for native RNP/Sm.

5. SSA (Ro) and SSB (La)

SSA is represented by particles that contain at least a 60-kDa polypeptide[12,13] plus one of four RNAs, termed hY RNAs (for human cYtoplasmic). Nevertheless, at least three other antigenically distinct SSA proteins have been identified (46, 52, and 54 kDa)[14-17] (see Chapter 5). SSB is a 46- to 48-kDa phosphorylated ribonucleoprotein involved in processing products of RNA polymerase III.[18]

For clinical laboratory testing, the source of SSA is bovine and human spleen.[19] Human SSA possesses epitopes that bovine SSA apparently lacks because a minor percentage of patient sera react with human and not with bovine SSA. This observation indicates that anti-SSA antibody activity is directed toward both highly conserved and toward specific human epitopes.[20] Certain SSA epitopes may be conformational, since the 60-kDa SSA polypeptide bound more anti-SSA sera by double diffusion than by immunoblotting.[21] Overall, however, purified native bovine SSA may provide more epitopes for the ELISA assay than a recombinant human form.

SSA and SSB are contained in the 60 to 80% ammonium sulfate cut of adult bovine spleen extracts.[22-24] Also, a 60 to 80% ammonium sulfate cut of calf thymus acetone powder contains SSB (see above for Sm and RNP).[24] Both SSA and SSB are purified by immunoaffinity chromatography, as described above for anti-Sm and anti-RNP.[22,23] Some studies suggest that recombinant SSB and probably SSA may be suitable for ELISA testing.[25,26]

6. Scl-70

This autoantigen, DNA topoisomerase I, is a 100-kDa enzyme that catalyzes the relaxation of superhelical DNA.[27] The antigen may be purified by immunoaffinity chromatography as described above from the 60 to 90% saturated ammonium sulfate precipitate cut of bovine thymus extracts. The cDNA for Scl-70 has been cloned and three linear epitopes have been identified.[28,29]

Hillebrandt et al.[30] have compared four methods for the detection of anti-Scl 70 antibodies using native topoisomerase: ELISA, immunoblotting, immunodiffusion, and inhibition of topoisomerase I activity. Using the inhibition of enzyme activity as the "gold standard" (i.e., sensitivity/specificity 100%/100%), they found that the sensitivity/specificity of the assays were as follows: immunodiffusion, 79%/100%; immunoblot, 100%/97%; ELISA, 100%/98%. Thus, the data suggest that ELISA is the method of choice for the clinical laboratory (see also Chapter 7).

7. Centromere Antigens

Three centromeric antigens (CENP) have been identified: CENP-A (17 kDa), CENP-B (80 kDa), and CENP-C (140 kDa).[31] CENP-B is the major centromeric antigen that is recognized by anti-centromere antibody reactive sera. Anti-centromere antibodies have been identified by indirect immunofluorescence (IFA) using dividing HEp-2, by immunoblotting, and most recently by ELISA using CENP-B fusion protein.[32] Currently, indirect immunofluorescence is most commonly used by clinical laboratories. For obvious reasons a negative F-ANA with HEp-2 cells does not exclude the presence of anti-centromere antibodies, unless mitotic figures are examined. The antibody appears as a fine speckle on these cells. ELISA is likely to supplant this technique in the immediate future.

8. ANCA

ANCA reactivity is routinely determined by IFA using fixed human neutrophils.[33] C-ANCA, a diffuse cytoplasmic distribution, and P-ANCA, a perinuclear distribution, describe the two dominant staining patterns. Although the main antigens for C-ANCA and P-ANCA are myeloperoxidase and proteinase 3, respectively, elastase as well as other autoantigens undoubtedly contribute to ANCA specificity (see Chapter 5).

A crude neutrophil extract has been used for ANCA solid-phase screening assays.[34,35] However, due to the loss of conformational epitopes during the coating process, the solid-phase assay is less sensitive than IFA.[36] The autoantigens for C-ANCA (proteinase 3 and elastase) and P-ANCA (myeloperoxidase) may be purified by immunoaffinity or traditional chromatographic methods from neutrophil extracts,[6] or may be prepared biochemically. To obtain a general ELISA screening "antigen", human neutrophils are isolated from whole blood by methyl cellulose/Hypaque gradient centrifugation and incubated in 0.2 *M* sodium acetate (pH 4.2) for 2 h at 4°C. The suspension is sonified and the efficiency of lysis is evaluated microscopically. This extract is stable when stored at −70°C and should be thawed immediately prior to the coating process.

B. COATING OF ANTIGENS TO PLASTIC (SEE ALSO CHAPTER 1)

1. Coating of ssDNA and dsDNA

Incubation of polystyrene microwells with ssDNA (2 μg/well) overnight produces satisfactory attachment. Unlike ssDNA, dsDNA binds poorly to plastic; therefore, a precoating step is necessary. However, if the laboratory plans to test simultaneously for anti-ssDNA and anti-dsDNA, the precoating procedure is essential for both DNA preparations.

To ensure that dsDNA attaches to commercially available plastic material, the microtiter plate is first incubated overnight with 0.01 to 0.1% methylated bovine serum albumin (BSA) (PBS, pH 7.4). After four washes with PBS, the wells are incubated overnight with the DNA solution at room temperature. Following another three washes with PBS, the wells are incubated for 3 to 4 h with a blocking solution (e.g., BSA or horse serum in PBS) at room temperature. The blocking solution is removed by washing with 0.05% Tween 20 (v/v) in PBS. The specimen diluent should contain all antigenic proteins that exist in the precoating buffer (e.g., BSA). This is necessary to competitively inhibit potential antiprotein antibodies (e.g., anti-BSA) that may exist in the test specimen. For example, when protamine sulfate served as precoating solution, its exclusion from the specimen diluent resulted in the detection of both anti-DNA and anti-protamine sulfate antibodies.[37]

2. Coating with Protein Nuclear Antigens

The wells are coated overnight at room temperature, washed, and the plastic is blocked or saturated with a protein solution: BSA, fetal bovine serum, or horse serum, as described above for DNA. If the antigen itself saturates the plastic, as determined experimentally, this step may not be necessary (see Chapter 1).

3. Coating for ANCA

As discussed above many of the ANCA autoantigens have conformationally dependent epitopes[38] that may be lost during the purification process or during interaction with the solid-phase support. The problem is partially obviated by using a capture antigen ELISA system (see Chapter 1).[3,39,40] For example, to detect P-ANCA, the wells are coated first with a goat anti-mouse IgG that captures added mouse monoclonal against human myeloperoxidase (MPO).

C. COMPONENTS OF ELISA TESTS

1. Standards

World Health Organization (WHO) standards for the total ANA[4] and anti-dsDNA are available from two sources: (1) Center for Disease Control (AF/CDC ANA Reference Laboratory, Center for Disease Control, Immunology Branch, 1600 Clifton Road, 1-1202 A25, Atlanta, Georgia) and (2) WHO, Laboratory of the Netherlands Red Cross Blood Transfusion Service (Department of Immune and Blood Group Reagents, P.O. Box 9190, 1006 AD, Amsterdam, The Netherlands). Commercial sources also offer standards (or calibrators) with a designated number of units, but they do not always correspond to the international standards. Internal laboratory standards and controls may be prepared from known serum specimens and diluted with normal human serum to match the external standard. The working calibrator or standard should be validated against a stored standard (external or internal) at a predetermined interval that is defined by testing volume (e.g., every 3 to 12 months).

To prepare an internal standard for F-ANA testing, F-ANA serum with a high level of antibody (homogeneous) is successively diluted with normal human serum until it reacts with HEp-2 cells at the same dilution as the standard (e.g., 1/160). Thus, if the international standard has 100 units/ml, any patient specimen that reacts at this dilution also contains 100 I.U./ml. However, if the sample reacts at 1/20, it contains eight times less antibody (i.e., 100 I.U. ÷ 8 = 12.5 I.U.). In various studies sera from 95% of normal subjects have less than 6.25 to 7.5 I.U./ml.

Generally, the activity of the working standard for ELISA (expressed as units) should be ± 15% of the value obtained for the original stored standard (tested in triplicate). If the deviation exceeds this value, the following adjustments warrant consideration: (1) the amount of antigen coated to microwells should be altered; (2) the concentration of enzyme conjugate should be changed; and (3) the amount of antibody in the working standard should be changed. For a one-point calibrator, too low an absorbance value often leads to a false-positive result while too high a value produces a false negative. A multi-point standard curve enhances test precision and thus the ability to provide better quantitative data for longitudinal observations.

2. Positive Controls

The positive control ensures that the assay functions as intended. Various antibody specificities are available from CDC and from commercial sources. In addition, controls are available for individual autoantibody (anti-dsDNA, -Sm, -RNP, -SSA, -SSA, -SSB, -Scl70. -centromere, -P-ANCA, and -C-ANCA). However, most of these positive controls are not monospecific when tested by ELISA. For panel testing, a single positive control that contains multiple specificities is desirable.

3. Negative Control

The negative control is human serum that provides a normal test result for the desired ANA specificity. Although the negative control is identified by its ability to produce absorbance values that fall within the range of normal values, it does not serve to define the normal limit the day the test is performed. Specimens with designated cut-off values may be identified to serve this function.

4. Blanks

The blank controls for factors, other than the specimen's specific antibody, that could generate a color reaction. The resultant value for the blank is then subtracted from absorbance value obtained for the test sample incubated in the antigen-coated microwell. This subtraction also obviates, at least in part, the need for dual-wavelength reading of absorbance. The blank has two forms: (1) the specimen diluent incubated in an antigen-coated well (conjugate blank), and (2) the specimen incubated in a well that lacks antigen (specimen blank). Patients with autoimmune diseases frequently have hypergammaglobulinemia; therefore, the specimen blank represents the best control for nonspecific binding of the patient's IgG to the solid phase (see also Chapter 1). At the same time the negative control provides ample reassurance that the conjugate does not react unacceptably with the antigen-coated well.

5. Specimen Diluent

Excluding specific antigen, the specimen diluent should contain all potentially antibody-reactive materials that are in the buffer used during the coating process. Simple salt buffers (e.g., PBS), buffers with nonionic detergents, and complex protein solutions that contain animal serum may be suitable specimen diluents. Rheumatoid factor (RF) activity in a test sample may frequently cause a false-positive screening ANA because it cross reacts with histone nucleoproteins.[41] Specimen diluents that contain adult animal serum may block such RF activity; therefore, such diluents function well for ANA and anti-cytoplasmic antibody assays.

6. Wash Solution

This solution, prepared from a powder or a concentrated solution, contains a nonionic detergent (e.g., Tween 20) that facilitates the release of Ig that has interacted hydrophobically with the microwell. The deionized water (CAP Type 1, USP or equivalent) should be devoid of interfering agents (e.g., trace metals for tetramethyl benzidine [TMB] substrate).

7. Developing System

For anti-nuclear and anti-cytoplasmic antibody testing, the developing or reporter system includes an enzyme-conjugated antibody solution, usually anti-IgG (Fcg specific), in a stabilizing buffer to enhance reproducibility and a substrate solution (see Chapter 1). Anti-IgG enzyme conjugate is preferred because the diagnostic value of IgM antibody against nuclear antigens has not been established. A large proportion of IgM-mediated reactions may represent nonpathogenic ''natural antibodies'' (see Chapters 2 and 5). The selection of the substrate solution depends on the enzyme chosen (see Chapter 1). For horseradish peroxidase TMB is the most sensitive and widely used substrate.

III. ASSAY PROCEDURE

A. TESTS FOR ANA SCREENING AND INDIVIDUAL ANTIBODIES

The procedures to screen for ANA reactivity and to measure a specific autoantibody are similar.

1. Depending on the sensitivity of the assay system, the controls, calibrators, and specimens are usually diluted in specimen diluent at either 1/50 or 1/100.
2. 100 μl of diluted specimen is added to antigen-coated and blank wells, incubated for 30 min at room temperature, and washed.
3. After adding the anti-IgG-specific antibody, the wells are incubated another 30 min, washed, and thoroughly blotted to remove residual wash buffer.
4. The substrate is dispensed and the reaction then is terminated with acid after a predetermined time (e.g., 10 or 15 min). For kinetic analysis, readings are taken at various time intervals until the color reaction reaches a predetermined value in the calibrator, usually the highest level for which the reaction is still linear (e.g., 1.2).

B. PANELS OF MULTIPLE AUTOANTIBODIES: THE ANA PROFILE

When a serum sample is positive by ANA screen, the sample may be reflexively tested against a panel of autoantigens to determine if it contains clinically relevant specificities.

The panel may include: ssDNA, dsDNA, Sm, RNP, SSA, SSB, histone, and/or Scl70. If the patient is considered to have scleroderma, a test for anti-centromere antibody may also be added. To measure multiple autoantibodies, microwells containing the desired autoantigens are constructed as a strip or are prearranged by the manufacturer (e.g., ANA/6[22]). The various specificities tested in the panel share the same "specimen blank" and the positive control contains all antibody specificities measured by the panel.

IV. MEASUREMENTS, DATA REDUCTION, AND PRESENTATION OF RESULTS

Most ELISA plate readers are interfaced with computers equipped with software to facilitate data reduction (see Appendix). The net absorbance is determined by subtracting the absorbance value of the desired blank (specimen blank or conjugate blank) from that obtained for calibrator, positive control, negative control, or patient specimens. The unit value for the controls and specimens are determined with either a one-point calibration curve or a standard curve (see Chapter 1).

Results should be reported in units/ml (I.U./ml for anti-dsDNA). The report form may include the normal limit and high laboratory value for each autoantibody. The high value is established by the experience of the individual laboratory (see Chapter 3, Section V.). Graphic display of results, particularly for multiple autoantibodies, is desirable because the presentation facilitates rapid interpretation in a clinical context (Figure 1) (see Chapter 1).

V. LIMITATION OF PROCEDURE

Since an abnormal test for specific autoantibody does prove the existence of disease and a negative result does not exclude disease, caveats such as "result valid only in clinical context" or "a negative test does not rule out SLE" should be included in the report. Beside limitations that are inherent to ELISA testing for autoantibodies (Chapter 1), the following should be considered for ANA tests:

1. Many normal subjects, particularly the elderly (upwards to 25%), may have a relatively high ANA titer. When tested by multi-antibody panels, most of these individuals have normal profiles or display low abnormal levels of two or less antibodies.
2. A positive test for one autoantibody in a profile, usually at a low level, may be observed in normal subjects (e.g., anti-SSA).
3. Borderline positive values should be interpreted cautiously and repeated 4 to 6 weeks later.
4. Diagnosis should not be made solely on the basis of a positive test result and a negative result does not exclude the diagnosis of a specific rheumatic disease.
5. The presence of C-ANCA and/or P-ANCA does not necessarily indicate the presence of vasculitis.

VI. QUALITY CONTROL (SEE CHAPTER 1 FOR GENERAL PRINCIPLES)

Prior to reporting the results of the assay, the performance of the ELISA test process should be analyzed to ensure that blanks, calibrators, positive controls, negative controls, and specimens have functioned predictably. The facets examined should include:

UIC RHEUMATOLOGY/IMMUNO LAB   Report: EL-ANA8 Analytical

Patient: PATIENT, PATIENT   Sample ID: 1415
Physician: DR. DOCTOR Inst: HOSPITAL USA
Drawn: 02/18/93   Reported: 02/18/93   Reported By: __________

Results expressed as Units/ml

Test (ELISA method-IgG)	Patient Result	Normal Max	High Value
ssDNA Quantitative	820	91	1000
dsDNA Quantitative (I.U.)	48	40	1000
Sm Quantitative	320	90	1200
RNP/Sm - Quantitative	450	74	1200
SSA (Ro) Quantitative	20	117	1200
SSB (La) Quantitative	18	66	1000
Histone - Quantitative	290	71	1000
Scl-70 Quantitative	23	37	500

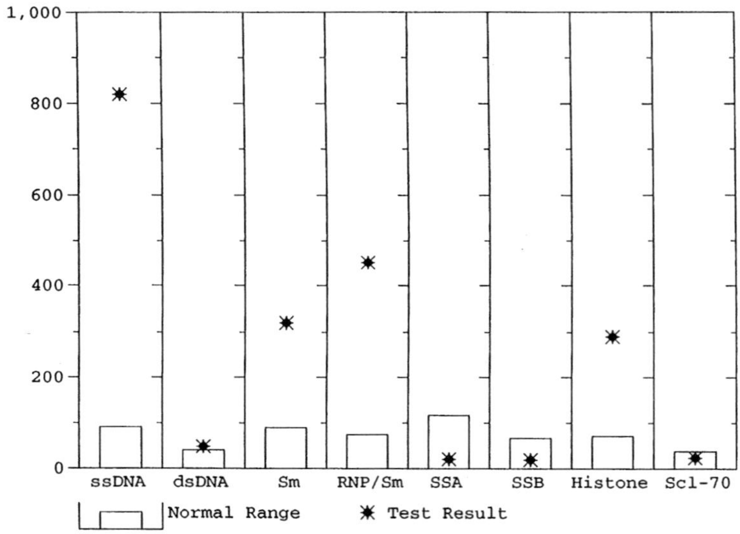

TheraTest Labs, Inc. EL-ANA profile (c) 1991
Interpretation (valid only in clinical context)

- [] Normal
- [] Chronic Inflammation
- [X] SLE
- [] Active Disease
- [] Sjogren's Syndrome
- [] MCTD
- [] Scleroderma
- [] Drug Induced SLE
- [] Some "normal"
- [] Suggest Retest in 4 to 6 weeks
- [] Interpretation deferred to clinician

Figure 1 A computer-generated report of a multi-autoantibody test (see Chapter 7 for interpretation of various autoantibody panels).

1. An unanticipated pronounced shift in absorbance value of a control or calibrator
2. A downward or upward trend in the value of a control or calibrator
3. Excessively high frequency of positive results for a particular antibody with low prevalence
4. Contiguous specimens that produce similar values for a particular autoantibody

Any deviation from the predicted behavior should initiate an action that includes repeat testing (see Table 1 and Figure 2).

Although this review process is sufficient for assays that measure individual ANAs, based on the interrelationships among different sets of autoantibodies, panel tests have another dimension that warrants scrutiny (Figure 2).

Table 1 **Corrective Actions for Review of ANA Test Results (Panels and Individual Test)**

Problems	Causes and Corrective Actions
1. Calibrator cannot be used for a particular test (e.g., its blank is high or calibrator Abs is low). Low blanks may cause false low positive results.	Review the absorbance for positive control from an earlier run (same lot #). If the value is ±25% of the present value and it was a valid run use the calibrator from that run. Repeat whenever possible.
2. Specimen blank for either positive or negative control is too high and the net absorbance is low.	If the absorbance value in the antigen-coated well is within 25% of a previous run, use the corresponding blank value from that run.
3. Specimen blank for one or a few specimens is high.	If the absorbance values in antigen-coated wells are abnormally high for multiple antigens, the specimen may contain high levels of IgG. Values as high as 0.5 are acceptable. Consider bacterially contaminated serum.
4. Absorbance for calibrators and positive controls show downward trend or sudden shift.	Determine if the change represents a trend or a shift. A trend suggests reduced antigen or enzyme conjugate activity. A sudden downward shift suggests reduced volume of specimen and/or conjugate or shortened incubation time.
5. Absorbance for controls, specimens, or blanks shows downward shift, generally low values.	Check water quality, pipettor accuracy, substrate volume and storage conditions (e.g., crystals in wash concentrate).
6. Absorbance for any control shows upward trend or shift.	Unusual. Check timer and volumes dispensed.
7. Levels of anti-dsDNA > anti-ssDNA, anti-Sm > anti-RNP/Sm, or if anti-SSB > anti-SSA by >30%. If both values in a pair are normal, or both abnormal, accept results.	If the values on the left of (>) sign in each pair is over 50% of the value on the right, or if only the value on the right is abnormal, repeat the test. Accept the test if both are normal or if anti-ssDNA > anti-dsDNA, anti-RNP/Sm > anti-Sm, and anti-SSA > anti-SSB.
8. The units for calibrator is preceded by (>) or their absorbance used in calculation is above a tolerated range (e.g., 1.5).	If the positive and negative controls are within the acceptable range accept the test.
9. The units for specimen value of units is above a tolerated range of calibration (e.g., 1.5).	Repeat the test at a preassay* dilution of 1:10, 1:100, 1:1000. Use the absorbance value that is closest to 1.0. Avoid the use values under 0.4. If

Table 1 **Corrective Actions for Review of ANA Test Results (Panels and Individual Test) (Continued)**

Problems	Causes and Corrective Actions
	after repeating the test the value is <0.4, use the absorbance value from the previous dilution or run for the final calculation.
10. The color intensity appears as usual but the values are much lower.	Check wavelength of filter. Reading at 405 for TMB gives about 3 × lower value.
11. No color change after adding stop solution.	A solution other than the stop solution was used. Check label. Add stop solution from another lot.
12. Contiguous specimens have very similar absorbance values or results in units.	Consider "double dipping" in the same specimen. Check tube rack organization. Repeat the test.

*Preassay: dilution before the serum is diluted 1/100 for ELISA.
Table constructed for a particular test system. It should be adapted to each particular test.

The main rules may be summarized as follows.

1. Anti-dsDNA antibody molecules almost always react with ssDNA; it is not unusual, however, to find specimens that react with ssDNA and not with dsDNA even in SLE patients.
2. Sera that contain abnormal levels of anti-Sm antibody, with rare exceptions, are expected to react at abnormal levels with both Sm and Sm/RNP complex. An anti-RNP-reactive specimen is expected to react with RNP/Sm and with RNP from recombinant DNA sources without reacting with Sm antigen (see above).
3. Sera containing anti-SSB also contain anti-SSA. During 10,000 ANA/6 and 8 panels over the last 5 years (Figure 1), we have seen only three specimens that had abnormal levels of anti-SSB and not anti-SSA.
4. Since the overlap of SLE and scleroderma is rare, anti-Scl-70 with high levels of anti-ssDNA is unusual. In the routine laboratory setting, it is unusual to observe several patients with abnormal levels of anti-Scl-70, anti-Sm, anti-dsDNA, or anti-SSB in the same run. It should always be assumed that a technical error has occurred and the data should be reviewed before reporting the result.

VII. TEST IMPLEMENTATION AND NORMAL LIMITS (SEE ALSO CHAPTER 1)

Prior to implementation of the test for a specific antibody, the upper limit of normal and a high value are established. If the kit is available commercially, these values may be provided by the manufacturer. Nonetheless, a small sample of normal subjects and patients (n = 30) should be tested by the laboratory performing the test in order to validate the manufacturer's specifications.

As discussed above (Chapter 1), the distribution of values for any autoantibody derived from either normal subjects or patients is non-gaussian. Therefore, it is invalid

Quality Control review for ANA panels and individual antibody tests

Date______ **Lot #**______ **Performed by** _________ **Verified by**___________

TEST PERFORMED (circle applicable): **Panels:** ANA/6, ANA/7, ANA/7S, ANA/8

Individual Ab test: anti-ssDNA, -dsDNA, -Sm, -RNP/Sm, -SSA, -SSB, -His, -Scl70

PERFORMANCE OF COMPONENTS (see Table 1, #1, 2, 3,5) (Mark acceptable values **or** values found):

Blanks: Calibrators [ ] < .... [ ] or.............. Negative control [ ] <.............or [ ] ....

Positive control [ ] < .... [ ] or........... Specimens [ ] < 0.4........... except............................

Calibrators (established or provided) (Table, # 1, 4, 5, 8)

[ ] ssDNA > .... [ ] dsDNA > .... [ ] Sm > .... [ ] RNP/Sm > ....

[ ] SSA > .... [ ] SSB >............ [ ] Hist > .... [ ] Scl70 > ....

Previous data of calibrator used (circle applicable): **ALL**; ssDNA; dsDNA; Sm; RNP; SSA; SSB; His; Scl70

Date(s) calibrator(s) previously used: ________________________

TREND ANALYSIS BY LONGITUDINAL GRAPHICS (see Table 1, #1, 4,5,6,10):

Tracking of calibrator (absorbance) __________ [ ] Acceptable behavior

[ ] Downward shift for _________ [ ] Downward trend for _________
[ ] Upward shift for _________ [ ] Upward trend for _________

*Tracking of Positive Controls (units)*__________ [ ] All in acceptable range
[ ] Downward shift for _________ [ ] Downward trend for _________
[ ] Upward shift for _________ [ ] Upward trend for _________

Tracking of Negative Control (units:) [ ] Accept ; [ ] ______________________________

ANALYSIS OF NUMERIC OR GRAPHIC DATA FOR ABNORMAL VALUES:

Relationships between paired antibodies (see Table 1, #7):

anti-ssDNA ≥ anti-dsDNA	[ ] YES = [ ] accept /	[ ] inverted =	[ ] repeat OR	[ ] accept
anti-RNP/Sm ≥ anti- Sm	[ ] YES = [ ] accept /	[ ] inverted =	[ ] repeat OR	[ ] accept
anti-SSA ≥ anti-SSB	[ ] YES = [ ] accept /	[ ] inverted =	[ ] repeat OR	[ ] accept

Two adjacent Specimens have similar unit values for particular antibody (see Table 1, #12):
[ ] None
[ ] YES: Specimen No. and tests____

FINAL DISPOSITION: [ ] Acceptable [ ] Repeat: [ ] All Specimens **OR** only

[ ] Specimen No. and tests____

Absorbance value for Specimen exceeds acceptable maximum (see Table 1, #8, 9):
[ ] None
[ ] YES: Specimen No. and tests____

Figure 2 Checklist for quality control for ANA tests by ELISA (see Table 2 for corresponding numbers). The checklist is only a model; it applies to a specific test kit.

to define the upper limit of normal based on mean and standard deviation (s.d.). Nevertheless, the uppermost normal value can be established by testing 100 normal blood bank donors and describing the upper limit at a defined percentile value. For example, the 95th percentile is defined by excluding the five highest values as being "potentially abnormal" (Table 1).

Other parameters should be considered to decide the cut-off percentile for normal. Since the predictive value of a positive test varies with the prevalence of false-positive tests, a high number of false positives will diminish the predictive value. If an antibody is relatively common in the "normal population", the number of false-positive tests may be reduced by choosing a cut-off level that is likely to exclude a reasonable percentage of the normal donors. This decision, however, is often arbitrary. Another method that may facilitate the decision making is to visualize a distribution curve of the antibody values (i.e., ranking) for the normal donors. The curve will be significantly skewed to the right (towards high values), because a relatively few normal donors will have distinctly higher antibody values than the majority, which will be clustered at a lower level on the scale. Therefore, for an antibody that is relatively prevalent among normal subjects (e.g., anti-SSA), exclusion of the values that are clearly disparate from the majority of the tested normal subjects (e.g., uppermost five or ten) would allow a decision to be made that the 95th or 90th percentile is the normal limit. On the other hand, for relatively uncommon antibodies, such as anti-dsDNA, -Sm, -SSB and -Scl-70, the exclusion of the highest value may be acceptable (99th percentile) (Table 2).

Compared to individual antibody testing, the advantage of panel testing is that the predictive value of the panel increases as the number of abnormal or high normal values in the panel increases. The result is a decrease in the number of "false positives". Although 14% of normal donors had a single abnormal value (shown in bold in Table 2), only 3% of normal donors had two antibodies above the cutoff and 1% had three (donors are represented by lower case letters). This is, in part, due to the inherent linkage of certain antibodies (e.g., anti-dsDNA almost always reacts with ssDNA, and anti-Sm with anti-RNP/Sm). No normal individuals were found to have elevated levels of four autoantibodies (Table 2).

As noted above, 14% of normal subjects may have an abnormal panel because a single antibody is detected at "high normal" levels. Thus, when a panel is examined two parameters are considered: the level of each individual antibody and the number of antibodies found above the established normal limit. For example, a panel may be considered abnormal by having only anti-ssDNA at 400 units, which exceeds all 100 normals, or by having high normal levels for three autoantibodies: anti-ssDNA at 195, anti-RNP at 110, and anti-SSA at 174. Computer analysis of the panel data collected from the ELISA plate for each patient may facilitate the calculation of probability that the patient's panel is normal. Nevertheless, the diagnosis is never made solely on the basis of an abnormal test result. The data provided by the patient history and other clinical information available to the physician are corroborated with laboratory data for an accurate diagnosis.

VIII. RADIOIMMUNOASSAY (FARR) FOR DETECTION OF ANTI-dsDNA ANTIBODY

A. PRINCIPLE OF THE ASSAY AND CLINICAL UTILITY

Although the Farr assay is the "gold standard" for the measurement of anti-dsDNA antibodies, the technique has liabilities that have dampened its desirability (radioisotopes, high relative cost, false positives in infectious diseases). The Farr assay is ideal for detecting high-affinity anti-dsDNA antibody. The assay is highly sensitive and specific, particularly for low levels of anti-dsDNA antibody, i.e., 0 to 40 I.U. range, where ELISA may not have sufficient precision (see Chapter 7). However, the clinical significance of such low levels is questionable, since even patients with long-term remis-

Table 2 **Determination of the Upper Limit of Normal for Eight Antinuclear Antibodies**[a]

ssDNA	dsDNA	Sm	RNP/Sm	SSA	SSB	Histone	Scl-70	Percentile
337-*a*	**48**-*b*	**131**-*d*	**123**-*f*	**210**-*d*	**96**-*k*	**154**-*l*	**38**-*n*	100
335-*b*	34-	101-	**100**-*g*	**187**-*a*	85-	**144**-*m*	36-	99
218-*c*	31-	79-	83-	**180**-*h*	62-	69-	32-	98
197-*d*	28-	75-	46-	**174**-*i*	38-	47-	32-	97
129-*e*	26-	72-	42-	**168**-*j*	*37-*	*41-*	*31-*	*96*
91-	19-	68-	39-	111-	37-	40-	28-	95

[a] Autoantibody levels (units/ml) were plotted in descending order for 100 normal blood donors. The upper limit of normal for each autoantibody was assigned based on the skewness of resultant graph (see Chapter 1, Figure 4) and the prevalence of the diseases in which the individual antibodies are found. The table shows the uppermost six values for each antibody with the "abnormal" values in bold and associated donor in italics. Anti-dsDNA is in I.U./ml. Values for each antibody were generated with one point calibrator.

sions may have such low levels of antibodies. The justification for using more than one method to detect anti-dsDNA is based on the maxim that all anti-dsDNA assays do not detect all anti-dsDNA antibodies (see Chapter 7).

B. MATERIALS

The general concepts for the Farr assay are similar to those described above for ELISA, with the following differences. Bacteriophage DNA or circular plasmid DNA, usually radiolabeled with ^{125}I is used for the Farr assay (see Appendix for resources). The DNA is incubated with patient serum, standards, or controls and antibody-bound radiolabeled DNA and free immunoglobulin are precipitated with 50% saturated ammonium sulfate. The high salt concentration dissociates the ^{125}I-labeled DNA from low-affinity antibody molecules, leading to the preferential detection of high-affinity anti-dsDNA antibodies. The precipitate is collected by centrifugation and the cpm counted. The results are expressed as percent DNA bound (ratio between cpm in the precipitate and total cpm/tube, or in I.U. by using a standard curve).

1. Kits containing radiolabeled DNA, sera to generate a standard curve, positive control, negative control, and precipitation material (ammonium sulfate).
2. All glassware, plasticware, and instruments are described in Chapter 1 with one exception: a gamma radiation counter substitutes for the ELISA reader.
3. The laboratory must be equipped to work with radioactive materials according to published guidelines.

C. PROCEDURE

1. Place aliquots of specimens, controls, and standards in tubes. If dilution is necessary, use normal human serum. For effective ammonium sulfate precipitation, all specimens must contain a level of IgG found in serum.
2. Add DNA and incubate at 37°C, precipitate with cold ammonium sulfate solution, and centrifuge.
3. Discard the supernatant and determine the cpm left in each tube.

D. CALCULATION AND REPORTING OF RESULTS

The values of duplicates are averaged and plotted on a linear-linear graph paper. The units per milliliter of the specimens and controls are determined from this curve. Calculation may also be performed by computer. Results are reported in I.U./ml with an upper limit of normal.

REFERENCES

1. **Fritzler, M.,** Antinuclear autoantibody testing, in *Manual of Clinical Laboratory Immunology,* Rose, N. R., deMacaro, E. C., Fahey, J. L., Friedman, H., and Penn, G. M., Eds., American Society of Microbiology, Washington, D.C., 1992, 724.
2. **Santos, M. E., Lopez, L. R., Jara, L. J., Espinoza, L. R., and La Rosa, F. G.,** Can ELISA have comparable clinical sensitivity for antinuclear antibody determinations, *Lupus,* 1 (S1), 66, 1992.

3. **Brouwer, E., Cohen Tervaert, J. W., Horst, G., Huitema, M. G., Van Der Giessen, M., Limburg, P. C., and Kallenberg, C. G. M.,** Predominance of IgG1 and IgG4 subclasses of anti-neutrophil cytoplasmic autoantibodies (ANCA) in patients with Wegener's granulomatosis and clinically related disorders, *Clin. Exp. Immunol.*, 83, 379, 1991.
4. **Hollingsworth, P. N., Bonifacio, E., and Dawkins, R. I.,** Use of standard curve improves precision and concordance of ANA measurement, *J. Clin. Lab. Immunol.*, 22, 197, 1987.
5. **Jitsukawa, T., Nakajima, S., Usui, J., and Watanabe, H.,** Detection of anti-nuclear antibodies from patients with systemic rheumatic diseases using Hep-2 cell nuclei, *J. Clin. Lab. Anal.*, 5, 49, 1991.
6. **Savige, J. A., Gallicchio, M., Georgiou, T., and Davies, D. J.,** Diverse target antigens recognized by circulating antibodies in anti-neutrophil cytoplasm antibody-associated renal vasculitides, *Clin. Exp. Immunol.*, 82, 238, 1990.
7. **Lange, A.,** Evaluation of the simultaneous detection of anti-dsDNA and ssDNA antibodies for clinical purposes, *Clin. Exp. Immunol.*, 31, 472, 1987.
8. **Rubin, R. L.,** EIA for anti-DNA and anti-histone antibodies including anti-(H2A-H2B), in *Manual of Clinical Laboratory Immunology,* Rose, N. R., deMacaro, E. C., Fahey, J. L., Friedman, H., and Penn, G. M., Eds., American Society of Microbiology, Washington, D.C., 1992, 735.
9. **Totoriis, M., Tan, E., McNally, E., and Rubin, R.,** Association of anti-histone (H2A-H2B) complex antibody with symptomatic procainamide-induced lupus erythematosus, *N. Engl. J. Med.*, 318, 1431, 1988.
10. **Buchanan, R., Venables, P., Morgan, A., Stains, N., Smith, P., and Maini, R.,** Separation of two species of the Sm antigen by affinity chromatography with murine monoclonal and human antinuclear antibodies, *Clin. Exp. Immunol.*, 51, 8, 1983.
11. **ter Borg, E., Horst, G., Limburg, P., van Venrooij, W., and Kallenberg, C. G. M.,** Changes in levels of antibodies against the 70kDa and A polypeptides of the U1RNP complex in relation to exacerbations of systemic lupus erythematosus, *J. Rheumatol.*, 18, 363, 1991.
12. **Deutscher, S., Harley, J. B., and Keene, J. D.,** Molecular analysis of the 60kD human Ro ribonucleoprotein, *Proc. Natl. Acad. Sci. U.S.A.*, 85, 9479, 1988.
13. **Ben-Chetrit, E., Gandy, B., Tan, E., and Sullivan, K.,** Isolation and characterization of cDNA encoding the 60kD component of the human SSA/Ro ribonucleoprotein, *J. Clin. Invest.*, 83, 1284, 1989.
14. **Ben-Chetrit, E., Fox, R., and Tan, E.,** Dissociation of immune responses to the SSA 52 kD and 60 kD polypeptides in SLE and Sjogren's syndrome, *Arthritis Rheum.*, 33, 349, 1990.
15. **McCauliffe, D. P., Lux, F. A., Lieu, T. S., Sanz, I., Hanke, J., Newkirk, M. M., Bachinski, L. I., Itoh, Y., Siciliano, M. J., Reichlin, M., Sontheimer, R. D., and Capra, J. D.,** Molecular cloning, expression, and chromosome localization of a human Ro/SSA autoantigen, *J. Clin. Invest.*, 85, 1379, 1990.
16. **Ben-Chetrit, E., Chan, E., Sullivan, K., and Tan, E.,** The 52kD protein is a novel component of the SSA/Ro antigenic particle, *J. Exp. Med.*, 167, 1560, 1988.
17. **Rader, M., O'Brien, C., Liu, Y., Harley, J., and Reichlein, M.,** Heterogeneity of the Ro/SSA antigen. Different molecular forms in lymphocytes and in red blood cells, *J. Clin. Invest.*, 83, 1293, 1989.
18. **Chan, E. K., Sullivan, K. F., Fox, R. I., and Tan, E.,** Sjogren's syndrome nuclear antigen (SSB): cDNA cloning, structural domains, and autoepitopes, *J. Autoimmun.*, 2, 321, 1989.

19. **Fields, R. A., Toubbeh, H., Searles, R. P., and Bankhurst, A. D.,** The prevalence of anticardiolipin antibodies in a healthy elderly population and its association with antinuclear antibodies, *J. Rheumatol.,* 16, 623, 1989.
20. **Reichlin, M. and Reichlin, M. W.,** Autoantibodies to the Ro/SSA particle react preferentially with the human antigen, in *Sjogren's Syndrome: A Model for Understanding Autoimmunity,* Talal, N., Ed., Academic Press, New York, 1989, 51.
21. **James, J., Dickey, W., Fujisaku, A., O'Brien, C., Deutscher, S., Keene, J., and Harley, J.,** Antigenicity of a recombinant Ro (SSA) fusion protein, *Arthritis Rheum.,* 33, 102, 1990.
22. **Froelich, C. J., Wallman, J., Skosey, J. L., and Teodorescu, M.,** Clinical value of an integrated ELISA system for the detection of 6 autoantibodies (ssDNA, dsDNA, Sm, RNP/Sm, SSA, and SSB), *J. Rheumatol.,* 17, 192, 1990.
23. **Maddison, P. J., Isenberg, D. A., Goulding, N. J., Leddy, J., and Skinner, R. P.,** Anti-SSB identifies a distinctive subgroup of systemic lupus erythematosus, *Br. J. Rheumatol.,* 27, 27, 1988.
24. **Nakamura, R. M., Peebles, C., Rubin, R., Molden, D., and Tan, E. M.,** *Autoantibodies to Nuclear Antigens (ANA),* American Society of Clinical Pathologists, New York, 1985.
25. **St.Clair, E. W., Burch, J. A., Jr., Ward, M. W., Keene, J. D., and Pisetsky, D. S.,** Temporal correlation of antibody responses to different epitopes of the human La autoantigen, *J. Clin. Invest.,* 85, 515, 1990.
26. **Veldhoven, C. H. A., Meilof, J. F., Huisman, J. G., and Smeenk, R. J. T.,** The development of a quantitative assay for the detection of anti-Ro/SS-A and anti-LA/SS-B autoantibodies using purified recombinant proteins, *J. Immunol. Meth.,* 151, 177, 1992.
27. **Juarez, C., Vila, J. L., and Gelpi, C.,** Characterization of the antigen reactive with Scl-70 antibodies and its application in an ELISA, *Arthritis Rheum.,* 31, 108, 1988.
28. **D'Arpa, P., Coper, H. W., and Cleveland, D.,** Use of molecular cloning methods to map the distribution of epitopes on Scl-70, *Arthritis Rheum.,* 33, 1501, 1990.
29. **Maul, G., Jimenez, S., and Riggs, E.,** Determination of an epitope of diffuse systemic sclerosis marker antigen DNA topoisomerase I: sequence similarity with retroviral p30 gag protein suggests a possible cause for autoimmunity in systemic sclerosis, *Proc. Natl. Acad. Sci. U.S.A.,* 86, 8492, 1989.
30. **Hillebrandt, S., Weiner, E., Senecal, J., and Rothfield, N.,** Autoantibodies to topoisomerase I (Scl-70): analysis by gel diffusion, immunoblot, and ELISA, *Clin. Immunol. Immunopathol.,* 57, 399, 1990.
31. **Earnshaw, W. and Rothfield, N.,** Identification of a family of human centromere proteins using autoimmune sera from scleroderma patients, *Chromosoma,* 91, 313, 1985.
32. **Rothfield, N., Whitaker, D., and Bordwell, B.,** Detection of anti-centromere antibodies using the cloned autoantigen, CENP-B, *Arthritis Rheum.,* 30, 1416, 1987.
33. **Roberts, D. E. and Rubin, R. L.,** Antineutrophil cytoplasmic antibodies, in *Manual of Clinical Laboratory Immunology,* Rose, N. R., deMacaro, E. C., Fahey, J. L., Friedman, H., and Penn, G. M., Eds., American Society of Microbiology, Washington, D.C., 1992, 781.
34. **Savage, C. O. S., Pottinger, B. E., Gaskin, G., Pusey, C. D., and Pearson, J. D.,** Autoantibodies developing to myeloperoxidase and proteinase 3 in systemic vasculitis stimulate neutrophil cytotoxicity toward cultured endothelial cells, *Am. J. Pathol.,* 141, 335, 1992.

35. **Jayne, D. R. W., Weetman, A. P., and Lockwood, C. M.,** IgG subclass distribution of autoantibodies to neutrophil cytoplasmic antigens in systemic vasculitis, *Clin. Exp. Immunol.,* 84, 476, 1991.
36. **Bini, P., Gabay, J. E., Teitel, A., Melchior, M., Zhou, J.-L., and Elkon, K. B.,** Antineutrophil cytoplasmic autoantibodies in Wegener's granulomatosis recognize conformational epitope(s) on proteinase 3, *J. Immunol.,* 149, 1409, 1992.
37. **Brinkman, K., Termaat, R., Van den Brink, H., Berden, J., and Smeenk, R.,** The specificity of the anti-dsDNA ELISA. A closer look, *J. Immunol. Meth.,* 139, 91, 1991.
38. **Halma, C., Daha, M. R., Schrama, E., Hermans, J., van Es, L. A., and Van der Woude, F. J.,** Value of anti-neutrophil cytoplasmic autoantibodies and other laboratory parameters in follow-up of vasculitis, *Scand. J. Rheumatol.,* 19, 392, 1990.
39. **Goldschmeding, O., van der Schoot, M. A., and van der Snoek, M. A.,** A monoclonal antibody against the 29kD ANCA antigen: application as catching antibody in a sandwich ELISA for ANCA detection, *Acta Pathol. Microbiol. Immunol. Scand.,* 97(S1), 47, 1989.
40. **Cohen, T., Goldschmeding, O., Elma, J. D., and Limburg, P. C.,** Autoantibodies to myeloperoxidase are associated with different forms of vasculitis, *Arthritis Rheum.,* 33, 1264, 1990.
41. **Hannested, R., Rekvig, O., and Husebekk, A.,** Cross reacting rheumatoid factors and lupus (LE) factors, *Springer Semin. Immunopathol.,* 4, 133, 1981.

Chapter 7

Clinical Significance and Interpretation of Anti-Nuclear Antibody Tests

Christopher J. Froelich and Marius Teodorescu

CONTENTS

I. THE RATIONALE FOR AN ALGORITHM APPROACH TO ANTI-NUCLEAR ANTIBODY TESTING

The immunofluorescent anti-nuclear antibody (ANA) screening test (F-ANA) and the subsequent measurement of specific anti-nuclear antibodies (ANAs) are essential steps in the evaluation of the patient suspected to have systemic lupus erythematosus (SLE) or a related connective tissue disease. The primary goal of ANA testing is to perform a screening test and then to identify the specific ANAs in the patient's serum. The clinical pathologist and the practitioner frequently have divergent expectations about ANA testing. While the laboratory focuses on efficient, cost-effective testing that provides accurate results, the clinician, being unaware of the methodology, desires a test that has high predictive value (i.e., differentiates the true from the false positive).

Most practitioners are familiar with the F-ANA technique. Some, however, may not appreciate that a normal result is the most valuable. The tendency exists, then, to

0-8493-5974-1/94/$0.00 + $.50

overestimate the predictive value of a F-ANA screen; this is a perception that leads to inadvertent misdiagnosis. The potential for diagnostic error increases as techniques that detect specific ANAs become more sensitive and complex. Combining disparate techniques with the large number of potentially detectable antibodies, the clinical laboratory may adopt one of more than a hundred different procedures, policies, or ''habits'' for antibody testing. Inasmuch as the milieu has engendered confusion about the proper approach for ANA testing, the clinical implications of accrued results often are ambiguous.

The overall approach entails first determining if the patient's serum has ANAs by performing a screening test (e.g., F-ANA or enzyme-linked immunosorbent assay [ELISA] for total ANA). If an abnormal level exists, additional assays are requested to determine if the patient's serum contains clinically relevant antibody specificities. In this regard, two diagnostic pathways are pursued: (1) the clinician, based on experience, will order a set of specific ANAs. Inasmuch as the results are frequently normal, the significance of the screening ANA remains equivocal and produces anxiety for both physician and patient. (2) An exhaustive search is undertaken to identify specific antibodies responsible for the abnormal ANA screen. This approach, albeit scientifically valid, is infeasible. Based on extant clinical studies, however, a limited number of ANAs are most frequently associated with different connective tissue disorders.[1,2] These are anti-ssDNA, -dsDNA, -Sm, -RNP, -SSA, -SSB, -Scl-70, -histone, and -centromere. Detection of the individual ANAs as a panel by a single technique offers a more robust predictive value than when measured individually by disparate techniques.[3,4] Although other clinically relevant ANAs are known, (e.g., anti-Ku and anti-ribosomal P ANAs in SLE or anti-PM1 and Jo1 in polymyositis), the antibody either coexists at a low prevalence with one or more of the aforementioned antibodies (i.e., provides redundant information) or the antibody rarely contributes to screening ANA reactivity (e.g., Jo1). Therefore, to evaluate the screening ANA, only a finite number of specific ANAs warrant routine testing.

The diagnosis of a ''connective tissue disorder'', albeit occasionally straightforward, more often requires validation by assessing the patient's ''ANA status''. Based on the history and physical, the clinician formulates a probability that the patient has SLE or another connective tissue disease. Then he orders an ANA screening test and the results are used to modify the initial prediction (Figure 1).

When the clinical probability is low, the ANA screening test functions to exclude the diagnosis of SLE or related conditions. Therefore, if it is normal (e.g., <6.2 I.U., see Chapter 6), the diagnosis is unlikely.[2] However, an abnormal ANA screen may suggest a bona fide connective tissue disease, an ''ANA'' induced condition (e.g., drug or paraneoplastic), or a ''false-positive'' result. To determine if the ANA screen reflects a true abnormality, an ANA specificity profile that includes anti-ssDNA, -dsDNA, -Sm, -RNP/Sm, -SSA, -SSB, -histone, and -Scl-70 may be performed. The vast majority of patients with ''positive'' ANA do not have abnormal levels of these specific autoantibodies; therefore, the probability of SLE or a related condition becomes remote. Using this approach, as many as 87% of patients referred to an arthritis center for evaluation of a ''positive ANA'' had negative ANA/6 specificity profiles (anti-ssDNA, -dsDNA, -Sm, -RNP/Sm, -SSA, -SSB).[4] In a minor percentage of patients with low probability of disease, one or, occasionally, more specific ANA(s) may be elevated. Consequently, these patients need further investigation and/or careful follow-up.

When the probability of SLE is high, the specificity profile is performed in conjunction with the ANA screening test rather than afterward (see case report #3 below). This

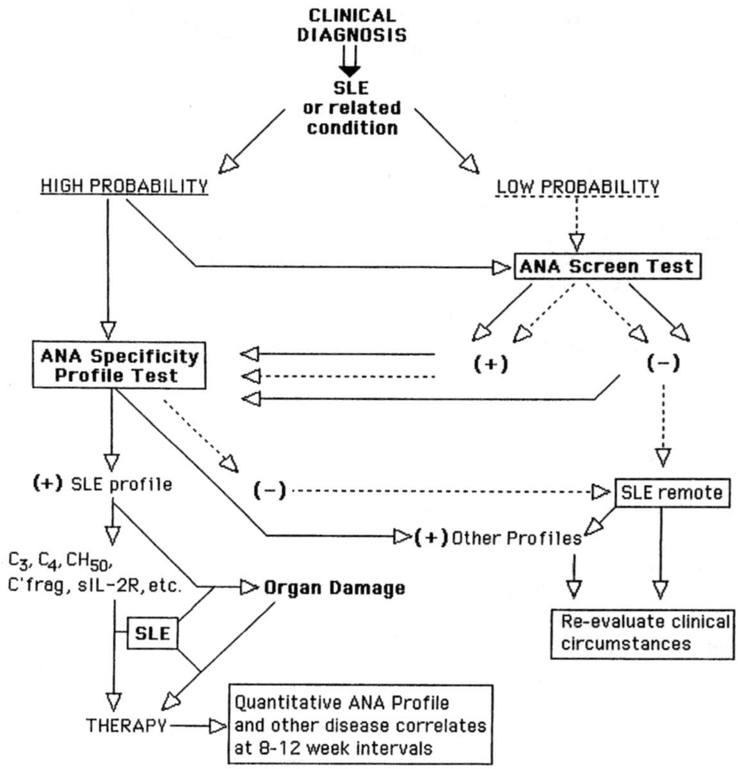

Figure 1 Algorithm for laboratory testing in a clinical rheumatology laboratory. The solid arrows for SLE indicate the pathways for high probability or confirmed SLE; the dotted lines indicate pathways for low probability — exclusion — of SLE.

concept is based on rationales that a positive ANA screening test does not provide, in isolation, sufficiently meaningful information and that a negative test is likely ignored. For example, if the clinical probability is high but the F-ANA is normal (e.g., "ANA-negative SLE"), the clinician disregards the result and orders the measurement of specific ANAs or an ANA profile. The request for the profile test, therefore, is not necessarily contingent on the result of a screening ANA test. The following laboratory scenarios may occur when the probability of SLE is high: (1) both the screening ANA and specific ANA profile test are positive (see Section IV, below); (2) the ANA screen is negative and specificity ANA profile identifies one or more specific antibodies; (3) the ANA screen is positive and the profile test is normal. The last instance suggests that the original clinical data should be reevaluated to generate alternate diagnoses.

The remainder of this chapter discusses the assets, liabilities, and clinical impact of techniques that measure screening ANAs and specific autoantibodies. Thereafter, attention focuses on the clinical applicability of multiparametric ANA testing for the diagnosis and management of connective tissue disorders.

II. CLINICAL SIGNIFICANCE OF ANA SCREENING TESTS

Reported by Friou in 1957,[5] the F-ANA test has become one of the most important tests to evaluate patients for the presence of connective tissue disorders. While extremely sensitive, the ANA test has low diagnostic specificity for SLE (40%).[6,7] Because a diagnosis of SLE is less than 3% in a patient with negative ANA, the test is used primarily to exclude this diagnosis.[2,8,9]

The method remains basically unchanged from its original description. The test result is reported as "negative" or "positive" at a defined screening or endpoint dilution (i.e., "titer of ANA"). Although patients with active SLE tend to have moderate to high titers,[10] titration of the screening ANA rarely provides additional information inasmuch as "normals" may also have "high" titers and some patients with active SLE have low or even a normal level.

Test are often "falsely positive" secondary either to poor precision, the inadvertent detection of IgM ANA, or the inappropriate selection of normal limits. The precision of the ANA screening test is affected by such factors as cell substrate, the fixative, quality of the second anti-Ig antibody, optics, and the examiner's experience. On the premise that "it is better to be safe than sorry", up to 50% of routine requests are reported "positive" by some laboratories. Consequently, observer bias makes the test meaningless. The percentage often drops to less than 20% of requests, however, when the laboratory implements the international World Health Organization (WHO) standard for IgG ANA (66/233 homogeneous pattern).[11]

The high sensitivity of the screening ANA leads to its detection among patients with diverse medical conditions, in healthy elderly (10 to 37%), and in 5% of nonelderly normal subjects.[12-15] In our experience as many as 87% of patients referred to a university-based rheumatology group for evaluation of a "positive ANA" did not have an autoimmune disorder.[4] In another analysis, ANA-positive patients referred to a rheumatologist fared substantially better. The patients had the following diagnoses: 18% SLE, 33% definable connective tissue disease, 16% organ-specific autoimmune disease (e.g., thyroiditis), and 22% miscellaneous nonautoimmune medical illness.[16] Although methodological differences and patient referral patterns may explain these divergent results, individuals without obvious autoimmune disorders frequently have ANAs. In fact, a sufficiently sensitive technique (e.g., immunoblotting) will detect ANAs in virtually all normal individuals.

Recent observations may provide a clue to the nature of ANAs in normal individuals.[17] When western blotting was employed to identify these antibodies,[1,8,18,19] substantial differences in the specificity of IgG antibodies for different protein bands in normal and SLE sera were found. SLE IgG antibodies reacted at various intensities with over 55 proteins (HeLa cell extract), whereas normal sera recognized only 17 proteins.[1] Most autoimmune IgG antibodies bind cellular enzymes, whereas "natural autoantibodies" bind to "structural" components of the cell.[20] Future studies with the immunoblotting technique may assist in the identification of the F-ANA-positive individual who has an abnormal immunoblot pattern and is perhaps destined to develop autoimmune diseases despite the lack of overt clinical signs.

The recognition pattern of the ANA (e.g., homogeneous, speckled) has been used to guide the subsequent testing for specific autoantibodies. Recent data, however, suggest that speckled or homogeneous patterns may be generated by any number and/or combinations of specific autoantibodies.[21,22] Thus, with the exception of anti-centromere antibodies,[23] the ANA pattern is a very poor predictor of the antibody specificity.

If a F-ANA is negative, testing for specific antibodies is justified when SLE or a related condition is still likely, inasmuch as some nuclear antigens are either present in low quantities (e.g., SSA) or absent (e.g., ssDNA). ELISA tests using either Hep2 nuclei, their extracts,[24] or purified antigen mixtures have been described[25] that are likely to supplant immunofluorescence (IFA) microscopic techniques. When combined with ELISAs for specific antibodies, the consequence will be an ELISA workstation that offers a complete ANA testing system.

III. DIAGNOSTIC IMPLICATIONS OF SPECIFIC ANTI-NUCLEAR ANTIBODY TESTING

A. FACTORS THAT AFFECT THE CLINICAL UTILITY OF ANA TESTS

Laboratories use a variety of techniques to detect specific ANAs: immunofluorescence, double diffusion, counterimmunoelectrophoresis, hemagglutination, liquid- and solid-phase radioimmunoassays, ELISAs, and, recently, western and dot/slot immunoblotting[26] (see Chapter 1). To select a method and properly interpret its results, the assets and pitfalls of the technique require thorough understanding. In addition to being sensitive, specific, and precise, the ideal method should also not be labor intensive and should be computer interfaced for efficient data analysis and retrieval.

Among these attributes, the assay's test sensitivity raises major concerns. This characteristic markedly influences the frequency at which a selected autoantibody is detected. Generally, dogma holds that a reciprocal relationship exists between test sensitivity and its diagnostic specificity. For example, the commonly used double diffusion technique has a low test sensitivity but relatively high diagnostic specificity. On the other hand, passive hemagglutination, immunoblotting, radioimmunoassay (RIA), and ELISA generally have high test sensitivities and, hence, may have low diagnostic specificity. High diagnostic specificity, however, may be achieved with sensitive assays, such as RIA or ELISA, if normal and abnormal control value ranges are established for different age groups and external standards are used to perform quantitative analysis[13,27] (see Chapter 6 Normal Levels).

The nature of the antigen (e.g., DNA or protein), its source (natural vs. recombinant), its degree of homogeneity, as well as the technique used to detect the antigen-antibody reaction, all significantly affect the reliability of the assay system. Native protein antigens are obtained from various sources, usually tissue or cultured cell extracts: bovine and rabbit thymus,[28,29] lymphoblastoid cell lines,[30] HeLa cells,[31] rat liver,[32] bovine and human spleen.[7] Since nuclear autoantigens, with rare exceptions,[33] are genetically conserved,[34] extracts from animal tissues, available in many commercial products, are suitable sources of antigen for routine laboratory testing.

The test method dictates the necessary degree of antigen "homogeneity".[35] For passive hemagglutination, ELISA, and RIA, purified antigen is essential. Residual IgG from the immunoaffinity columns may create a false-positive result that is amplified by the presence of rheumatoid factor. Recombinant antigens, isolated from bacterial expression systems, may have contaminant bacterial antigens that react with anti-bacterial antibodies present in test sera. Also, the presence of β-galactosidase from the fusion protein may either cause false-positive reactions or "mask" antigenic determinants.[36]

Whether recombinant antigens are as reliable for autoantibody detection as natural antigens needs further evaluation in both liquid- and solid-phase assays.[33] The tertiary structure of the recombinant protein may be perturbed secondary to incomplete glycosylation or expression of the primary sequence. Moreover, certain autoantigens consist of multimeric protein complexes (e.g., Sm antigen); therefore, the relative proportions present in natural preparations may be difficult to mimic. Furthermore, all the proteins in the complex may not possess autoepitopes necessary to define the ANA specificity. For example, data are available suggesting that the primary autoantigenic proteins of Sm are B/B′, therefore an assay that uses only these constituents may be sufficient to identify most "anti-Sm"-positive sera.[37] Additional studies are also needed to clarify the autoantigenic potential contributed by protein-RNA interactions (e.g., the SSA protein). When these issues are resolved for each autoantigenic complex, recombinant proteins should offer a consistent and reliable source of nuclear antigens.

The physical state of the antigen in the assay dictates the epitopes available for antibody binding (i.e., conformational vs. linear). Soluble-phase assays (double diffusion, counterimmunoelectrophoresis) minimally influence tertiary structure, therefore these assays preferentially detect antibodies directed toward conformational epitopes. The binding to a solid phase denatures the antigen and reduces the number of conformational epitopes. Linear epitopes, consequently, are generated and antibodies toward these determinants are preferentially detected.[38] Another effect of denaturation is the generation of new unpredicted (cross-reactive) epitopes that could bind low-affinity antibodies (particularly polyreactive natural IgM).[2]

High-affinity IgG antibodies are most often associated with clinically active disease.[2,39-41] Antigen-antibody reactions detected by immunoprecipitation, hemagglutination, solid-phase RIA, and ELISA are dependent on the affinity of the involved antibodies. For immunoprecipitation and hemagglutination, low-affinity IgG and IgM antibodies did not contribute significantly to the reaction. On the other hand, solid-phase RIA and ELISA may detect antibodies with various affinities.[42] If the epitope density on the solid phase is sufficiently low, however, only high-affinity antibody binding occurs.[43] Thus, solid-phase conditions that reduce the number of antigenic epitopes can influence not only the amount of antibody bound but also the affinity of the interaction antibody. Since most clinically relevant autoantibodies in SLE are high-affinity IgG, and since ELISAs can be designed monospecific for IgG antibodies, this technique is well suited for the clinical laboratory.

The precision and accuracy of a quantitative test for a specific ANA are influenced fundamentally by two factors: (1) the detection system for the reaction and (2) the intrinsic differences in antibody heterogeneity of the standard (calibrator) and the analyte.[44] The reaction parameters (e.g., type of enzyme and substrate, amount of secondary antibody, period of incubation, etc.) can markedly reduce the sensitivity of such techniques as ELISA, RIA, and immunoblotting. Differences in the diversity of epitopes identified either on the same protein or on different proteins of a complex antigen (e.g., Sm, RNP, etc.) and the "affinity heterogeneity" of an antibody population make standardization a *relative* process. Thus, any "quantitative" test that measures autoantibodies should be used primarily to compare serum samples obtained longitudinally from the same individual. During such observations if the value for the test result does not exceed 30% of the previous value(s), then the apparent change is probably not significant.

B. TESTS FOR ANTI-ssDNA AND ANTI-dsDNA ANTIBODIES

The association of SLE with the presence of anti-DNA antibodies was first recognized in 1957; their correlation with disease activity, particularly renal, was not appreciated, however, until the next decade.[45] Although the measurement of anti-DNA antibodies is now routine in clinical laboratories, a consensus as to the most suitable technique(s) for their detection is still not available. When interpreting the results of anti-dsDNA antibody testing, two main issues deserve consideration: (1) the antibody specificity recognized, i.e., dsDNA vs. dsDNA contaminated with ssDNA; and (2) class and/or affinity (or avidity) of the antibody measured.

High-affinity IgG anti-dsDNA antibodies are specific for SLE,[46] whereas patients with a variety of autoimmune conditions have anti-ssDNA.[2,47,48] To reliably measure anti-dsDNA antibodies, the preparation of dsDNA must be free of ssDNA. Manufacturers of diagnostic reagents and clinical laboratories have routinely employed calf thymus, *Escherichia coli,* bacteriophage, or circular plasmid DNA to detect anti-dsDNA. Irrespective of the source, extracted dsDNA undergoes a step to remove ssDNA (S1 nuclease treatment). The manufacturer then provides reasonable assurance that the dsDNA lacks ssDNA. However, the instability of certain DNA preparations, notably calf thymus, requires that the DNA be redigested with S1 nuclease prior to assay. For unclear reasons, lambda bacteriophage DNA remains stable in double-stranded form.[4]

The likelihood that ssDNA contaminates dsDNA is also influenced by assay conditions (i.e., soluble vs. solid phase). For soluble assays, small single-stranded ends of linear DNA (available with calf thymus, *E. coli,* and bacteriophage) may be sufficient to react with anti-ssDNA antibody. However, the single-stranded ends of phage λ DNA (12 single nucleotides or 0.0002% of the DNA molecule at the 5′ end) may have minimal consequences for either Farr or ELISA assays.[4] Since adsorption of dsDNA to a solid phase may generate ssDNA epitopes, it should be assumed that dsDNA is contaminated with ssDNA. Therefore, control serum monospecific for anti-ssDNA should be periodically tested against the DNA preparation.

Beside functioning as a tool to assess the integrity of dsDNA (i.e., quality control testing), the measurement of anti-ssDNA has clinical utility. Although anti-ssDNA antibody lacks diagnostic specificity, it sensitively indicates disease activity.[49,50] To determine the level of anti-ssDNA in a test specimen, anti-ssDNA (denatured) and anti-dsDNA antibodies should be detected simultaneously with ssDNA and dsDNA. Virtually all anti-dsDNA antibodies react with ssDNA but anti-ssDNA does not react with dsDNA.[2,51] The magnitude of the antibody reaction with ssDNA is either greater or equal to that for anti-dsDNA antibody. The difference reflects anti-ssDNA antibody activity. Finally, single-stranded DNA may serve to screen for all ''anti-DNA antibodies''. Thus, the measurement of anti-ssDNA (and anti-dsDNA) with both ssDNA and dsDNA preparations offers significant advantages for the clinical laboratory (Figure 2).

High-affinity IgG anti-DNA antibodies participate in the pathogenesis of SLE,[39,41,52] hence techniques that preferentially measure high- and not low-affinity anti-dsDNA antibodies may have greater clinical value. In the Farr assay, hypertonic ammonium sulfate solution precipitates antigen-antibody complexes that contain primarily high-affinity IgG anti-dsDNA antibodies (Chapter 1). Solid-phase assays, particularly ELISA, detect both high- and low-affinity antibodies. Most IgG anti-dsDNA, however, are high-affinity; therefore, if the solid phase assay is designed to measure IgG anti-dsDNA, then the assay preferentially detects high-affinity antibodies.[40,53,54] Furthermore, the ionic strength of the specimen diluent and wash solution may influence the affinity of the bound antibody.[55]

Despite these assurances, the test specificity of ELISA is debated. When we tested 74 specimens from SLE patients by Farr (DuPont Chemical Co., phage 1 DNa) and by

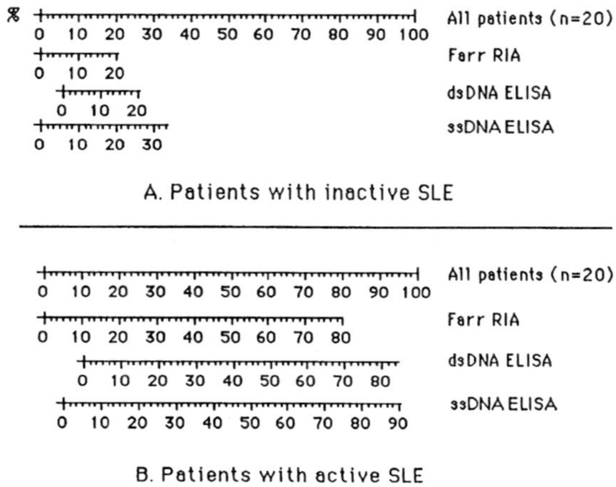

Figure 2 Percentages of specimens with abnormal levels of anti-DNA by radioimmunoassay (RIA, Farr assay) and by ELISA. Percentages of patients with SLE (active and inactive) with abnormal levels of anti-ssDNA detected by ELISA (TheraTest method) and of anti-dsDNA by radioimmunoassay (DuPont method).

IgG ELISA (TheraTest, Inc., phage 1 DNA), a high correlation ($R = 0.84$) existed. The sensitivity and specificity of ELISA with bacteriophage λ dsDNA was essentially the same as that of RIA for patients with either active or inactive disease (Figure 2). Therefore, ELISA, under the appropriate conditions, also detects primarily IgG anti-dsDNA of high affinity (unpublished).

The conditions employed for antibody binding may have other consequences for the measurement of anti-DNA antibodies. A pitfall of tests that use soluble radiolabeled DNA (Farr, polyethylene glycol (PEG), and nitrocellulose filter assays) is that all DNA-binding proteins, not only antibodies, are detected. For example, during infections there may be an increase in nonimmunoglobulin DNA-binding proteins, which produces false-positive results.[56]

A *Crithidia luciliae* kinetoplast IFA is highly specific (56 to 60%), but insensitive (40 to 45%), implying that a large number of patients have antibodies that do not react with this DNA substrate. We have encountered highly reactive sera from SLE patients (2500 I.U.) (by RIA and ELISA) that were negative in the *C. luciliae* assay.

Based on available information, the ability of various assays to detect high-affinity specific IgG anti-dsDNA antibodies (i.e., *diagnostic* value) ranks as follows: Farr RIA (with plasmid or bacteriophage DNA) > solid-phase ELISA (IgG) > filter binding assay > PEG assay >> *C. luciliae* IFA.[4,40,53,56,58,59,61-72]

C. DETECTION OF ANTI-Sm AND ANTI-RNP ANTIBODIES

Anti-Sm and anti-RNP antibodies are distinct sets of antibody specificities (Chapters 5 and 6). Native purified Sm antigen is suitable for ELISA when isolated by affinity chromatography[4,73,74] (Chapter 6). Native RNP antigen, however, is isolated as RNP/Sm complex. Therefore, two broad antibody specificities, anti-Sm and anti-RNP/Sm, are identified. A reaction with RNP/Sm but not Sm indicates that the specimen contains only anti-RNP antibody (e.g., MCTD, Figure 3j and k). If the serum sample reacts with both antigen preparations, both antibody specificities are present (Figure 3b, c, e). The level of anti-RNP, however, cannot be accurately determined with RNP/Sm complex.

Virtually all anti-Sm-containing sera have anti-RNP antibodies.[2,4,73,75] Indeed, the binding of anti-Sm reactive sera (individual or pooled) to RNP/Sm-coated wells is

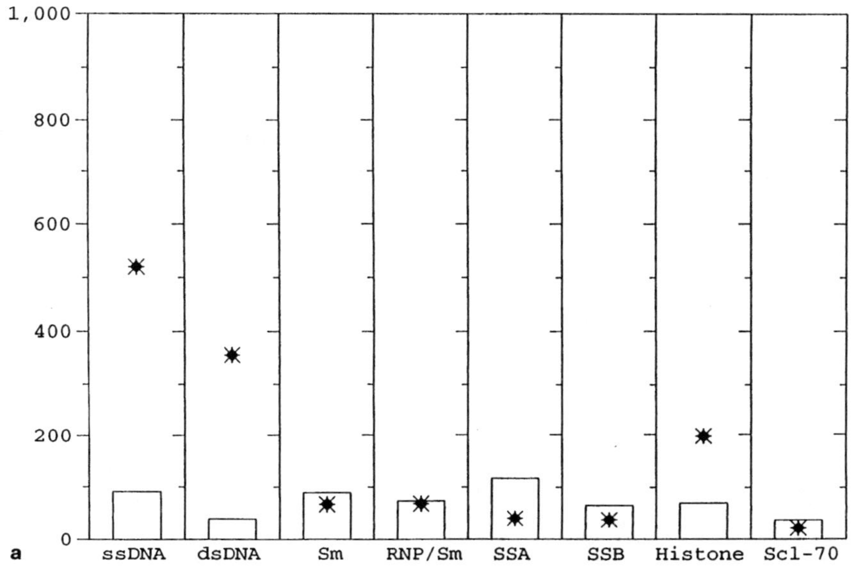

Figure 3 Profile of six or eight autoantibodies (ANA/8) in patients with positive ANA and suspected of SLE (TERIS© program, TheraTest Labs Inc., Chicago, IL). The values in the small open columns represent normal range. The "spiked" diamond represents patient's values. The results for anti-dsDNA are expressed in I.U./ml. The results for the remaining antibodies are expressed in units related in value with anti-dsDNA. The antigens on solid phase were ssDNA, denatured, single-stranded calf thymus DNA; dsDNA, double-stranded bacteriophage lambda DNA; Sm, Sm antigen from calf thymus; RNP, RNP/Sm complexes from bovine thymus; SSA, antigen from bovine spleen; SSB, antigen from bovine thymus; histone, total bovine thymus histone; Scl-70 was obtained from bovine thymus. The significance of each profile is described in the text.

effectively inhibited by purified Sm antigen by as much as 20%.[4] Therefore, if we assume that all anti-Sm-positive samples contain anti-RNP, native RNP/Sm complex may be used to detect anti-RNP antibodies as long as anti-Sm and anti-RNP antibodies are measured simultaneously with both Sm and RNP/Sm complex. With this approach, anti-Sm-positive serum must react with RNP/Sm antigen complex before a specimen is considered ''anti-Sm positive''. Comparable to the simultaneous detection of anti-ssDNA and -dsDNA with ssDNA- and dsDNA-coated wells, the coincident measurement of anti-Sm and anti-RNP with Sm and RNP/Sm offers inherent quality control (Chapter 6).

In lieu of RNP/Sm complex, anti-RNP antibodies can be detected with recombinant ''RNP'' proteins. In an investigative ELISA that contained recombinant 68-kDa and A proteins, the majority of anti-RNP reactive sera among patients with SLE and MCTD were detectable.[36] Using a commercial product that contained recombinant 68-kDa-coated wells, we observed a predictive value of 75% for MCTD patients. Therefore, commercial ''recombinant RNP'' ELISA is not, as yet, equivalent to ELISA that uses

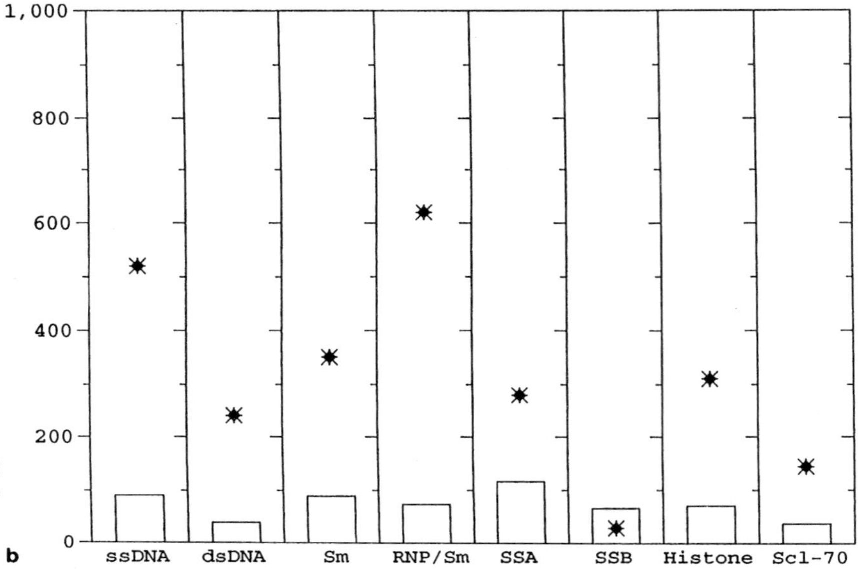

b

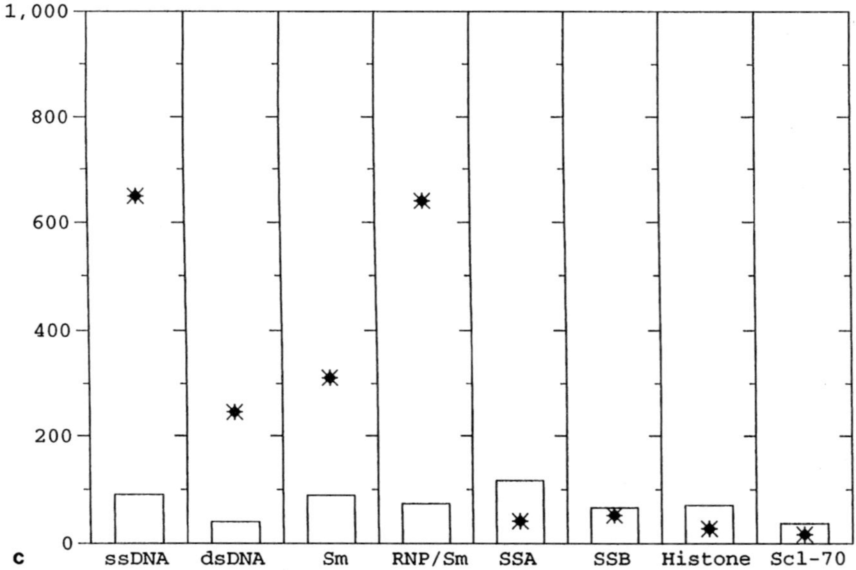

c

Figure 3 (continued).

native RNP/Sm. Moreover, detection of anti-RNP without also measuring anti-SM has no demonstrated clinical value.

The presence of anti-Sm is considered highly diagnostic for SLE.[7] Nevertheless, this perception is not entirely correct. The test sensitivity of the assay that measures anti-Sm markedly influences the frequency at which anti-Sm is detected among various

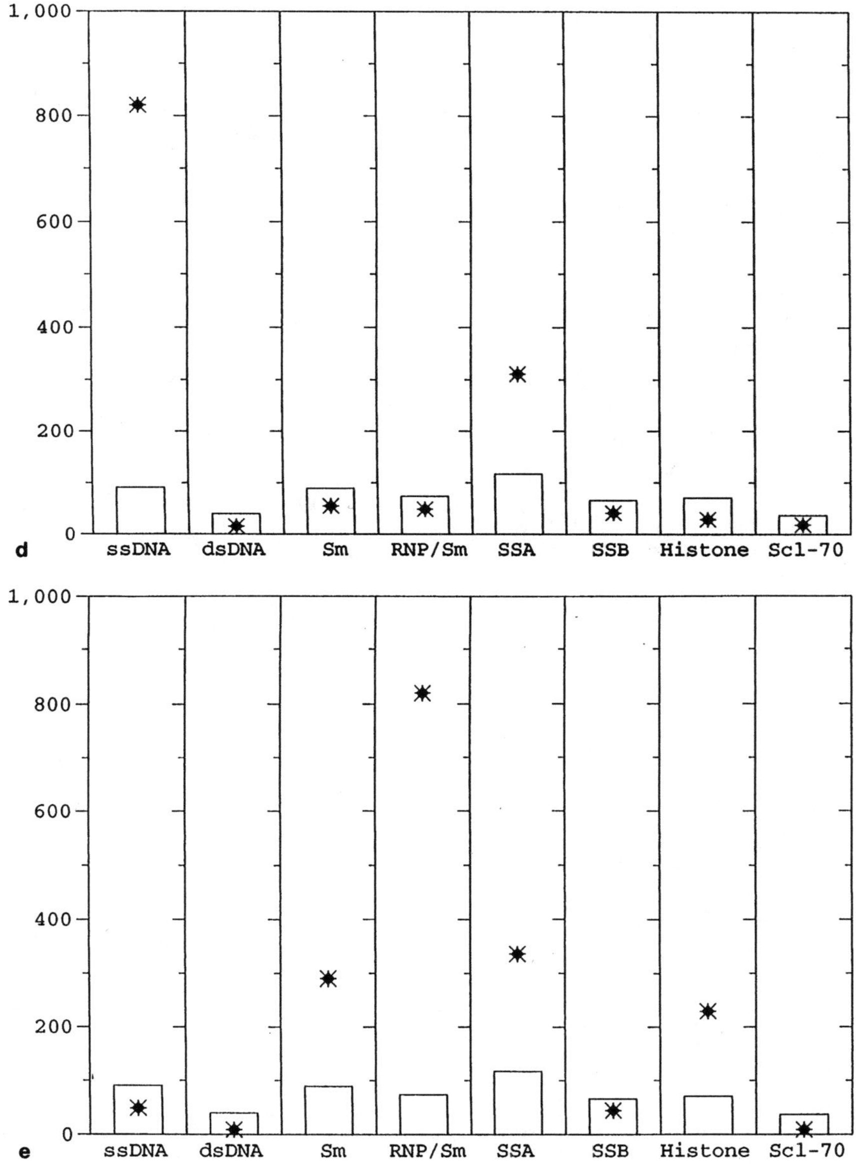

Figure 3 (continued).

connective tissue diseases. By immunodiffusion, anti-Sm is limited to SLE. However, when detected by immunoblotting or ELISA, patients with MCTD, undifferentiated connective tissue disease (UCTD), or progressive systemic sclerosis (PSS), will have detectable, albeit lower, levels of anti-Sm antibodies than SLE patients.[4,73,76]

The frequency of anti-Sm and anti-RNP in SLE patients also depends on the demographics of the patient population. When determined by immunodiffusion and ELISA,

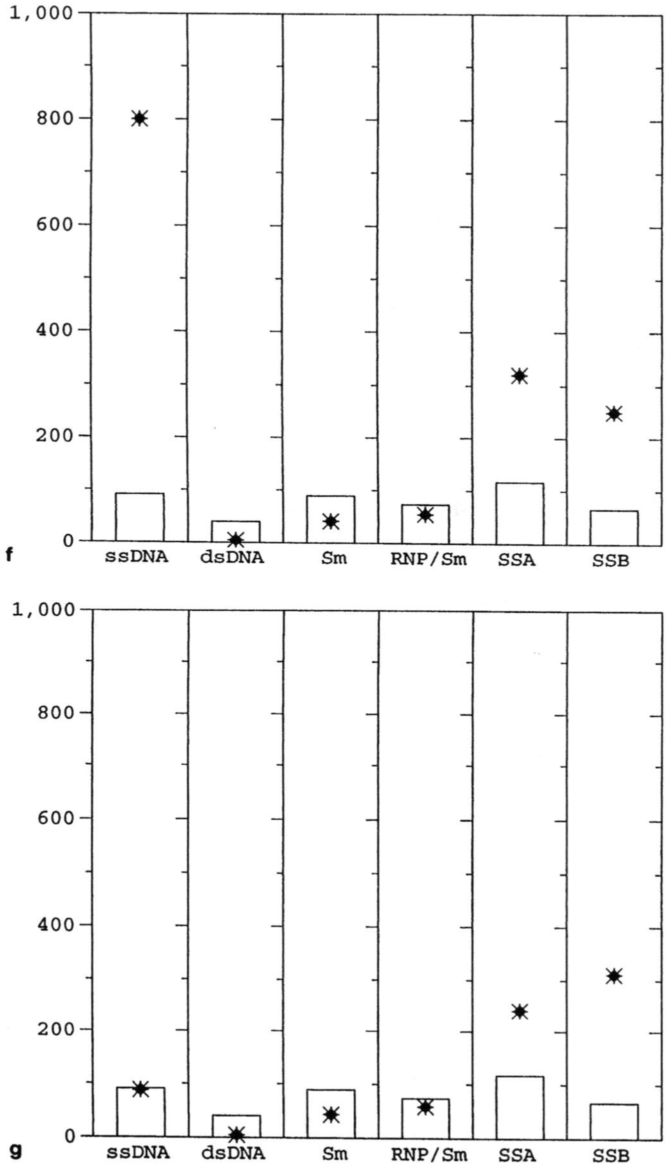

Figure 3 (continued).

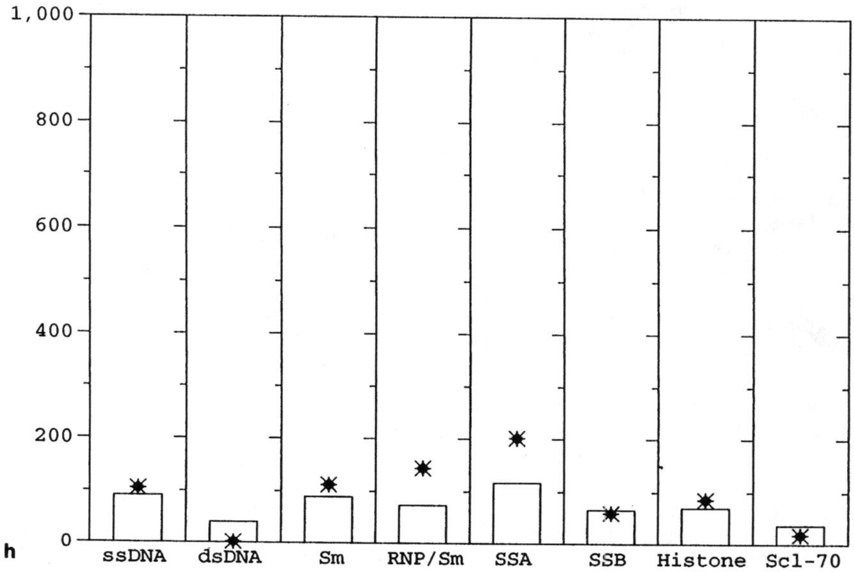

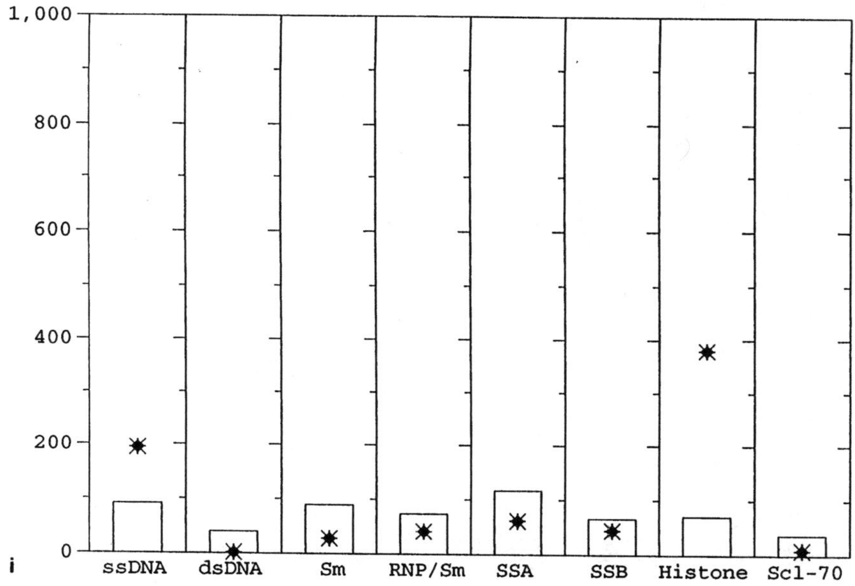

Figure 3 (continued).

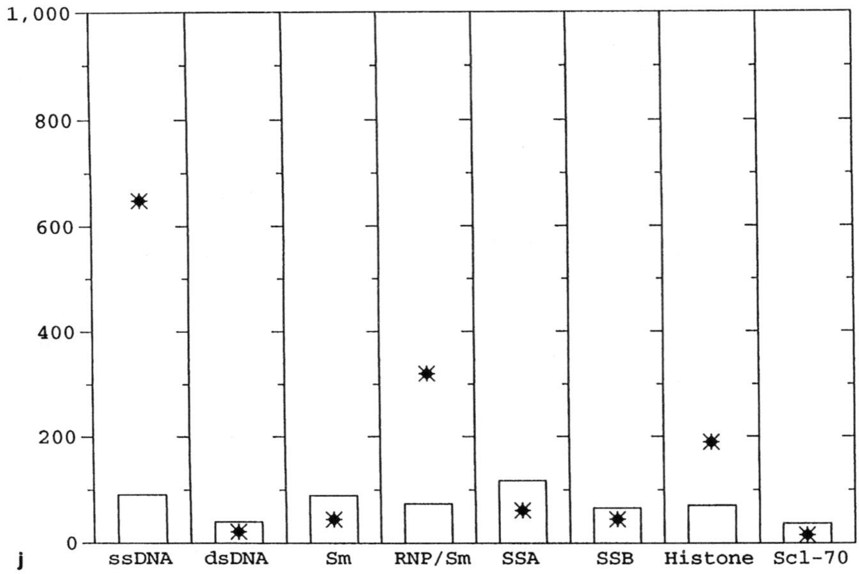

j

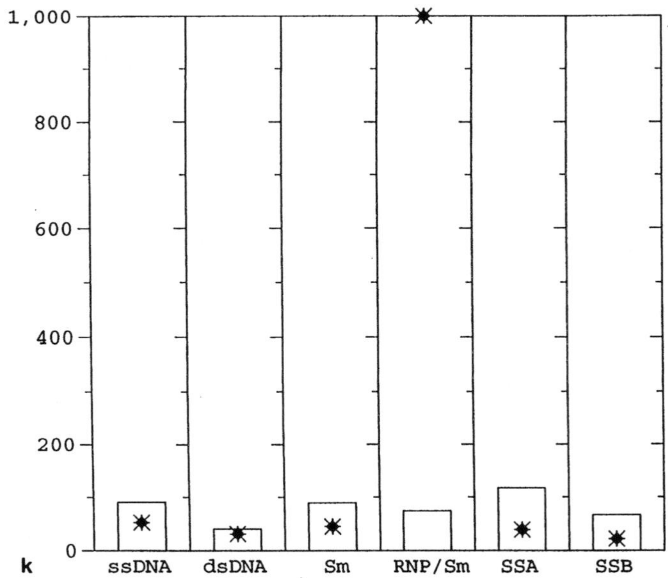

k

Figure 3 (continued).

30 and 50% of a racially mixed SLE population have anti-Sm.[2,4,77] Irrespective of the technique, however, compared to Caucasians, the frequency of anti-Sm is twice as high in Afro-Caribbean patients.[75,78]

Anti-RNP, although observed frequently in SLE, commonly occurs in other connective tissue diseases. Anti-RNP has been reported in rheumatoid arthritis, scleroderma, and dermatomyositis.[73,79] If anti-RNP is detected at high levels in isolation, the antibody

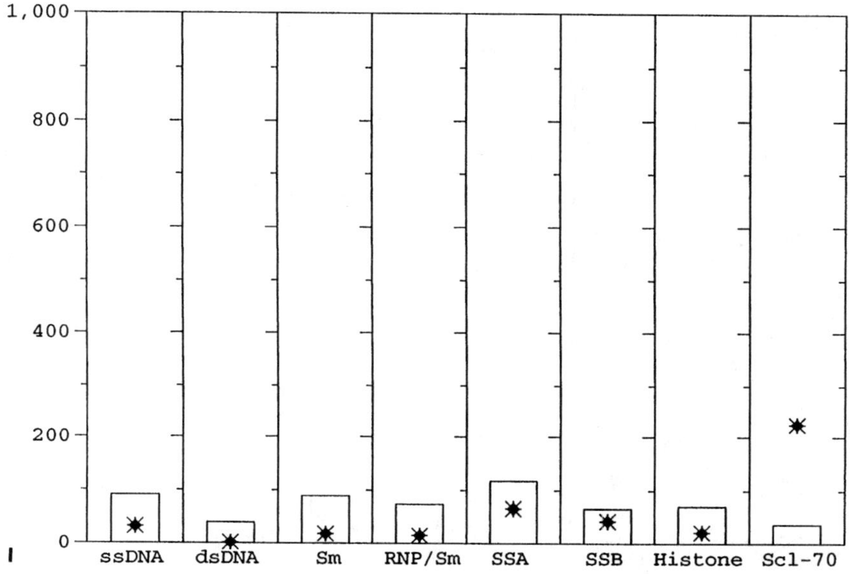

l

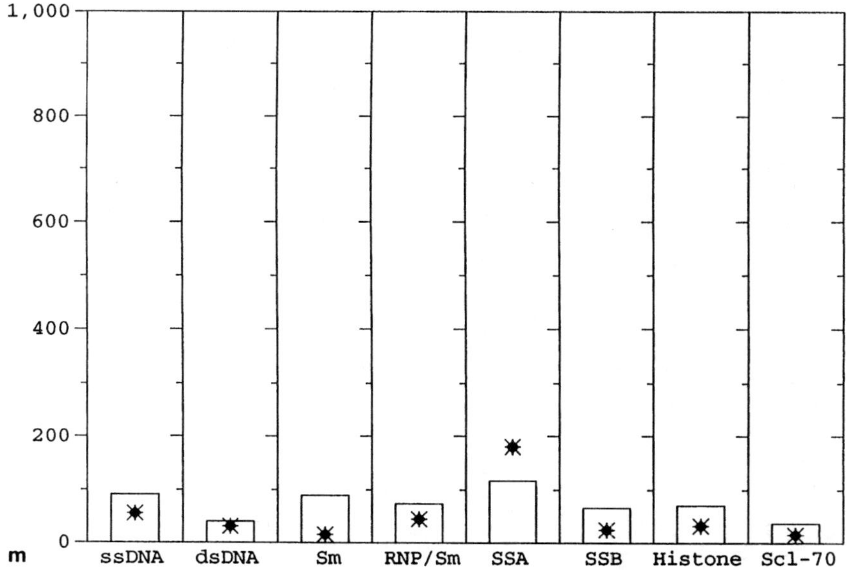

m

Figure 3 (continued).

is diagnostic for MCTD (Figure 3).[80,81] Thus, the conspicuous absence of the other antibodies is just as important as the presence of a high level of anti-RNP antibody.

D. DETECTION OF ANTI-SSA AND ANTI-SSB ANTIBODIES

Patient serum should be evaluated in tandem for anti-SSA and anti-SSB antibodies. Their presence, either together or alone, has both clinical and laboratory ramifications.

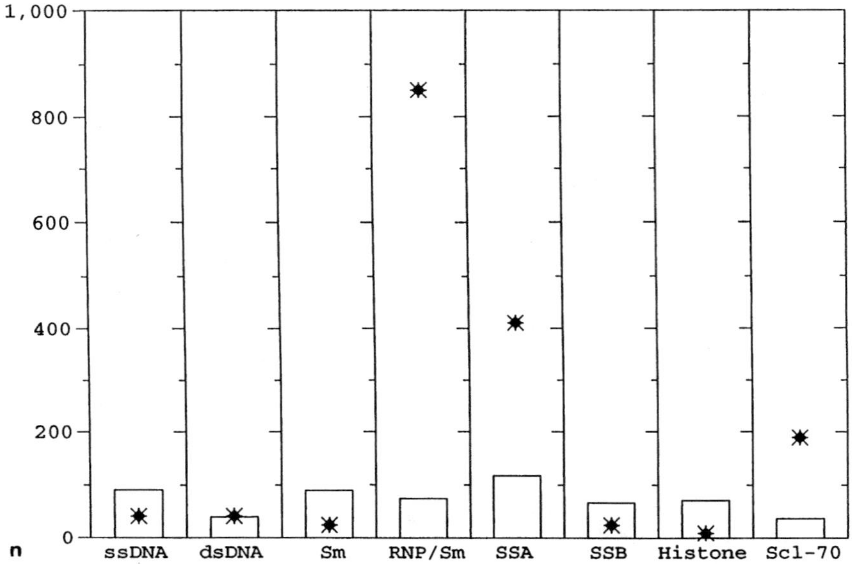

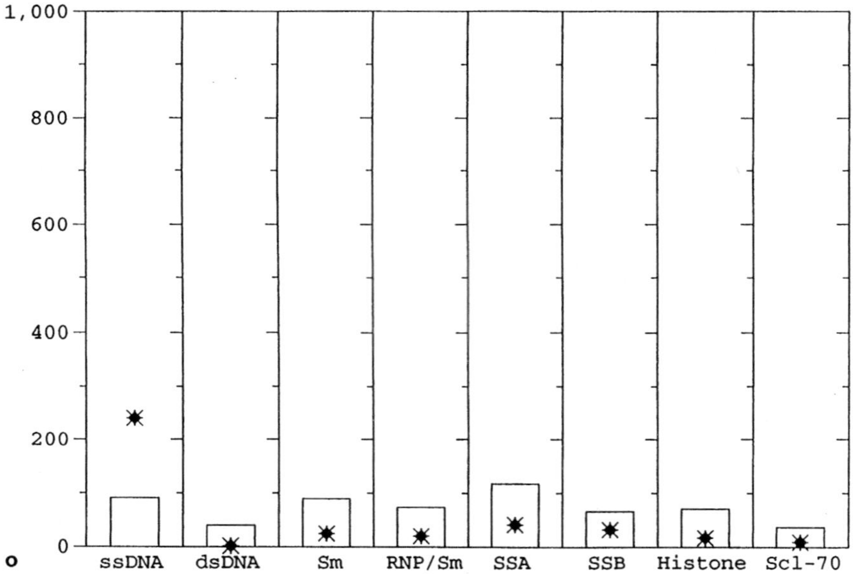

Figure 3 (continued).

In SLE and related conditions, if anti-SSB antibody exists, anti-SSA antibody is invariably present.[82,83] However, the opposite is not necessarily true: a large proportion of SLE patients may have anti-SSA without detectable anti-SSB. Recent work may clarify why anti-SSA and anti-SSB frequently, but not always, coexist.[84,85] SSA ribonucleoprotein particles segregate into three discrete subpopulations with characteristic physicochemical properties: one contains hY4 RNA (SSA^{hY4}), another has hY5 RNA (SSA^{hY5}), and the third has hY1, hY3, and hY4 RNAs ($SSA^{hY1\text{-}hY4}$).[85] Apparently the SSB protein associates with hY5 RNA (SSA^{hY5}) and not the other SSA snRNPs. Hence, one may postulate that SSA^{hY5} stimulates an immune response that generates both anti-SSA and anti-SSB antibodies, while other autoimmunogenic SSA particles induce primarily an anti-SSA antibody response. If a specimen has anti-SSB but lacks anti-SSA, the following should be considered: (1) test error (see chapter 6), (2) test sensitivity for anti-SSB exceeds anti-SSA, and (3) certain SSA epitopes may not exist in the test system.

By ELISA, anti-SSA antibody is present among 10% of random normal blood bank donors. This prevalence dictates the need for caution when tested sera only contain this antibody. The prevalence of anti-SSA and -SSB antibodies in SLE also varies according to the method of detection. By immunodiffusion and ELISA the frequency of anti-SSA and anti-SSB were 35 and 15%, vs. 60 and 50%, respectively. Anti-SSA and anti-SSB antibodies are often associated with primary Sjögren's syndrome, suggesting a significant overlap between these two syndromes. Indeed, about 30% of SLE patients have lymphocytic infiltration of the salivary glands that is similar to the histopathology in Sjögren's syndrome.[86] In the presence or absence of clinically manifest Sjögren's syndrome, a subset of patients with rheumatoid arthritis also may have these autoantibodies. In our experience, this subset is quite small.

SLE patients with nephritis have been described who have anti-SSA but lack anti-dsDNA antibodies.[87,88] Anti-SSA by ELISA occurs in 53% of nephritis patients, whereas only 9% had coexistent anti-SSB. Moreover, SSA antigen has been identified as immune complexes in glomeruli.[89] In primary Sjögren's syndrome, where nephritis is rare, the coincidence of anti-SSA and anti-SSB is high.[90,91] Consequently, the detection of both antibodies may have prognostic implications wherein the presence of anti-SSA alone increases the likelihood of kidney disease.[89,92]

Cutaneous SLE, primarily subacute SLE (i.e., ANA-negative lupus)[93] or neonatal rash,[94] is associated with anti-SSA. This relationship is perhaps due to the observation that exposure of cells to ultraviolet light causes expression of "SSA antigen" on the cell surface of keratinocytes.[95] Anti-SSA antibodies have also been connected with congenital heart block.[96] A large proportion of babies born to anti-SSA-positive mothers, however, do not have cardiac dysfunction; therefore, the pathogenic significance of this observation is unclear.[97]

E. DETECTION OF ANTI-HISTONE ANTIBODIES

Anti-histone antibodies have been routinely measured by immunofluorescence on acid-treated section of mouse tissue, a technique that preferentially identifies anti-H2a/H2b antibodies. By this method, almost all patients with drug-induced SLE (procainamide) and about 30% of patients with SLE have elevated levels of anti-histone antibodies.[98] Sensitive solid-phase RIA and ELISA detect antibodies either against total histones or against histone fractions (H1, H2a, H2b, H3, and H4).[99-101] In active SLE, 80% of patients have anti-histone antibodies,[102] whereas they exist in 55% of randomly selected SLE patients.[101] Antibody levels are higher in drug-induced than idiopathic SLE and are mainly directed against H2a/H2b complex.[103,104] The presence of anti-ssDNA at low to moderate levels, plus the absence of other autoantibodies differentiates the drug-induced variant from idiopathic SLE (see Section IV).

F. DETECTION OF ANTI-Scl-70 (TOPOISOMERASE I) AND ANTI-CENTROMERE ANTIBODIES

Anti-Scl-70 antibodies bind to a 100-kDa, DNA topoisomerase I[105] that catalyzes the relaxation of superhelical DNA. The cDNA for Scl-70 has been cloned and three linear epitopes have been identified.[106,107] For immunodiffusion and blotting, the prevalence is 20 and 28%, respectively. Hillebrandt et al. have compared four methods for the detection of anti-Scl-70 antibodies: ELISA, immunoblotting, immunodiffusion, and inhibition of topoisomerase I activity.[108] Using the enzyme inhibition as the "gold standard", they found that the sensitivity/specificity of the assays were as follows: immunodiffusion, 79%/100%, immunoblot, 100%/97%, and ELISA, 100%/98%. The data suggest that ELISA is the method of choice for the clinical laboratory.

Three centromeric antigens (CENPs) are known: CENP-A (17 kDa), CENP-B (80 kDa), and CENP-C (140 kDa).[109] CENP-B is the major centromeric antigen recognized by anti-centromere antibody-reactive sera. Anti-centromere antibodies have been identified by indirect immunofluorescence, using dividing Hep-2, as well as by immunoblotting and, most recently, by ELISA using CENP-B fusion protein as the antigen.[110] Dividing cells have to be examined to detect anti-centromere antibody. Therefore, a "negative" F-ANA with Hep-2 cells does not always exclude the presence of anti-centromere antibodies. An anti-centromere antibody test should be specifically requested. Currently, indirect immunofluorescence is most commonly used by clinical laboratories; however, ELISA is likely to supplant this technique.

Although fairly insensitive, anti-centromere antibody appears to be specific for patients with Raynaud's syndrome, with or without a connective tissue disease. The prevalence of anti-centromere antibodies is higher in secondary (32%) than in the primary (20%) forms of Raynaud's syndrome.[111] The presence of anti-centromere antibodies occurs in patients with diagnoses ranging from Raynaud's disease to diffuse systemic sclerosis. The antibody, however, arises most frequently in the CREST variant of scleroderma (calcinosis, Raynaud's, esophageal dysmotility, sclerodactyl, telangiectasia).[111] Further, anti Sel-70 and anti-centromere antibodies appears to be mutually exclusive.

G. ANTI-NEUTROPHIL CYTOPLASMIC ANTIBODIES (ANCA)

Anti-neutrophil cytoplasmic antibodies, directed toward proteins in the primary granules of neutrophils and lysosomes of monocytes, have been reported to assist in the diagnosis and management of various forms of vasculitis.[112] The most frequently reported technique to detect ANCA-positive serum is a variant of the F-ANA test. Two dominant patterns are observed: cytoplasmic-ANCA (C-ANCA) and perinuclear ANCA (P-ANCA). The C-ANCA pattern has been associated with antibodies that bind proteinase 3, whereas the P-ANCA pattern defines antibodies to myeloperoxidase (MPO) and, less frequently, to elastase, cathepsin G, and lactoferrin.[113,114] Crude neutrophil extract has been used for ANCA solid-phase screening assays.[114,115] Nevertheless, due to the loss of conformational epitopes during the coating process, the solid-phase assay is less sensitive than IFA.[116] Commercial kits also are available to measure anti-myeloperoxidase by ELISA.[113]

ANCA reactivity is most commonly associated with vasculitic disorders: Wegener's granulomatosis, polyarteritis nodosa, Churg-Strauss vasculitis, leukocytoclastic angiitis, and crescenteric glomerulonephritis. Among pulmonary-renal syndromes, ANCA positivity is much more common than either immune complex or anti-glomerular basement membrane disease-mediated diseases. The predictive value of C-ANCA (i.e., anti-proteinase 3) is highest for Wegener's granulomatosis.[117] For other vasculitic disorders, the diagnostic/prognostic values of ANCAs or detection of individual ANCA antibody specificities require further study.

In a useful analysis, Gross et al. evaluated the prevalence of ANCA in connective tissue diseases.[118] While the C-ANCA was not detected among SLE, MCTD, scleroderma, or polymyositis patients, 4% of the SLE patients were P-ANCA positive. In another study, 30% of SLE sera were P-ANCA but not C-ANCA positive. The primary antibody of the ANA+, P-ANCA+ SLE patients was toward lactoferrin and much less commonly to myeloperoxidase.[119] For other rheumatologic disorders C-ANCA reactivity also was not identified, whereas P-ANCA reactivity was as follows: rheumatoid arthritis (RA), 2.5%; Felty's syndrome, 21%; Still's disease, 15%; Sjögren's syndrome, 26%; psoriatic arthritis, 15%.[118] No patients with reactive arthritis, Reiter's syndrome, or ankylosing spondylitis had P-ANCA. Therefore, P-ANCA is associated with a number of different diseases. What remains to be determined is whether the ANA identified in patients who do not have a defined connective tissue disease (i.e., "false positives"), also are likely to be P-ANCA positive.

IV. INTERPRETATION OF SPECIFIC MULTIPARAMETER ANA PROFILES

A. INTRODUCTION

ANA specificity profiles that consist of six or more autoantigens (e.g., anti-ssDNA, -dsDNA, -Sm, -RNP/Sm, -SSA, -SSB, -histone, and -Scl-70) can be performed using ELISA-based kits (Figure 3). The antigens and the blank microwells are configured in a plate so that each column or row serves as a multitest panel for each individual patient. The system eliminates the errors introduced during the dispensing of a patient's serum specimens for various ANAs (e.g., immunodiffusion, IFA, and RIA). When combined with software that processes the generated data, the result is a cost-effective, non-labor-intensive assay system that reports both normal and abnormal autoantibody levels, and, when presented graphically, provides a composite of specific ANAs in the patient's serum (Figure 3) (see also Chapter 6). Finally, the panel offers a more robust predictive value than the measurement of individual antibodies.[3,4]

Inasmuch as the screening ANA frequently occurs in patients who have equivocal evidence of a connective tissue disorder,[16] the ANA profile test primarily acts to discount such diagnoses. In this regard, 87% of "ANA+" patients referred to a university rheumatology group did not have an autoimmune disorder.[140] On the other hand, an analysis of more than 10,000 ANA-positive sera has revealed that an ELISA panel (ANA/6, 7, and 8) is never completely normal in patients with active SLE (unpublished data). This sensitivity clearly exceeds that for any individual antibody (e.g., anti-dsDNA antibody are positive in 45 to 75% of patients with SLE). Moreover, if the autoantibody profile demonstrates the presence of more than one ANA *(vide infra)*, the probability that the patient has a connective tissue disease significantly increases (see Chapter 6, Normal Limits). In summary, ELISA ANA profile testing:

1. Identifies specific antibodies that have diagnostic value (e.g., anti-DNA, anti-Sm)
2. Serves as an index of disease activity (e.g., multiple autoantibodies at high levels)
3. Provides quantitative data to follow during treatment and remission

4. Stimulates, when the profile suggests SLE, the request for additional tests that may identify other indicators of disease activity (e.g., measurement of complement fragments)
5. Identifies the SLE patient who has quiescent or ''burned out'' disease

B. DESCRIPTION OF ANA SPECIFICITY PROFILES IN CONNECTIVE TISSUE DISEASES

A certain profile may be primarily associated with a particular connective tissue disease or may occur among several related conditions (Figure 3). Nevertheless, the ANAs identified by a profile test act as a ''motif'' that defines the individual's autoantibody status. Changes in the ''motif'' may indicate either clinical worsening or improvement and may guide therapeutic intervention.

For idiopathic SLE — ANA profiles are extremely protean, but certain general patterns have emerged. Interpretation of these profiles chronologically may be particularly useful to characterize the flare and remission status for the patient (see case report #1). Profiles frequently appear as:

1. Moderate to high levels of multiple autoantibodies[4] which include both anti-ssDNA and anti-dsDNA in most cases (Figures 3A, B, C)
2. Moderate elevation of only anti-ssDNA and anti-dsDNA
3. High levels of anti-ssDNA and one or two antibodies (Figures 3D, J)
4. High levels of anti-Sm and anti-RNP/Sm, with or without anti-ssDNA or dsDNA antibodies (Figures 3C, E)
5. Anti-ssDNA with moderate to high levels of anti-SSA and anti-SSB (Figure 3F)
6. Only anti-SSA and anti-SSB (very rare and more typical of Sjögren's syndrome) (Figure 3G)

While the presence of multiple autoantibodies at high levels (Figure 3B) is usually associated with active SLE, we have occasionally observed this pattern in patients with minimal organ involvement. SLE patients in remission may continue to have low levels of multiple autoantibodies (Figure 3H). This pattern, however, is rarely observed in other inflammatory conditions.

Drug-induced SLE — Appears as: (1) moderate to high levels of anti-histone, (2) low to moderate amounts of anti-ssDNA, (3) low to moderate levels of anti-ssDNA plus anti-histone (Figure 3I). All other ANAs are usually normal.

Mixed connective tissue disease — Appears as a marked elevation of anti-RNP/Sm without other ANAs (Figure 3K). If anti-Scl-70 is also increased, the development of scleroderma is probable.

Scleroderma — Appear as follows: (1) only anti-Scl-70 is elevated (Figure 3L), (2) only anti-SSA is elevated (Figure 3M) (this antibody exists in as many as 50% of scleroderma patients), (3) anti-Scl-70, anti-RNP, and/or anti-SSA (Figure 3N), and (4) normal profile (ANA/8, 40%). Anti-centromere antibody may exist alone or with anti-RNP, anti-SSA, but not with anti-Scl-70. Testing for anti-centromere antibody is indicated in scleroderma because it identifies the relatively benign CREST variant.[111] The serology as well as the clinical manifestations and organ involvement of scleroderma may overlap with SLE.

Sjögren's syndrome — Patients may have: (1) anti-SSA and anti-SSB at various levels (Figure 3G), (2) low anti-ssDNA plus anti-SSA and anti-SSB, (3) only anti-SSA

(Figure 3M), and (4) a normal profile. High levels of rheumatoid factor are frequently detected in these patients (Chapters 2 and 4).

Rheumatoid arthritis — Sera may appear as follows:

1. Most frequently normal even despite abnormal levels of F-ANA
2. ssDNA at low levels (Figure 3O)
3. Anti-RNP at low to moderate levels
4. Anti-SSA and/or anti-SSB, mainly in patients with secondary Sjögren's (Figure 3M, G)
5. Anti-histone due mainly to a cross reaction between histone and rheumatoid factor[99,100,120]
6. P-ANCA is present in a large minority of patients with RA, particularly those with vasculitis (49%)[121]

Primary anti-phospholipid syndrome — Appears frequently as anti-ssDNA at low to moderate levels (Figure 3O). This is most likely due to a cross reaction between anti-ssDNA and phospholipids antibodies (see Chapter 13). Thus, patients who have only anti-ssDNA should be routinely tested for anti-cardiolipin antibodies. In our experience, this subset is quite small.

V. FOLLOW-UP OF AUTOANTIBODY LEVELS IN PATIENT MANAGEMENT

Once the diagnosis of a connective tissue disease is accepted, the laboratory must answer two questions: (1) what is the magnitude of tissue damage in affected organs? and (2) what test(s) can act to monitor the severity of their destruction?

Nonquantitative results obtained for anti-dsDNA *(C. luciliae)* and for other ANAs by double diffusion have minimal value in the treatment of SLE patients. With the advent of quantitative antibody testing, however, the utility of serially measuring autoantibody levels has been validated in numerous research studies. The application of this information to the bedside is now feasible with the availability of ELISA testing (see the Appendix).

The potential clinical value of measuring anti-dsDNA antibodies has been demonstrated in numerous reports that showed a correlation between antibody levels and disease activity.[52,54,55,77,122-126] Notably, an elevation in anti-dsDNA antibodies may predict a clinical flare,[127,128] suggesting that serial measurements of anti-dsDNA could provide sufficient evidence to intervene early in the disease process. Anti-Sm antibody levels also fluctuate with changes in disease activity.[4,129-132] These antibodies, however, may increase after, rather than before, a disease exacerbation.[130] In our experience, anti-DNA antibody decreases more rapidly than anti-Sm during steroid therapy, coincident with clinical improvement. This observation suggests that anti-DNA levels correlate well with disease activity. Nevertheless, the rapid reduction in anti-DNA levels may not reflect the inflammatory process. The slower reduction in anti-Sm antibody levels (Figure 4) may more accurately reflect chronicity of organ damage and recovery in SLE.

Elevation of anti-RNP antibodies also may precede flares in SLE[133] and MCTD.[79,134,135] In most instances this antibody is the last to normalize during long therapy.[132] The levels of anti-SSA also varies with disease activity, and, analogous to anti-dsDNA, may increase significantly prior to exacerbation of lupus nephritis.[87] However, unlike the

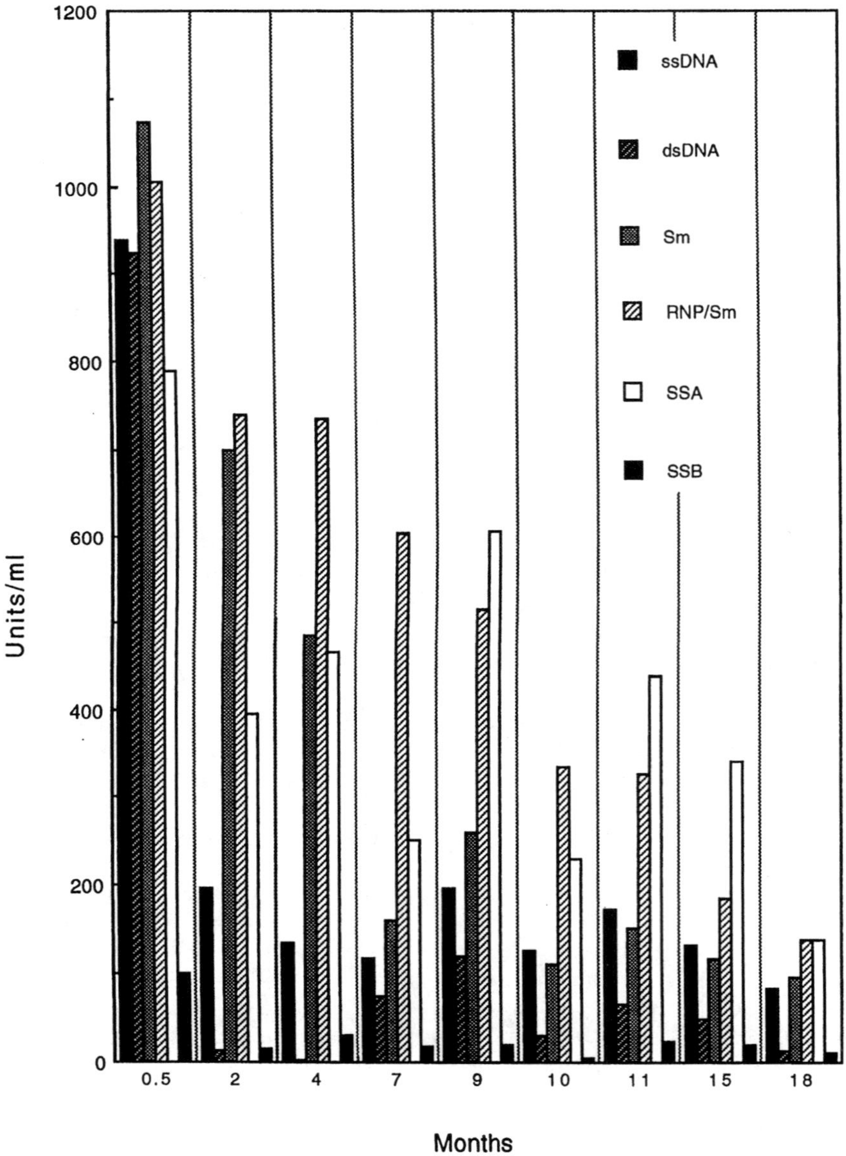

Figure 4 Longitudinal autoantibody observations in a patient with SLE and proliferative glomerulonephritis during treatment with high-dose steroids. The antibody levels were determined by ELISA as previously described[4] (Chapter 6). Anti-dsDNA is presented in international units. The patient was treated successfully and remission was obtained.

anti-dsDNA, anti-SSA antibody has a tendency to persist or decrease very slowly during effective treatment[132] (Figure 4). Similarly, anti-SSB has been reported to fluctuate with disease activity.[91,136] Anti-histone antibody increases along with anti-dsDNA during flares. Anti-Scl-70 has not been reported to vary with disease activity.

When a serological parameter that correlates with tissue damage is identified, it may assist in the evaluation of the patient's disease activity. Virtually any autoantibody associated with SLE could increase with a flare and may persist for a variable period of time after treatment. An increase in multiple autoantibodies strongly indicates active disease.[4] For the SLE patient with quiescent disease, repeated profile testing at 6- to 12-week intervals may lead to therapeutic intervention prior to another cycle of organ damage. In our experience, if a particular profile is observed during an exacerbation, the reappearance of a similar profile likely heralds another flare that will damage the same organ. Moreover, serologic monitoring during remission may distinguish a flare from an infectious process (case report #1 below). Although prospective studies are needed to validate this concept, available data demonstrate that prevention of a clinical flare by timely therapeutic intervention improves outcome. Survival in SLE is directly proportional to the number of flares experienced by the patient. Patients with a single flare have almost 100% survival after 10 years, whereas patients who have two or more flares have significantly reduced survival rates.[137]

VI. CASE REPORTS

Case report #1 — A 26-year-old black woman was referred to the Arthritis Center of the University of Illinois with the diagnosis of SLE. Her main complaints were chest pain, photosensitivity, arthralgias of hands, prolonged morning stiffness, insomnia, shortness of breath, and fatigue. She also had symptoms consistent with fibrositis. Her objective manifestations were arthritis, skin rash, alopecia, pleuropericarditis, and occasional fever; trigger points characteristic of fibrositis were also elicited. Significant laboratory changes included: high levels of F-ANA, westergren ESR-62, and chronically reduced levels of C3, C4, and CH50. She responded to steroid treatment. Six months after presentation she developed psoriasis and uveitis. During flares, chiefly polyserositis, her ANA/6 profiles were clearly abnormal (Figure 5A). For about 2 years, her disease was controlled with low-dose prednisone and azathioprine and her autoantibody profile was normal (Figure 5B)

The patient was admitted to the hospital with intensified chest pains, fatigue, and fever. The chest X-ray revealed a pleural effusion and an area of increased density. The clinical impression was another flare with pulmonary involvement. An ANA/8 profile, however, showed no increase in antibody activity (Figure 5B) that would be in keeping with her previous flares (Figure 5A). An infection rather than a lupus flare therefore was considered most likely. She was treated successfully with I.V. antibiotics.

Conclusion: ANA profile testing in SLE may differentiate a flare from an infection.

Case report #2 — A 32-year-old woman (L. W.) was seen at the University of Illinois Arthritis Center for complaints of fatigue, hair loss, night sweats, tremor, weakness, shortness of breath, and palpitations. She also complained of arthralgias, hand swelling, and Raynaud's phenomenon. She was told repeatedly by different clinicians that she had lupus. Past history revealed partial thyroidectomy 10 years ago for "a thyroid nodule". Clinical examination revealed an anxious female with synovitis pri-

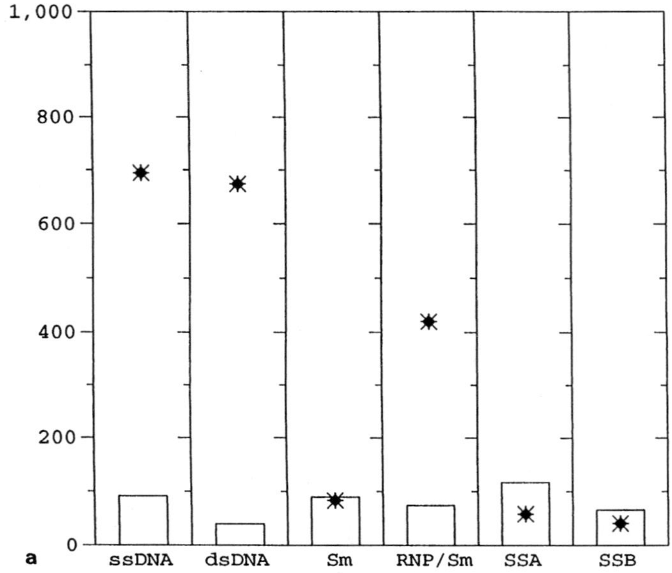

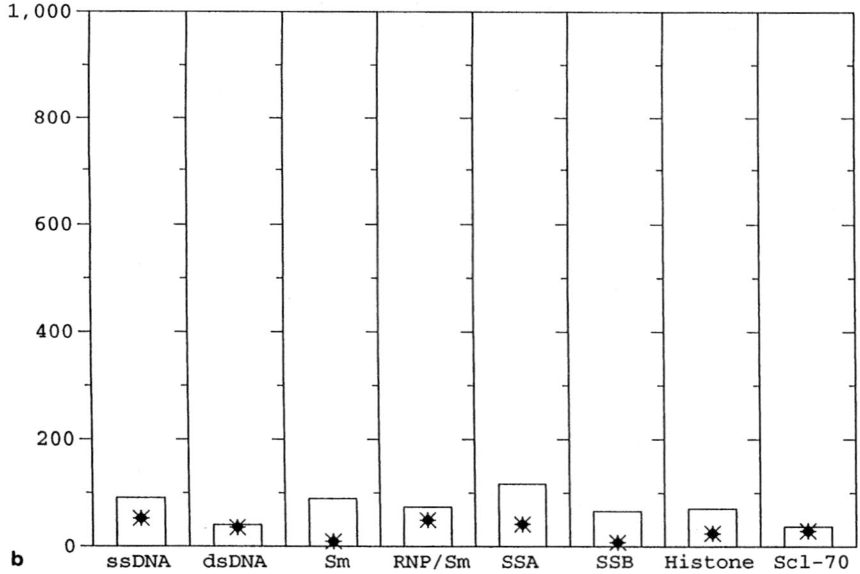

Figure 5 ANA/6 and 8 profiles of patients described as case reports. See text for explanations. Antibodies for each column described in Figure 3.

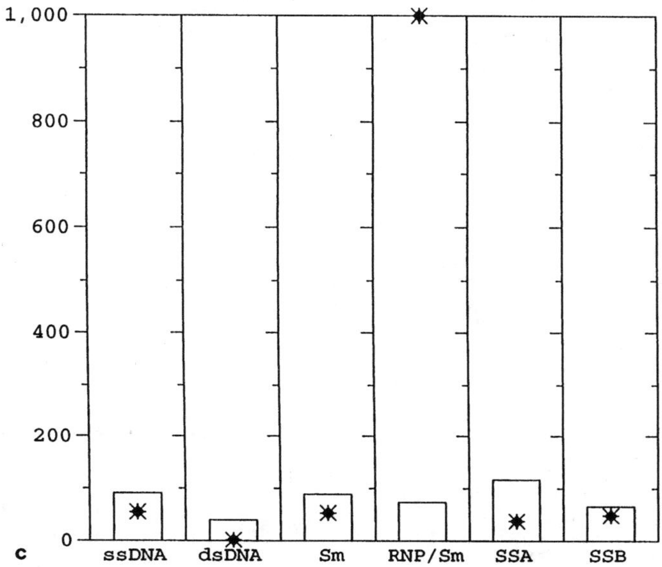

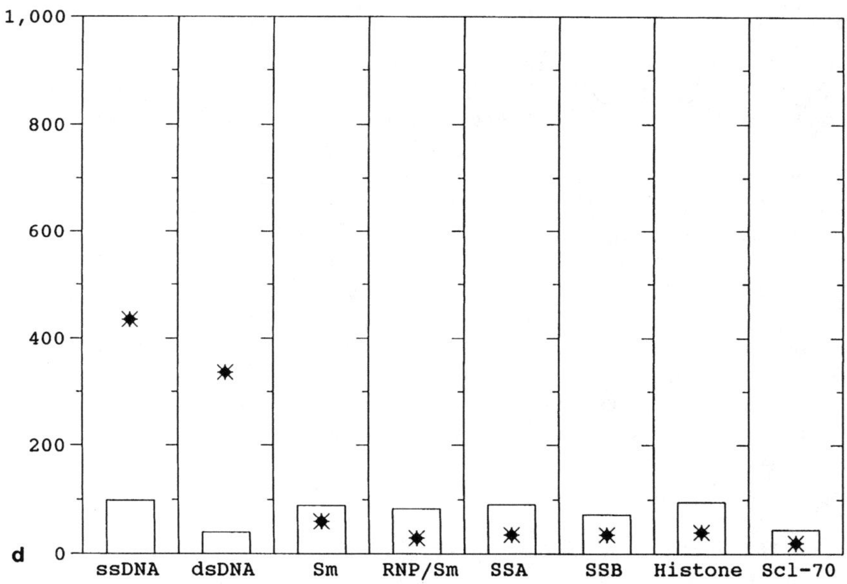

Figure 5 (continued).

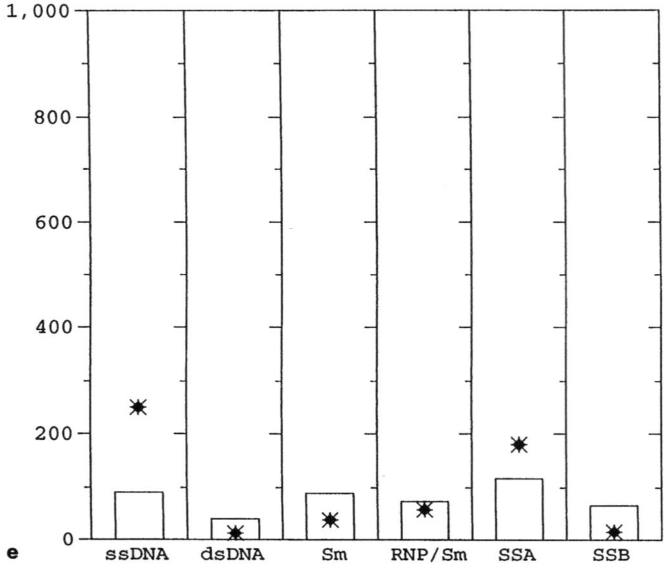

Figure 5 (continued).

marily in her hands and ankles, sausage-like swelling of digits, alopecia, and skin rash. She had proximal muscle weakness and a small nodule in the right lobe of her thyroid. Laboratory showed Hb-10.6, borderline thrombocytopenia, F-ANA - 1:1280 (speckled), and increased thyroxine level (T_4). An ANA/6 profile (Figure 5C) revealed only high levels of anti-RNP. The diagnosis of MCTD and Graves disease was rendered. She was treated with a nonsteroidal anti-inflammatory agent and referred to an endocrinologist.

Before reaching the endocrinologist, the patient, a health care worker, experienced alteration in her mental status and was admitted to a different hospital. There she again volunteered the past history of SLE. Based on the clinical picture and a high-titer F-ANA, a diagnosis of lupus cerebritis was entertained and she was treated with high-dose prednisone and I.V. cyclophosphamide for 3 months. Her clinical manifestations continued to deteriorate and she returned to the Arthritis Center. The steroid/cyclophosphamide treatment was discontinued and she was treated successfully for Graves disease with radioactive iodine. After 2 years she developed scleroderma.

Conclusion: The characteristic ANA ELISA profile of MCTD is particular useful because it displays a high level of anti-RNP and conspicuously lacks other autoantibodies.

Case report #3 — A 54-year-old white man was admitted to the hospital with complaints of skin rash, morning stiffness, and pain in his fingers. Physical examination showed a symmetrical synovitis of metacarpophalangeal joints and a maculopapular rash over arms and legs that subsequently progressed to bullae and necrosis. Laboratory tests demonstrated a normocytic normochromic anemia, and a westergren sedimentation rate of 110/h. Blood urea nitrogen (BUN), serum creatinine, and urinalysis were normal. Rheumatoid factor and F-ANA cryoglobulins were negative. Serum protein electrophoresis showed a normal pattern. Complement (C3, C4, and CH50) were normal. A skin biopsy revealed leukocytoclastic vasculitis with lymphocytic infiltration of thickened dermal capillaries.

During the next 5 days, the arthritis subsided with prednisone (100 mg/day) but the skin lesions persisted. Urinalysis now revealed proteinuria of 6.4 g/24 h, 50 to 100 red blood cells per high-power field and granular casts. Serum creatinine increased from 80 to 354 (nl-133 μmol/l). The F-ANA was repeated in another laboratory and again was "negative". An ANA/6 test showed a profile consistent with SLE (Figure 5D). A kidney biopsy revealed diffuse epithelial proliferation and necrosis as well as mesangial and subendothelial IgA deposits.

An incidental finding was a mediastinal mass; biopsy showed Hodgkin's lymphoma. He was treated with local irradiation and pulse cyclophosphamide and steroids. Thereafter, kidney function, skin lesions, arthritis, and proteinuria rapidly improved. The anti-DNA antibody decreased to normal and increased with subsequent relapses. During the last relapse of nephritis, anti-SSA antibody also increased.

Conclusion: When the probability of SLE is high, testing the F-ANA causes unnecessary delays in diagnosis; only the autoantibody profile is useful (Figure 1). This case offers several distinctive features: (1) association of SLE and Hodgkin's,[138,139] (2) F-ANA nonreactive despite relatively high levels of anti-dsDNA by ELISA (bacteriophage dsDNA) (>200 I.U./ml), and (3) normal complement levels during active renal disease.

Case report #4 — A 12-year-old boy was evaluated by a dermatologist for skin rash, alopecia, photosensitivity, malaise, fatigue, low-grade fever, and arthralgias. The westergren sedimentation rate was elevated (45 mm/h). Rheumatoid factor and F-ANA (Hep-2 cell) were negative. All routine laboratory tests were unremarkable. The skin biopsy was initially interpreted as granulomatous reaction. An ANA/6 showed elevation of anti-ssDNA and anti-SSA consistent with subacute SLE (Figure 5E).

Conclusion: As shown in the algorithm described above (Figure 1), when the clinical suspicion suggests SLE both F-ANA and an ANA profile should be ordered simultaneously.

REFERENCES

1. **Gharavi, A. E., Chu, J.-L., and Elkon, K.,** Autoantibodies to intracellular proteins in human systemic lupus erythematosus are not due to random polyclonal B cell activation, *Arthritis Rheum.,* 31, 1337, 1988.
2. **Tan, E. M.,** Antinuclear antibodies: diagnostic markers for autoimmune diseases and probes for cell biology, *Adv. Immunol.,* 44, 93, 1989.
3. **James, K. and Meek, G.,** Evaluation of commercial enzyme immunoassays compared to immunofluorescence and double diffusion for autoantibodies associated with autoimmune diseases, *Am. J. Clin. Pathol.,* 97, 559, 1992.
4. **Froelich, C. J., Wallman, J., Skosey, J. L., and Teodorescu, M.,** Clinical value of an integrated ELISA system for the detection of 6 autoantibodies (ssDNA, dsDNA, Sm, RNP/Sm, SSA, and SSB), *J. Rheumatol.,* 17, 192, 1990.
5. **Friou, G.,** Clinical application of lupus nucleo-protein reactions using fluorescent antibody technique, *J. Clin. Invest.,* 36, 890, 1957.
6. **Wiik, A.,** The value of specific ANA determination in rheumatology, update 1986, *Allergy,* 42, 241, 1987.
7. **Reichlin, M. and Arnett, F.,** Multiplicity of antibodies in myositis sera, *Arthritis Rheum.,* 27, 1150, 1984.

8. **Westgeest, A. A. A., van den Brink, H. G., de Jong, J., Swaak, A. J. G., and Smeenk, R. J. T.,** Routine testing for antinuclear antibodies: a comparison of immunofluorescence, counterimmunoelectrophoresis, and immunoblotting, *J. Autoimmmun.,* 1, 159, 1988.
9. **Speransky, A. I., Ivanova, M. I., Rjazantceva, T. A., Piven, V. A., and Bulanova, T. D.,** Antinuclear antibodies in lupus erythematosus and Sjogren's syndrome: clinical and immunological investigations, *Scand. J. Rheumatol. Suppl.,* 67, 39, 1988.
10. **Feltkamp, T. E., Janssens, M. B., and Kallenberg, C. G.,** Antinuclear antibody determinations in daily practice, in *Antibodies to Nuclear Antigens,* Kalden, J. R. and Feltkamp, T. E., Ed., Excerpta Medica, Amsterdam, 1982, 11.
11. **Feltkamp, T. E. W., Klein, F., and Janssens, M. B. J. A.,** Standardisation of the quantitative determination of antinuclear antibodies with a homogeneous pattern, *Ann. Rheum. Dis.,* 47, 906, 1988.
12. **Goshen, E., Livne, A., Krupp, M., Hammarstrom, L., Dighiero, G., Slor, H., and Shoenfeld, Y.,** Antinuclear and related autoantibodies in sera of healthy subjects with IgA deficiency, *J. Autoimmun.,* 2, 51, 1989.
13. **Tomer, Y. and Shoenfeld, Y.,** Ageing and autoantibodies, *Autoimmunity,* 1, 141, 1988.
14. **Fields, R. A., Toubbeh, H., Searles, R. P., and Bankhurst, A. D.,** The prevalence of anticardiolipin antibodies in a healthy elderly population and its association with antinuclear antibodies, *J. Rheumatol.,* 16, 623, 1989.
15. **Hooper, B., Whittingham, S., and Mathews, J.,** Autoimmunity in a rural community, *Clin. Exp. Immunol.,* 12, 79, 1972.
16. **Shiel, W. C. and Jason, M.,** Diagnostic associations of patients with antinuclear antibodies referred to community rheumatologist, *J. Rheumatol.,* 16, 782, 1989.
17. **Kallenberg, C. G. M., Wouda, A. A., Hoet, M. H., and Venrooij, W. J. V.,** Development of connective tissue disease in patients presenting with Raynaud's phenomenon: a six year followup with emphasis on the predictive value of antinuclear antibodies as detected by immunoblotting, *Ann. Rheum. Dis.,* 47, 634, 1988.
18. **Francoeur, A.-M.,** Analysis of autoantibody specificities in selected systemic lupus erythematosus sera, *J. Clin. Immunol.,* 9, 248, 1989.
19. **Shapiro, P., McAllister, G., Lerner, E., and Lerner, M.,** Healthy individuals and patients with systemic lupus erythematosus have unique, person-specific spectra of antibodies detectable on immunoblots, *Clin. Immunol. Immunopathol.,* 59, 129, 1991.
20. **Cohen, I. and Young, D.,** Autoimmunity, microbial immunity, and the immunological homunculus, *Immunol. Today,* 12, 105, 1991.
21. **Kioke, T. and Ichikawa, K.,** Proc. 2nd Int. Conf. on SLE, Professional Postgraduate Services Int. U.S.A., U.K., Mexico, Singapore, 1989, 146 pp.
22. **Radic, M., Mascelli, M., Erikson, J., Shan, H., and Weigert, M.,** Ig H and L chain contributions to autoimmune specificities, *J. Immunol.,* 146, 176, 1991.
23. **Fritzler, M. J.,** Antinuclear antibodies in the investigation of rheumatic diseases, *Bull. Rheum. Dis.,* 35, 1, 1985.
24. **Jitsukawa, T., Nakajima, S., Usui, J., and Watanabe, H.,** Detection of antinuclear antibodies from patients with systemic rheumatic diseases using Hep-2 cell nuclei, *J. Clin. Lab. Anal.,* 5, 49, 1991.
25. **Santos, M. E., Lopez, L. R., Jara, L. J., Espinoza, L. R., and La Rosa, F. G.,** Can ELISA have comparable clinical sensitivity for antinuclear antibody determinations, *Lupus,* 1 (S1), 66, 1992.

26. **Vertosick, F. T. and Kelly, R. H.,** Antibodies to native and denatured DNA: quantitation using an immuno-slot-blot technique, *J. Immunol. Meth.*, 102, 15, 1987.
27. **Ruffati, A., Calligaro, A., Del Ross, T., Bertaol, M. T., Doria, A., Rossi, L., and Todesco, S.,** Anti-double-stranded DNA antibodies in the healthy elderly: prevalence and characteristics, *J. Clin. Immunol.*, 10, 300, 1990.
28. **Northway, J. and Tan, E.,** Differentiation of anti-nuclear antibodies giving speckled staining patterns in immunofluorescence, *Clin. Immunol. Immunopathol.*, 1, 140, 1972.
29. **Kurata, N. and Tan, E.,** Identification of antibodies to nuclear acidic antigens by counterimmunoelectrophoresis, *Arthritis Rheum.*, 19, 574, 1976.
30. **Alspaugh, M. and Tan, E.,** Antibodies to cellular antigens in Sjogren's syndrome, *J. Clin. Invest.*, 55, 1067, 1975.
31. **Hollingsworth, P. N., Bonifacio, E., and Dawkins, R. I.,** Use of standard curve improves precision and concordance of ANA measurement, *J. Clin. Lab. Immunol.*, 22, 197, 1987.
32. **Douvas, A., Achten, A., and Tan, E.,** Identification of a nuclear protein (Scl-70) as a unique target of human antinuclear antibodies, *J. Biol. Chem.*, 254, 1051, 1979.
33. **Reichlin, M. and Reichlin, M. W.,** Autoantibodies to the Ro/SSA particle react preferentially with the human antigen, in *Sjogren's Syndrome: A Model for Understanding Autoimmunity.*, Talal, N., Ed., Academic Press, New York, 1989, 51.
34. **Provost, T. T., Levin, L., Watson, R., Mayo, M., and Ratrie, H., III,** Detection of anti-Ro (SSA) antibodies by gel double diffusion and a 'sandwich' ELISA in systemic and subacute cutaneous lupus erythematosus and Sjogren's syndrome, *J. Autoimmun.*, 4, 87, 1991.
35. **Kyriatsoulis, A., Manns, M., Roth, U., Gerken, G., Lohse, A., Wollensak, S., Reske, K., and Meyer zum Buschenfelde, K.-H.,** Strategy for the characterization of autoantigens in autoimmune disease: investigation of the target antigens of antimitochondrial antibodies by RIA, immunoblotting, monoclonoal antibodies and affinity chromatography, *J. Immunol. Meth.*, 109, 113, 1988.
36. **Habets, W. J. A., Hoet, M. H., Sillkens, P. T. G., de Rooij, D. J. M., van de Putte, L. B. A., and van Venrooij, W. J.,** Detection of autoantibodies in a quantitative ELISA using recombinant ribonucleoprotein antigens, *Clin. Exp. Immunol.*, 76, 172, 1989.
37. **Hines, J. J., Danho, W., and Elkon, K. B.,** Detection and quantification of human anti-Sm antibodies using synthetic peptide and recombinant SmB antigens, *Arthritis Rheum.*, 34, 572, 1991.
38. **Burghardt, T. and Axelrod, D.,** Total internal reflection fluorescence study of energy transfer in surface-adsorbed and dissolved bovine serum albumin, *Biochemistry,* 22, 979, 1983.
39. **Sabbaga, J., Pankewycz, O. G., Lufft, V., Schwartz, R. S., and Madaio, M. P.,** Cross-reactivity distinguishes serum and nephritogenic anti-DNA antibodies in human lupus from their natural counterparts in normal serum, *J. Autoimmun.*, 3, 215, 1990.
40. **Preud'homme, J. I., Rochard, E., Gouet, D., Danon, F., Alcalay, M., Touchard, G., and Aucouturier, P.,** Isotypic distribution of anti-dsDNA antibodies: a diagnostic evaluation by ELISA, *Diag. Clin. Immunol.*, 5, 256, 1988.
41. **Winfield, J., Faiferman, I., and Koffler, D.,** Avidity of anti-DNA antibodies in serum and glomerular eluates from patients with SLE, *J. Clin. Invest.*, 59, 90, 1977.

42. **Peterfy, F., Kuusela, P., and Makela, O.,** Contribution of antibody affinity in the determination of antibody reactions by different immunoassays, *J. Immunol.*, 130, 1809, 1983.
43. **Steward, M. W. and Lew, A. M.,** The importance of antibody affinity in the performance of immunoassay for antibody, *J. Immunol. Meth.*, 78, 173, 1985.
44. **Steward, M. and Steensgaard, J.,** *Antibody Affinity, Thermodynamic Aspects and Biological Significance,* CRC Press, Boca Raton, FL, 1983.
45. **Rothfield, N. and Stollar, B.,** The relation of Ig class pattern of ANA and complement fixing antibodies to DNA in sera from patients with SLE, *J. Clin. Invest.*, 46, 1785, 1967.
46. **Tan, E., Cohen, A., Fries, J., Masi, A., McShane, D., Rothfield, N., Schaller, J., Talal, N., and Winchester, R.,** The 1982 revised criteria for the classification of systemic lupus erythematosus, *Arthritis Rheum.*, 25, 1271, 1982.
47. **Gripenberg, M., Linder, E., Kurki, P., and Engvall, E.,** A solid phase enzyme-linked immunoabsorbent assay (ELISA) for the demonstration of antibodies against ssDNA in patient sera, *Scand. J. Immunol.*, 7, 151, 1978.
48. **Albani, S., Massa, M., Vioila, S., Pellegrini, G., and Martini, A.,** Antibody reactivity against single stranded DNA of various species in normal children and in children with diffuse connective tissue diseases, *Autoimmunity,* 8, 77, 1990.
49. **Misra, R., Malaviya, A. N., Kumar, R., and Kumar, A.,** Clinical relevance of the estimation of antibodies to single stranded DNA in SLE, *Indian J. Med. Res.*, 87, 463, 1988.
50. **Koffler, D., Agnello, V., and Winchester, R.,** Occurrence of single-stranded DNA in serum of patients with SLE and other diseases, *J. Clin. Invest.*, 52, 198, 1973.
51. **Nakamura, R. M., Peebles, C., Rubin, R., Molden, D., and Tan, E. M.,** *Autoantibodies to Nuclear Antigens (ANA),* American Society of Clinical Pathologists, New York, 1985.
52. **Leon, S., Green, A., Ehrlich, G., Poland, M., and Shapiro, B.,** Avidity of antibodies in SLE: relation to severity of renal involvement, *Arthritis Rheum.*, 20, 23, 1977.
53. **Halliday, M., Salaman, M. R., Seifert, M. H., Johnson, K. J., and Malcolm, J.,** Evaluation of an ELISA system for determination of class-specific antibodies to dsDNA and ssDNA in man, *Ann. Rheum. Dis.*, 44, 507, 1985.
54. **Devey, M. E., Lee, S. R., LePage, S., Feldman, R., and Isenberg, D. A.,** Serial studies of IgG subclass and functional affinity of anti-dsDNA antibodies in systemic lupus erythematosus, *J. Autoimmun.*, 1, 483, 1988.
55. **LePage, S. H., Dudney, C., Shall, S., Shoenfeld, Y., and Isenberg, D. A.,** Disease specificity of antibodies to poly(ADP ribose): their relationships to anti-DNA antibodies and to disease activity in SLE, *Autoimmunity,* 169, 177, 1990.
56. **Monier, J. C., Sault, C., and Bringuier, J. P.,** Discrepancies between 2 procedures for dsDNA antibody detection: Farr test and indirect immunofluorescence on *Crithidia luciliae, J. Clin. Lab. Immunol.*, 25, 149, 1988.
57. **Deng, J.-S., Sontheimer, R. D., Lipscomb, M. F., and Gilliam, J. N.,** The binding of anti-histone antibodies to *Crithidia luciliae* kinetoplasts is growth cycle dependent, *Arthritis Rheum.*, 28, 163, 1985.
58. **Tipping, P. G., Buchanan, R. R. C., Riglar, A. G., and Dimech, W. J.,** Detection of anti-DNA antibodies: a comparison between two Farr assays, *Crithidia luciliae* and a human chromosomal substrate assay, *Br. J. Rheumatol.*, 27, 206, 1988.

59. **Henderson, T., Medsger, T. A., Sontheimer, R. D., Harmon, C. E., and Deng, J. S.,** Specificity of the hydrochloric-acid-modified *Crithidia luciliae* immunofluorescence assay for detection of anti-dsDNA, *Diag. Clin. Immunol.*, 5, 20, 1987.
60. **Aarden, L., de Groot, E., and Feltkamp, T.,** Immunology of DNA. III. *Crithidia luciliae,* a simple substrate for the determination of anti-dsDNA with immunofluorescent technique, *Ann. N.Y. Acad. Sci.*, 254, 505, 1975.
61. **Rauch, J., Massicotte, H., Wild, J., and Tannebaum, H.,** Sensitive solid phase radioimmunoassay (RIA) for the detection of anti-dsDNA autoantibodies, *J. Rheumatol.*, 12, 482, 1985.
62. **Burdash, N., Teti, G., and Papadopoulos, V.,** The *Crithidia luciliae* and Farr assay for the detection of systemic lupus erythematosus, *Ann. Clin. Lab. Sci.*, 13, 49, 1983.
63. **Kavai, M., Banyai, A., Zsindely, A., Sonkoly, I., and Szegedi, G.,** ELISA for antibodies to dsDNA on sera of SLE, *J. Immunol. Meth.*, 48, 169, 1982.
64. **Turner Stokes, L.,** Meeting report: methods of detection and clinical relevance of anti-DNA/ENA antibodies, *Autoimmunity,* 1, 317, 1988.
65. **Eilat, D.,** The measurement of anti-DNA activity in the sera of patients with systemic lupus erythematosus: theoretical and practical considerations, *Autoimmunity,* 3, 299, 1989.
66. **Moses, S. and Barland, P.,** Laboratory criteria for a diagnosis of systemic lupus erythematosus, *JAMA,* 242, 1039, 1979.
67. **Isenberg, D. A., Dudney, C., Williams, W., Addison, I., Charles, S., Clarke, J., and Todd-Pokropek, T.,** Measurement of anti-DNA antibodies: a reappraisal using five different methods, *Ann. Rheum. Dis.*, 46, 448, 1987.
68. **Sarvas, H., Gripenberg, M., and Lerissalo-Repo, M.,** Anti-DNA antibodies: the choice of assays for routine diagnostic work, *Acta Pathol., Microbiol. Immunol. Scand.*, 93, 13, 1985.
69. **Valentijin, R. M., van Overhagen, H., Hazevot, H. M., Hermans, J., Cats, A., Daha, M. R., and van Es, L. A.,** The value of complement and immune complex determinations in monitoring disease activity in patients with systemic lupus erythematosus, *Arthritis Rheum.*, 28, 904, 1985.
70. **Preud'homme, J. I., Danon, F., Rochard, E., Gouet, D., Touchard, G., Aucouturier, P., and Alcalay, M.,** Measurement of anti-dsDNA antibodies by an immunoglobulin class-specific ELISA: comparison with the Farr assay and indirect immunofluorescence, *Presse Med.*, 17, 1401, 1988.
71. **Kumar, V., Krasny, S., and Beutner, E. H.,** Specificity of the *Crithidia luciliae* method for detecting anti-DNA antibodies. Effect of absorption for lipoproteins, *Immunol. Invest.*, 14, 199, 1985.
72. **Orr, K. B. and Foerster, J.,** An ELISA procedure to detect anti-double stranded and anti-single stranded DNA binding antibodies in connective tissue disorders, *J. Clin. Lab. Anal.*, 4, 328, 1990.
73. **Maddison, P. J., Skinner, R. P., Vlachoyiannopoulos, P., Brennand, D. M., and Hough, D.,** Antibodies to nRNP, Sm, Ro(SSA) and La(SSB) detected by ELISA: their specificity and inter-relations in connective tissue disease sera, *Clin. Exp. Immunol.*, 62, 337, 1985.
74. **Buchanan, R., Venables, P., Morgan, A., Stains, N., Smith, P., and Maini, R.,** Separation of two species of the Sm antigen by affinity chromatography with murine monoclonal and human antinuclear antibodies, *Clin. Exp. Immunol.*, 51, 8, 1983.

75. **Field, M., Williams, D. G., Charles, P., and Maini, R. N.,** Specificity of anti-Sm antibodies by ELISA for systemic lupus erythematosus: increased sensitivity of detection using purified peptide antigens, *Ann. Rheum. Dis.*, 47, 820, 1988.
76. **Lazaro, M., Cocco, J., Catoggio, L., Babini, S., Messina, O., and Morteo, O.,** Clinical and serologic characteristics of patients with overlap syndrome: is mixed connective tissue disease a distinct clinical entity?, *Medicine (Baltimore)*, 68, 58, 1989.
77. **Boey, M. L., Peebles, C. L., Tsay, G., Feng, P. H., and Tan, E. M.,** Clinical and autoantibody correlations in orientals with systemic lupus erythematosus, *Ann. Rheum. Dis.*, 47, 918, 1988.
78. **Arnett, F., Hamilton, R. G., Roebber, M. G., Harley, J. B., and Reichlin, M.,** Increased frequencies of Sm and nRNP autoantibodies in American blacks compared to whites with systemic lupus erythematosus, *J. Rheumatol.*, 15, 1773, 1988.
79. **Guldner, H., Lakomek, H., Szostecki, C., and Bautz, F.,** Autoantibody profiles in patients with SLE, scleroderma, and overlap syndromes, *Scand. J. Immunol.*, 56, 287, 1985.
80. **Sharp, G., Irvin, W., Tan, E., Gould, R., and Holman, H.,** Mixed connective tissue disease: an apparently distinct rheumatic disease syndrome associated with a specific antibody to an extractable nuclear antigen, *Am. J. Med.*, 52, 148, 1972.
81. **Kasukawa, T.,** Diagnostic criteria for MCTD, *Adv. Immunol.*, 21, 1989.
82. **Maddison, P. J., Isenberg, D. A., Goulding, N. J., Leddy, J., and Skinner, R. P.,** Anti-SSB identifies a distinctive subgroup of systemic lupus erythematosus, *Br. J. Rheumatol.*, 27, 27, 1988.
83. **Harley, J., Yamagata, H., and Reichlin, M.,** Anti-La(SSB) antibody is present in some normal sera and is coincident with Ro (SSA) precipitins in SLE, *J. Rheumatol.*, 11, 309, 1984.
84. **Mamula, M., Siverman, E., Laxer, R., Bentur, L., Isacovics, B., and Hardin, J.,** Human monoclonal anti-La antibodies: the La protein resides on a subset of Ro particles, *J. Immunol.*, 143, 2923, 1989.
85. **Boire, G. and Craft, J.,** Human Ro ribonucleoprotein particles: characterization of native structure and stable association with the La polypeptide, *J. Clin. Invest.*, 85, 1182, 1990.
86. **Ramos-Neimbo, F. and Alarcon-Segovia, D.,** Development of Sicca symptoms in systemic lupus erythematosus patients with existing subclinical abnormalities of lacrimal and/or salivary glands, *Arthritis Rheum.*, 22, 935, 1979.
87. **Scopelitis, E., Biundo, J., and Alspaugh, M.,** Anti-SSA antibody and other antinuclear antibodies in SLE, *Arthritis Rheum.*, 23, 287, 1980.
88. **Maddison, P., Provost, T., and Reichlin, M.,** Serologic findings in patients with "ANA" negative lupus, *Medicine (Baltimore)*, 60, 87, 1981.
89. **Wasicek, C. and Reichlin, M.,** Clinical and serological differences between SLE patients with antibodies to Ro and La, *J. Clin. Invest.*, 69, 835, 1982.
90. **Weiss, R., Mogavers, H., Synkowski, D., and Provost, T.,** Diagnostic tests and clinical subsets in SLE, *Ann. Allergy*, 51, 135, 1983.
91. **Harley, J., Reichlin, M., Arnett, F., Alexander, E., Bias, W., and Provost, T.,** Gene interactions at HLA-DR worsens the serologic abnormalities of primary Sjogren's syndrome, *Arthritis Rheum.*, 29, 538, 1986.
92. **Maddison, P. and Reichlin, M.,** Deposition of antibodies to a soluble cytoplasmic antigen in the kidneys of patients with SLE, *Arthritis Rheum.*, 22, 858, 1979.

93. **Gohill, J., Cary, P., Couppez, M., and Fritzler, M.,** Antibodies from patients with drug-induced and idiopathic lupus react with epitopes restricted to the amino and carboxy termini of histone, *J. Immunol.,* 135, 3116, 1985.
94. **Franco, H., Weston, W., Peebles, C., Forstot, S., and Phanuphak, P.,** Autoantibodies directed against Sicca syndrome antigens in the neonatal lupus syndrome, *J. Am. Acad. Dermatol.,* 4, 67, 1981.
95. **Furaukawa, F., Kashihara-Sawami, M., Lyons, M., and Norris, D.,** Binding of autoantibodies to the extractable nuclear antigens SSA/Ro and SSB/La is induced on the surface of human keratinocytes by ultraviolet light: implications for the pathogenesis of photosensitive cutaneous lupus, *J. Invest. Dermatol.,* 94, 77, 1990.
96. **Provost, T.,** Neonatal lupus, *Arch. Dermatol.,* 4, 67, 1983.
97. **Woolsey, R., Drager, D., Reidenberg, M., Nies, A., Carr, K., and Oates, J.,** Effects of acetylator phenotype on the rate at which procainamide induces antinuclear antibodies and the lupus syndrome, *N. Engl. J. Med.,* 298, 1157, 1987.
98. **Fritzler, M. J. and Tan, E.,** Antibodies to histone in drug-induced and idiopathic lupus erythematosus, *J. Clin. Invest.,* 62, 550, 1978.
99. **Rubin, R., Joslin, F., and Tan, E.,** A solid-phase radioimmunoassay for antihistone antibodies in human sera: comparison with immunofluorescence, *Scand. J. Immunol.,* 15, 63, 1982.
100. **Aitkaci, A., Monier, J., and Mamelle, N.,** Enzyme-linked immunosorbent assay for anti-histone antibodies and their presence in SLE sera, *J. Immunol. Meth.,* 44, 311, 1981.
101. **Fellows, G., Gottoes, N., Scott, D. G. I., Coppock, J. S., Wainwright, A., Goodall, M., and Turner, B. M.,** Individual variation in the isotype profile of antihistone autoantibodies in systemic lupus erythematosus, *Clin. Exp. Immunol.,* 72, 440, 1988.
102. **Gioud, M., Aitkaci, M., and Monier, J. C.,** Histone antibodies in systemic lupus erythematosus, *Arthritis Rheum.,* 35, 407, 1982.
103. **Rubin, W. and Waga, S.,** Anti-histone antibodies in systemic lupus erythematosus, *J. Rheumatol.,* 14(S-3), 118, 1987.
104. **Totoriis, M., Tan, E., McNally, E., and Rubin, R.,** Association of anti-histone (H2A-H2B) complex antibody with symptomatic procainamide-induced lupus erythematosus, *N. Engl. J. Med.,* 318, 1431, 1988.
105. **Juarez, C., Vila, J. L., and Gelpi, C.,** Characterization of the antigen reactive with Scl-70 antibodies and its application in an ELISA, *Arthritis Rheum.,* 31, 108, 1988.
106. **D'Arpa, P., Coper, H. W., and Cleveland, D.,** Use of molecular cloning methods to map the distribution of epitopes on Scl-70, *Arthritis Rheum.,* 33, 1501, 1990.
107. **Maul, G., Jimenez, S., and Riggs, E.,** Determination of an epitope of diffuse systemic sclerosis marker antigen DNA topoisomerase I: sequence similarity with retroviral p30 gag protein suggests a possible cause for autoimmunity in systemic sclerosis, *Proc. Natl. Acad. Sci. U.S.A.,* 86, 8492, 1989.
108. **Hillebrandt, S., Weiner, E., Senecal, J., and Rothfield, N.,** Autoantibodies to topoisomerase I (Scl-70): analysis by gel diffusion, immunoblot, and ELISA, *Clin. Immunol. Immunopathol.,* 57, 399, 1990.
109. **Earnshaw, W. and Rothfield, N.,** Identification of a family of human centromere proteins using autoimmune sera from scleroderma patients, *Chromosoma,* 91, 313, 1985.
110. **Rothfield, N., Whitaker, D., and Bordwell, B.,** Detection of anti-centromere antibodies using the cloned autoantigen, CENP-B, *Arthritis Rheum.,* 30, 1416, 1987.

111. **Weiner, E., Earnshaw, W., Senecal, J., Rothfield, N., Medsger, H., and Steen, V.,** Clinical associations of anti-centromere antibodies and antibodies to topoisomerase I: a study of 355 patients, *Arthritis Rheum.*, 31, 378, 1988.
112. **Venning, M. C., Quinn, A., Broomhead, V., and Bird, A. G.,** Antibodies directed against neutrophils (C-ANCA and P-ANCA) are of distinct diagnostic value in systemic vasculitis, *Q. J. Med.*, 77, 1287, 1990.
113. **Savige, J. A., Gallicchio, M., Georgiou, T., and Davies, D. J.,** Diverse target antigens recognized by circulating antibodies in anti-neutrophil cytoplasm antibody-associated renal vasculitides, *Clin. Exp. Immunol.*, 82, 238, 1990.
114. **Savage, C. O. S., Pottinger, B. E., Gaskin, G., Pusey, C. D., and Pearson, J. D.,** Autoantibodies developing to myeloperoxidase and proteinase 3' in systemic vasculitis stimulate neutrophil cytotoxicity toward cultured endothelial cells, *Am. J. Pathol.*, 141, 335, 1992.
115. **Jayne, D. R. W., Weetman, A. P., and Lockwood, C. M.,** IgG subclass distribution of autoantibodies to neutrophil cytoplasmic antigens in systemic vasculitis, *Clin. Exp. Immunol.*, 84, 476, 1991.
116. **Bini, P., Gabay, J. E., Teitel, A., Melchior, M., Zhou, J.-L., and Elkon, K. B.,** Antineutrophil cytoplasmic autoantibodies in Wegener's granulomatosis recognize conformational epitope(s) on proteinase 3, *J. Immunol.*, 149, 1409, 1992.
117. **Goeken, J. A.,** Antineutrophil cytoplasmic antibody — a useful serological marker for vasculitis, *J. Clin. Immunol.*, 11, 161, 1991.
118. **Gross, W. L., Schmitt, W. H., and Csernock, E.,** Antineutrophil cytoplasmic autoantibody-associated diseases: a rheumatologist's perspective, *Am. J. Kidney Dis.*, 18, 175, 1991.
119. **Lawton, J. W. M. and Lee, S. S.,** Anti-neutrophil cytoplasmic antibodies in SLE, *Am. J. Kidney Dis.*, 18 (Abstr.), 201, 1991.
120. **Hannested, R., Rekvig, O., and Husebekk, A.,** Cross reacting rheumatoid factors and lupus (LE) factors, *Springer Semin. Immunopathol.*, 4, 133, 1981.
121. **Lassoued, S., Sixou, L., Oksman, F., Pages, M., and Fournie, A.,** Antineutrophil cytoplasmic antibodies and antibodies to myeloperoxidase in rheumatoid arthritis, *Arthritis Rheum.*, 34, 1069, 1991.
122. **Cronin, M. E., Leair, D. W., Jaronski, S., and Lightfoot, R. W.,** Simultaneous use of multiple serologic tests in assessing clinical activity in systemic lupus erythematosus, *Clin. Immunol. Immunopathol.*, 51, 99, 1989.
123. **Swaak, A. J. G., Aarden, L. A., Statius van Eps, L. W., and Feltkamp, T. E. W.,** Anti-dsDNA and complement profiles as prognostic guides in systemic lupus erythematosus, *Arthritis Rheum.*, 22, 226, 1979.
124. **Isenberg, D. A., Dudney, C., Williams, W., Todd-Pokropek, T., and Stollar, B. D.,** Disease activity in systemic lupus erythematosus related to range of antibodies binding DNA and synthetic polynucleotides, *Ann. Rheum. Dis.*, 47, 717, 1988.
125. **Nossent, J. C., Huysen, V., Smeenk, R. J. T., and Swaak, A. J. G.,** Low avidity anti-dsDNA antibodies as a diagnostic tool, *Ann. Rheum. Dis.*, 48, 677, 1989.
126. **Ward, M. M., Pisetsky, D. S., and Christenson, V. D.,** Anti-dsDNA antibody assays in systemic lupus erythematosus: correlations of longitudinal antibody measurements, *J. Rheumatol.*, 16, 609, 1989.
127. **ter Borg, E., Horst, G., Hummel, E., Limburg, P., and Kallenberg, C. G. M.,** Predictive value of rises in double-stranded DNA antibody levels for disease exacerbations in SLE: a long term prospective study, *Arthritis Rheum.*, 33, 634, 1990.

128. **ter Borg, E., Horst, G., Hummel, E., Limburg, P., and Kallenberg, C. G. M.,** Rises in anti-double stranded DNA antibody levels prior to exacerbations of systemic lupus erythematosus are not merely due to polyclonal B cell activation, *Clin. Immunol. Immunopathol.*, 59, 117, 1991.
129. **Combe, B., Rucheton, M., Graafland, H., Lussiez, V., Brunel, C., and Sany, J.,** Clinical significance of anti-RNP and anti-Sm autoantibodies as determined by immunoblotting and immunoprecipitation in sera from patients with connective tissue diseases, *Clin. Exp. Immunol.*, 75, 18, 1989.
130. **ter Borg, E., Horst, G., Limburg, P., and Kallenberg, C. G. M.,** Shifts of anti-Sm specific antibodies in patients with systemic lupus erythematosus: analysis by counter-immunoelectrophoresis, immunoblotting, and RNA-immunoprecipitation, *J. Autoimmun.*, 4, 155, 1991.
131. **Yasuma, M., Takasaki, Y., Matsumoto, K., Kodama, A., Hashimoto, H., and Horose, S.-I.,** Clinical significance of IgG anti-Sm antibodies in patients with SLE, *J. Rheumatol.*, 17, 469, 1990.
132. **Dau, J., Callahan, J., Parker, R., and Golbus, J.,** Immunologic effects of plasmapheresis synchronized with pulse cyclophosphamide in SLE, *J. Rheumatol.*, 18, 270, 1991.
133. **ter Borg, E., Horst, G., Limburg, P., van Venrooij, W., and Kallenberg, C. G. M.,** Changes in levels of antibodies against the 70kDa and A polypeptides of the U1RNP complex in relation to exacerbations of systemic lupus erythematosus, *J. Rheumatol.*, 18, 363, 1991.
134. **Takeda, Y., Wang, G. S., Wang, R. J., Anderson, S. K., Pettersson, I., Amaki, S., and Sharp, G.,** ELISA using isolated (U) small nuclear ribonucleoprotein polypeptides as antigens to investigate the clinical significance of autoantibodies to these polypeptides, *Clin. Immunol. Immunopathol.*, 50, 213, 1989.
135. **Houtman, P., Kallenberg, C. G. M., Limborg, T., van Rijswijk, M., and The, T.,** Are anti-nRNP levels specific guides for assessing disease activity in patients with mixed connective tissue disease?, in *Protides of the Biological Fluids,* Peters, H., Ed., Pergamon Press, Oxford, 1985, 357.
136. **Venables, P., Smith, P., and Maini, R.,** Purification and characterization of the Sjogren's syndrome A and B antigens, *Clin. Exp. Immunol.*, 54, 731, 1983.
137. **Swaak, A. J. G., Nossent, J. C., Bronsveld, W., van Rooyen, A., Nieuwenhuys, E. J., Theuns, L., and Smeenk, R. J. T.,** Systemic lupus erythematosus. I. Outcome and survival: Dutch experience with 110 patients studied prospectively, *Ann. Rheum. Dis.*, 48, 447, 1989.
138. **Houssiau, F. A., Kirkove, C., and Asherson, R. A.,** Malignant lymphoma in systemic rheumatic diseases. A report of five cases, *Clin. Exp. Rheumatol.*, 9, 515, 1991.
139. **Nielsen, L. B., Missal, M. E., and Condemi, J. J.,** Appearance of Hodgkin's disease in a patient with systemic lupus erythematosus, *Cancer,* 20, 1930, 1967.
140. **Froelich, C. et al.,** unpublished observation.

IV. Complement and Immune Complexes

Chapter 8

Complement Cascade and Activation by Immune Complexes

Linda Cook

CONTENTS

I. INTRODUCTION

The complement system was originally recognized as a group of proteins that functioned together to mediate cell lysis.[1] Subsequent research, however, has shown that this system encompasses a large number of proteins and polypeptide fragments that participate in a variety of biological activities[2] (see Tables 1 and 2). Operationally, complement proteins can be divided into five groups: (1) proteins of the classical pathway, (2) proteins of the alternate pathway, (3) the membrane lysis complex, (4) regulatory proteins, either soluble or cell bound, and (5) complement receptor proteins that bind complement cleavage products. In addition, complement fragments generated through activation of the proteolytic cascade mediate numerous biologic processes through receptor-ligand interactions.

A number of laboratory assays have been designed to measure the serum or fluid concentration of complement proteins,[2] to measure their functional activity, or to detect activation complexes.[3] These assays can be used to detect activation of the complement system in a variety of clinical conditions and to monitor clinical autoimmune and immunodeficiency diseases.[4]

II. CLASSICAL PATHWAY OF ACTIVATION

Complement activation of the classical pathway generally is initiated by immune complexes. The acute-phase reactant C-reactive protein (CRP), behaving like an immunoglobulin molecule, may also trigger the cascade. The classical activation proteins are C1q, C1r, C1s, C2, C4, and C3 (Figure 1). Following antigen interaction, the antibody molecule, either IgG1, IgG2, IgG4, or IgM, undergoes a conformational change that exposes the C1q binding site in the Fc region of the heavy chain. Bound C1q becomes activated and generates proteolytic activity in the C1r molecule. C1r then cleaves C1s generating the first major enzyme in the complement system, C1 Esterase. Two C1r, two C1s, and a C1q molecule form C1 esterase. C1 esterase then cleaves C2 and C4

0-8493-5974-1/94/$0.00+$.50

Table 1 **Proteins of the Complement System**

Classical Pathway	Alternate Pathway
C1q	C3
C1r	Factor B
C1s	Factor D
C4	Properdin
C2	
C3	

Terminal Components	Regulatory Proteins
C5	C1 INH
C6	C4 binding protein
C7	Factor I
C8	Factor H
C9	Anaphylatoxin inactivator
	Vitronectin (S)

Table 2 **Cell Membrane Complement Receptor Proteins**

Protein	C′ Bound Protein	Protein Function	Cell Type
CR1	C3b, C4b, iC3b	Control of C3 breakdown immune complex binding	PMNs, RBCs, lymphocytes, monocytes, macrophages, dendritic cells, glomerular podocytes, eosinophils
CR2	C3d, C3dg, C3b, iC3b	Regulation of B cell EBV receptor	Lymphocytes, thymocytes, dendritic cells, NK cells
CR3	iC3b, C3d	Mediates phagocytosis, enhances Ab synthesis	PMNs, monocytes, macrophages, NK cells, dendritic cells, cytotoxic T cells
CR4	iC3b, C3dg	Unknown	PMNs, monocytes, macrophages, NK cells, cytotoxic T cells
MCP	C3b, C4b, iC3b	Control of C3 cleavage	PMNs, lymphocytes, monocytes, platelets, endothelial cells, epithelial cells, fibroblasts

Table 2 **Cell Membrane Complement Receptor Proteins (Continued)**

Protein	C′ Bound Protein	Protein Function	Cell Type
DAF	C4b2a, C3bBb	Decay of C3 and C5 convertase	PMNs, lymphocytes, monocytes, platelets, endothelial cells, epithelial cells, fibroblasts, erythrocytes
p150,95	iC3b, C3b	Unknown	Unknown
C3a/C4a R	C3a, C4a	Binding anaphylatoxin	PMNs, mast cells, macrophages, basophils, eosinophils, T cells
C5a R	C5a, C5a-des-arg	Binding anaphylatoxin	PMNs, mast cells, macrophages, monocytes
C3e R	C3e	Release of PMNs from marrow	PMNs, monocytes
C1q R	C1q	Unknown	PMNs, B cells, monocytes, macrophages, platelets, fibroblasts, lymphocytes
Factor H R	H	Unknown	PMNs, B cells, macrophages
Factor B R	Ba, Bb	Unknown	PMNs, B cells, macrophages

EBV, Epstein Barr virus; PMN, polymorphonuclear leukocytes; RBCs, red blood cells; NK, natural killer cell.

molecules whose major cleavage products form C4b2a or C3 convertase. The C4b2a complex is a magnesium-dependent serine protease which then cleaves the C3 protein, generating C3b and C3a fragments. C3b combines with C4b2a to produce the trimolecular complex C4b2a3b (C5 convertase activity). The C5 convertase activates the lytic function of the complement system (i.e., the membrane attack complex). This pathway is subject to amplification inasmuch as C1qrs and C4b2a3b cleave multiple C4 and C3 molecules. C3 and C4 molecules contain labile thioester bonds. When these bonds are cleaved, the sulfhydryl groups form covalent amide or ester linkage with adjacent cell surface proteins and carbohydrates. This reaction anchors the C4b2a3b complex to the membrane and ensures that the subsequent steps of the complement cascade focus at this site.

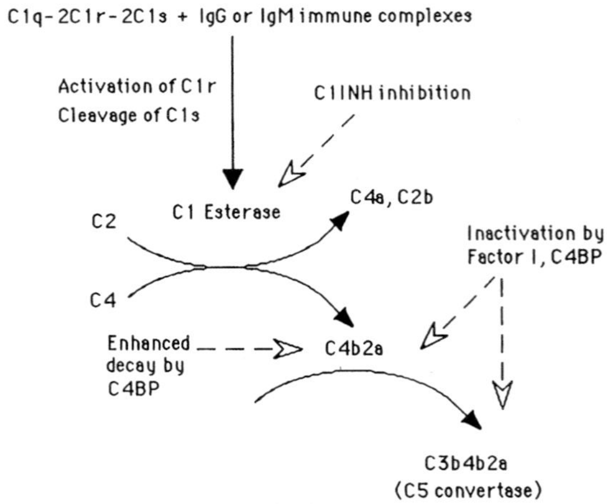

Figure 1 The classical pathway of activation.

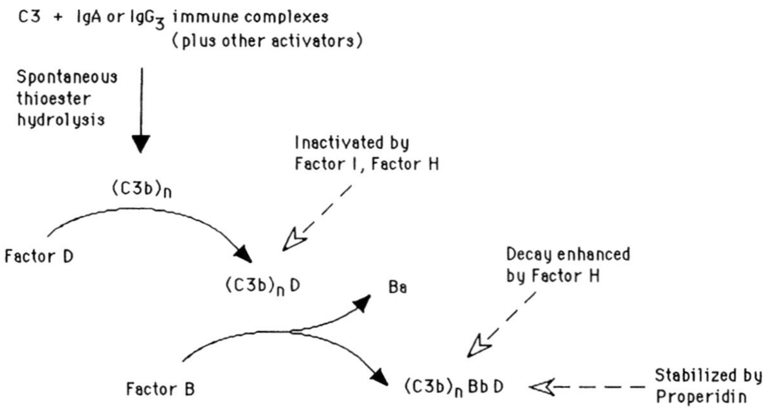

Figure 2 The alternate pathway of activation.

III. ALTERNATE PATHWAY OF ACTIVATION

The proteins of the alternate pathway are factors B, D, and C3 (Figure 2). Alternate pathway activation is initiated by the interaction of C3 with IgA or IgG3 immune complexes. Polysaccharides or lipopolysaccharide structures on the surface of fungi, bacteria, and viral-infected cells initiate activation. The interaction of C3 with repetitive molecular structures yields spontaneous hydrolysis of the thioester bond, converting C3 to a C3b-like molecule. The C3b-like molecule then interacts with factor D to cleave factor B, creating the fragment Bb. Stabilized by magnesium and Properdin, the Bb fragment then combines with C3b to form a complex ($[C3bBb]_n$) that is functionally comparable to C3 convertase. The C3 convertase then cleaves additional C3 molecules, which also bind factor B, ultimately forming the C5 convertase.

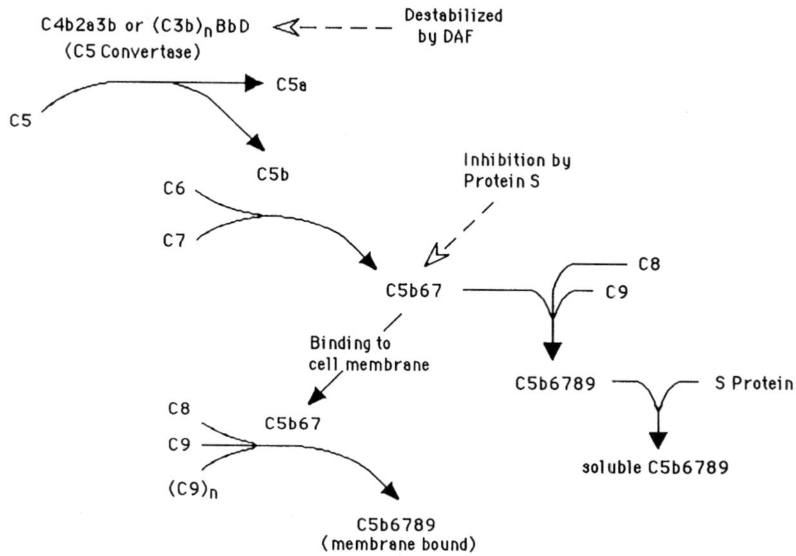

Figure 3 The terminal component assembly.

Although the two pathways use different proteins, the final result of both is the production of C3 convertase and C5 convertase. The C3 convertases, C4b2a and C3bBb, contain structurally related molecules in that C2 and B proteins as well as C4 and C3 have been found to share similar amino acid sequences. Inasmuch as C2 and factor B genes are closely linked on chromosome 6, this apparent redundancy is probably a consequence of gene duplication.

IV. TERMINAL COMPONENT ASSEMBLY AND LYSIS

C5 convertase, derived from either C4b2a3b (classical) or $[C3bBb]_n$ (alternate), cleaves C5 to produce C5b and the small fragment C5a (Figure 3). C5b then complexes with C6 and C7 and either remains in solution or binds to cellular membranes. The fluid-phase C5b-7 complex is inhibited by the S protein (vitronectin) while the membrane-bound form readily adsorbs C8 and C9 to complete the membrane attack complex [C5b-9(n)]. This self-assembly occurs without enzymatic processing of the proteins. Once a single C9 molecule binds to the complex, additional molecules undergo polymerization to form a cylindrical structure with a central hole that perforates the lipid membrane bilayer. The pore formation produced by the membrane attack complex culminates with osmotic lysis of the cell.

V. REGULATORY MOLECULES AND COMPLEMENT MEMBRANE RECEPTORS

The regulatory proteins, operating in the aqueous phase and at the membrane level, modulate the rate of complement activation or control the biological actions of generated fragments (Table 1). Properdin, by stabilizing C3 and C5 convertase complexes, en-

Table 3 **Biological Activities of Complement Components**

Complement Component	Biological Activity
C3b	Enhancement of phagocytosis (Opsonization)
C1C4b	Viral neutralization
C1q	Viral lysis initiation
C5b	Enhancement of yeast phagocytosis
C3, B, D, P, H, I	Solubilization of immune complexes
C3b, CR1	Clearance of immune complexes
C8, C9	Cell lysis
C4b, C3b, C3d	Modulators of immune response
Ba, Bb	Modification of lymphocyte proliferation
Bb	Activation of monocytes and macrophages
	Mediators of Inflammation
C3a, C5a, C5b67	Chemotactic factor
C3a, C5a	Anaphylatoxin
C2 kinin	Enhancer of vascular permeability
C3e	Marrow leukocyte release

hances activation. The inhibitory proteins of the classical pathway are (1) C1 esterase Inhibitor (C1-INH), which binds activated C1r and C1s, inhibiting C1 esterase; (2) factor I, which inactivates C4b and C3b cleavage products; and (3) C4 binding protein (C4bp) which augments decay of C4b2a and cleavage of C4 by factor I. In the alternate pathway, soluble factor H enhances the ability of factor I to decay C3bB and to cleave C3b. Vitronectin (S protein) binds soluble C5b-7, preventing interaction of the complex with cell membranes. Soluble decay accelerating factor (DAF) accelerates the decay of C3 and C5 convertases irrespective of the pathway. Finally, the anaphylatoxin inactivator protein depresses the biological effects of C3a, C4a, and C5a.

Complement receptors are distributed on a variety of cell types and primarily interact with complement fragments[5-7] (Table 2). CR1, CR2, CR3, CR4, MCP, p150/95, and the C3e receptor are cell membrane receptors that bind various cleavage fragments of C3 while C3a/4a, Factor H, Factor Bb, C1q, and C5a receptors bind activation fragments derived from other complement components. One receptor, decay accelerating factor (DAF), destabilizes the C5 convertase complexes of C4b2a and C3bBb. Secreted forms of factor H and DAF have been identified which may exert inhibitory effects on complement activation in the soluble plasma phase (see above).

VI. BIOLOGICAL ACTIVITIES OF THE COMPLEMENT SYSTEM

Although best known for its cytolytic function, the complement system has many other biologic actions that act in concert to modulate the inflammatory response (Table 3). The mechanism of action primarily involves the binding of the specific complement component (or fragment) to its high-affinity receptor on a subset of white blood cells. The binding transduces a signal that culminates in a specific, highly regulated cellular response (Table 2). Activation fragments C3a, C5a, and C5b67 are chemotactic factors that bind to their respective receptors on neutrophils and stimulate influx to the site where the fragments are generated. C3a and C5a also manifest anaphylatoxic activity that induces degranulation of cells that contain C3a and C5a receptors. The activation factors, Ba and Bb, modify lymphocyte proliferation and activate macrophages and monocytes. C2 kinin alters vascular permeability and factors C1 and C4b inhibit viral infectivity by binding and neutralizing invasive viral particles. A variety of C3 fragments bind to CR2 receptors modulating B cell function, and the C3e receptor and its ligand regulate lymphocyte migration. CR4 and the receptors for C1q, factor H, and factor I have been identified but their ligands and the functional significance are not well characterized.

Perhaps to favor phagocytic clearance from the circulation, alternative pathway components C3, B, D, P, H, and I solubilize otherwise insoluble immune complexes. The immune complexes then are cleared by a receptor-dependent mechanism. Removal occurs by binding of the immune complexes to red cells that are subsequently eliminated from the circulation. Finally, C3b acts as an opsonin that enhances phagocytic removal of coated particles or cells by macrophage and polymorphonuclear leukocytes that bear CR1 or CR3 receptors.

Complement deficiency diseases, either genetic or acquired, have been closely associated with the development of autoimmune diseases and with increased susceptibility to infections.[4,8] Susceptibility to *Neiserria* and other encapsulated organisms is common in patients with deficiencies of C3, C5, C6, C7, or C8. Patients with these deficiencies are unable to form the membrane attack complex and thus cannot mount the antibody-complement-mediated cell lysis necessary to clear the bacterial organisms from their bodies. The likelihood that complement-deficient patients will develop SLE and SLE-like illnesses is relatively high, especially for individuals who lack an early component of the classical activation pathway. The reasons why these complement-deficient patients develop rheumatologic disease are not well understood, but defective clearance of soluble and insoluble immune complexes is postulated to play a role in the genesis of the autoimmune diathesis.

VII. IMMUNE COMPLEXES AND COMPLEMENT ACTIVATION

Immune complexes consist of noncovalently interacting antigen and antibody molecules that frequently bind complement proteins, activation fragments, and/or rheumatoid factors. The physiochemical properties of clinically relevant immune complexes are as follows: (1) in antigen excess, small complexes are formed by the binding of a single antibody to two antigens; (2) in antibody excess, small complexes of a single antigen bind two or more antibodies; and (3) when the antibody and antigen concentrations are near equivalence, large complexes of many antigens and antibodies are formed in a lattice structure. Immune complexes may contain IgG, IgA, or IgM, or have a mixture of antibody classes. They may contain rheumatoid factors and by activating the cascade contain complement components and/or fragments. Immune complex assays either measure physiochemical attributes of the complex (differential solubility) or are detected by identifying activated complement components neoantigens on either the antibody or activation products in the complexes. Numerous assays have been developed to detect immune complexes; however, the quantities detected in plasma often do not correlate with disease activity.

The biological effects of immune complex formation vary according to the size and constituents of the complex, the sites of complex deposition, and the ability of the complex to activate complement. If immune complexes activate the complement system, the consequence is inflammatory tissue damage. Since immune complex assays are difficult to standardize, and insofar as the pathologic significance of immune complex formation depends on complement activation, techniques that measure complement levels or complement activation products are now widely used in clinical practice to assess immune complex-mediated disease processes.

REFERENCES

1. **Frank, M. M.,** New developments in immunopathology with special reference to complement and immune complexes, *Int. Arch. Allergy Appl. Immunol.,* 77, 89, 1985.
2. **Ruddy, S.,** Complement, in *Manual of Clinical Laboratory Immunology,* 4th ed., Rose, N. R., DeMacario, E. C., Fahey, J. L., Friedman, H., and Penn, G. M., Eds., American Society for Microbiology, Washington, D.C., 1992, 114.
3. **Cook, L. and Agnello, V.,** Detection of immune complexes, in *Manual of Clinical Laboratory Immunology,* 4th ed., Rose, N. R., DeMacario, E. C., Fahey, J. L., Friedman, H., and Penn, G. M., Eds., American Society for Microbiology, Washington, D. C., 1992, 110.
4. **Cook, L. and Agnello, V.,** Complement deficiency and systemic lupus erythematosus, in *Systemic Lupus Erythematosus,* 2nd ed., Lahita, R. G., Ed., Churchill Livingstone, New York, 1992, 569.
5. **Hourcade, D., Holers, V. M., and Atkinson, J. P.,** The regulators of complement activation (RCA) gene cluster, *Adv. Immunol.,* 45, 381, 1988.
6. **Ahern, J. M. and Fearon, D. T.,** Structure and function of the complement receptors CR1 (CD35) and CR2 (CD21), *Adv. Immunol.,* 46, 183, 1989.
7. **Gaither, T. A. and Frank, M. M.** Complement receptors, in *Manual of Clinical Laboratory Immunology,* 4th ed., Rose, N. R., DeMacario, E. C., Fahey, J. L., Friedman, H., and Penn, G. M., Eds., American Society for Microbiology, Washington, D.C., 1992, 142.
8. **Colten, H. R.,** Complement deficiencies, *Annu. Rev. Immunol.,* 10, 809, 1992.

Chapter 9

Measurement of Complement Consumption, Complement Components, and Immune Complexes in Body Fluids

Linda Cook

CONTENTS

I. INTRODUCTION

A variety of immunoassays are clinically available that assess the functional capacity of the complement cascade or determine the concentration of individual complement components, various complexes, and activation products. Although studies in patients with systemic lupus erythematosus have demonstrated that levels of CR1 and CR2 are significantly decreased during active disease,[1,2] assays for complement receptors remain experimental. Numerous immune complex assays have also been developed by research laboratories. However, in most instances a positive assay does not have diagnostic utility or measure disease activity.[3,4] Thus, techniques that measure levels of immune complexes have been supplanted by assays that quantify the levels of complement fragments or complement-containing immune complexes.[5] Since active complement-mediated disease will generate fragments or complexes as byproducts of the activation reactions, these newer assays may offer better correlates of disease activity.

II. FUNCTIONAL ASSAYS FOR TOTAL COMPLEMENT

Clinical labs use either the Meyer assay[5] or the Kent and Fife assay[6] to measure the functional capacity of the complement cascade. In both systems, sheep red cells are coated with IgG and mixed with dilutions of patient serum. The suspension then incubates to allow complement activation and attendant hemolysis. The amount of hemolysis at each dilution is measured spectrophotometrically by quantifying the hemoglobin released. To determine the volume of serum that causes 50% lysis, an aliquot that contains a fixed number of erythrocytes is mixed with various dilutions of patient serum. The amount of hemolysis vs. serum dilution is graphed and the volume of patient serum that is necessary for 50% hemolysis is determined. CH50 units represent the reciprocal

0-8493-5974-1/94/$0.00 + $.50

Table 1 **Commercial Sources for Complement Component Measurements**

Manufacturer	Methodology	Components Assayed	Instruments
Beckman	Nephelometry	C3, C4, factor B	Array 360, Auto-ICS
Behring	Nephelometry	C3c, C4	BN, BN100
	Turbidimeter	C3c, C4	Turbidtimer
	Immunodiffusion	C3/C3c, C4	—
Institute Pasteur	Nephelometry	C3, C4	QM300
	Radial Diffusion	Total complement	—
Roche	Turbidimeter	C3, C4	Cobas
Binding Site	Nephelometer	C1INH, factors B, H, C3, C4	Array 360, BN, BN100
	Turbidimeter	C1 INH, factors B, H	Turbidtimer
		C3, C4	Cobas
	Immunodiffusion	C1 INH, C1q, C1r, C1s, factors B, H, I, C4BP, Properdin, C2, C3, C4, C3d, C5, C6, C7, C8, C9, C1 INH functional activity	—
	Radial Diffusion	Total complement	
Diamedix	Hemolysis	Total complement	
Sigma	Hemolysis	Total complement	

of serum volume (μl) that yields 50% lysis. Normal serum values are in the range of 25 to 50 U/ml and 150 to 250 U/ml, respectively, for the Meyer[5] and for the Kent and Fife[6] versions. Normal ranges must be established for each laboratory performing the assay. Commercially prepared red blood cells (RBCs) are available (Table 1). Comparison of the precision and accuracy of freshly prepared RBCs vs. commercial reagents is not available, but limited analysis suggests that the quality of commercial preparations may vary considerably.[17]

Functional assays have also been developed to measure the activity of the alternate pathway.[7] The AP50 method uses rabbit red blood cells to directly activate the alternate pathway. A buffer with ethylene glycol tetraacetic acid (EGTA) and high magnesium concentration inhibits classical pathway activation and facilitates activation and assembly of the alternate pathway C3Bb complex. Procedurally, the AP50 assay is similar to the CH50 method.

Several commercial manufacturers produce agar plates that contain sensitized red cells for the semiquantitative screening of complement activity by radial diffusion (Table 1). These plates are most commonly used to screen for total deficiencies and are not sufficiently sensitive to quantitate changes in total hemolytic activity.

III. QUANTITATIVE ASSAYS FOR COMPLEMENT PROTEINS

The concentrations of complement components are determined by either radial immunodiffusion, turbidimetry, or nephelometry. Inasmuch as nephelometry offers rapid and

Table 2 **Complement Fragments and Complexes Measured with Monoclonal Antibodies**

Biologic Activity Measured	Complement Component Measured
Terminal complement activation	SC5b-9, C5b-9(m), poly C9
Initial terminal activation	C5b
Anaphylaxis	C5a, C3a, C4a, C4a-desArg, C5a-desArg, C3a-desArg
Initiation of classical pathway	C1rC1sC1INH
Classical pathway activation	C4d, C3dg
Alternate pathway activation	Ba, Bb, C3BbP

accurate results, this method is preferred by most clinical laboratories. Antisera to C3, C4, C1, C1INH, C2, and factor B are available and can be used to measure levels of these factors with commercial nephelometers (Table 1). The antisera is mixed with a dilution of patient serum in the reaction cuvette precipitating the desired antigen. The amount of light scatter produced by the complexes is compared to light scatter by known quantities of the specific complement proteins that are reacted with the antiserum. Interpolation of the standard curve yields the quantity of each complement component in the test sample. World Health Organization (WHO) and U.S. standardized preparations of C3 and C4 exist, but the values differ slightly. International reference standards for C3 and C4 values are forthcoming. Turbidimetric and radial diffusion methods are also used to quantitate complement components (Table 1). Compared to nephelometry, the turbidimetric assay is procedurally similar but less sensitive, whereas radial diffusion is less precise and more labor intensive.

IV. ELISA TESTING FOR COMPLEMENT COMPONENTS AND FRAGMENTS

The availability of monoclonal antibodies that react with a variety of activation fragments[9-15] has resulted in the development of assays that may have significant clinical utility. The monoclonal antibodies can be categorized as follows: (1) antibodies to epitopes restricted to the native complement protein, (2) antibodies that react with activation-induced (neoepitopes) on activation products (Table 2), and (3) antibodies to activation-independent epitopes (epitopes shared by native components and their cleavage products). Efforts have focused on the development of assays that use monoclonals that are specific for activation-induced epitopes. Capture antibody enzyme-linked immunosorbent assays (ELISA) for iC3b, C3dg, C4d, Ba, Bb, or C9(poly) are available.[13,14] In these systems, bound activation fragments are subsequently detected by an enzyme-conjugated monoclonal antibody that reacts with another epitope on the same molecule.

ELISA assays have also been developed to measure complement complexes. These assays are sandwich ELISAs where the first monoclonal antibody binds one complement protein in the complex. Binding then is assessed with an enzyme-labeled monoclonal antibody for another component in the complex. Soluble C5b-9 complexed to the S regulatory protein can be measured by ELISAs that use anti-C9 or anti-C6 as the capture antibody.[13,15] Binding of the complex is then detected with an anti-C5, S, or C9 enzyme-labeled monoclonal antibody. Early events in the classical activation pathway have been

Table 3 **Commercial ELISA Complement Fragment and Complexes Assays**

Manufacturer	Component Measured	Capture Reagent	Detection Reagent	Enzyme
Quidel	Bb	Mouse monoclonal anti-Bb	Mouse polyclonal anti-Bb	HRP[a]
Quidel	C4d	Mouse monoclonal anti-C4d	Mouse polyclonal anti-C4d	HRP
Quidel	C9(poly)	Mouse monoclonal anti-C9(poly)	Goat polyclonal anti-C7 and -C6	HRP

[a]HRP, horseradish peroxidase.

detected by measuring the C1r-C1s-C1INH complex. In this assay, an anti-C1s monoclonal is the capture antibody and the detection antibody is an enzyme-labeled anti-C1INH monoclonal.[16] Early alternate pathway activation has been detected by measuring the C3BbP complex. The ELISA method captures the complex with an anti-properdin and detects the complex by an enzyme-labeled anti-C3 monoclonal antibody.

In limited studies, complement fragment and complex assays have been used to accurately measure disease activity in patients with systemic lupus erythematosus (SLE), and a variety of other autoimmune diseases.[4] These assays have monitored complement activation during cardiac bypass surgery, kidney dialysis, massive trauma, sepsis, and ischemia. More work is necessary, however, to determine if these techniques warrant implementation by the clinical laboratory.

Few complement ELISA-based assays are marketed. Quidel (San Diego, CA) distributes tests for Bb, C4d, and the soluble C5b-9 complex (see Table 3). These kits contain a positive and negative control, but no standard. In-house assays for other complement components, complexes, or fragments must be developed using reported techniques. Since these assays have been used primarily for research purposes, the individual clinical laboratory must develop the standard, assign a unit system of measurement, and establish the normal range.

V. TEST PROCEDURE FOR C4d COMPLEMENT COMPONENT DETECTION (Quidel)

Specimens, supplies, reagents, and equipment: The blood sample is collected in ethylene diamine tetraacetate (EDTA) inasmuch as coagulation generates complement fragments. The plasma is cooled immediately to 4°C and stored at −70°C within 4 h of collection. Some authors suggest adding 1 to 5 m*M* benzamidine or synthetic protease inhibitors like nafamstat mesilate (Futhan) to minimize consumption.

Necessary supplies include adjustable pipets, pipet tips, multichannel pipettors and reagent reservoirs, microtiter plates (either plates or 8- or 12-well strips), a microtiter plate reader, test tubes, timer, Erhlenmeyer flasks, graduated cylinders, pH meter, and an automated plate washer if desired.

A. Reagents present in kit:

1. 96-well microtiter plate (8-well strips) coated with monoclonal anti-C4d
2. 20× wash solution concentrate, diluted to yield a 0.01 *M* phosphate-buffered saline (PBS), 0.05% Tween-20 solution

3. C4d standards, three vials with different quantities of C4d
4. C4d-positive control lyophilized human serum
5. C4d-negative control lyophilized human serum
6. Specimen diluent 0.01 *M* PBS, 0.05 *M* Tween-20, protein stabilizers
7. C4d conjugate, anti-human C4d conjugated to horseradish peroxidase
8. Substrate buffer, 0.1 *M* citrate buffer, and hydrogen peroxide
9. Substrate concentrate (azino-di-3-ethylbenzthiazoline sulfonic acid diammonium salt)
10. Stop solution, oxalic acid
11. Hydrating reagent

B. Test procedure:

1. Prepare the wash solution by diluting it 1:20 with distilled water.
2. Remove the appropriate number of strips needed from the sealed package and place in the plate frame. Reseal the bag containing unused strips and store them at 2 to 8°C.
3. Reconstitute the standard and control vials with hydrating reagent. Allow to rehydrate for 15 min and then mix thoroughly. These standard and controls are then stable at 2 to 8°C for 30 d.
4. Dilute each patient solution to be tested as desired depending on the assay range and adsorbance to be desired. For this kit, the manufacturer suggests a 1:25 to a 1:200 dilution for patient serum that must be determined by the user.
5. Prewash the microtiter plates three times with wash solution. To do this, add 200 to 300 μl of wash solution to each well and allow to incubate for 1 min at room temperature. Aspirate the wells and then add additional buffer, incubate, and aspirate two more times. When completed, invert the plate and tap firmly on absorbent paper to remove all residual liquid.
6. Add diluent buffer to duplicate wells to serve as the blank, and then add 100 μl of the three standards, two controls, and patient dilutions to duplicate microtiter wells. Incubate the plate at room temperature for 30 min.
7. Aspirate the contents of the wells, then wash and aspirate all wells five times. Blot dry on absorbent paper.
8. Add 50 μl of C4d conjugate to all wells and incubate at room temperature for 30 min.
9. During the incubation prepare the substrate solution by adding 50 μl of substrate concentrate to each milliliter of substrate diluent needed. About 10 ml of diluent is needed for an entire 96-well plate; i.e., for an entire plate add 500 μl of substrate concentrate to 10 ml of substrate diluent. When prepared this solution should be colorless or have just a faint green color. If the color becomes dark green, discard it and prepare fresh reagent.
10. Aspirate the conjugate from all wells, and wash and aspirate the plate five times. Then blot dry and add 100 μl of freshly prepared substrate solution to all wells.
11. Incubate the plate at room temperature for 30 min. Then add 50 μl of stop solution to each well.
12. Read the adsorbance for each well at 405 nm within 1 h of stopping the reaction.
13. Examine the blank wells to ensure that the optical density (O.D.) for each is <0.3. If not the assay results are not valid. If the blank background is acceptable, subtract the mean O.D. of the two blank wells from all other wells on the plate.

Table 4 **Commercial ELISA Immune Complex Assays**

Manufacturer	Capture Reagent	No. of Standards	Detection Antibody	Normal Range (μg eq/ml)
Quidel	Human C1q	3	Goat anti-human IgG	<10
Quidel	Mouse anti-iC3b, C3dg, C3d	3	Mouse anti-human IgG	<15
Diamedix (Sigma)	Goat C1q	1	Goat anti-human IgG	<20
Immunomedix	Mouse anti-C1q	3	Mouse anti-human IgG	<34
Immunomedix	Mouse anti-C3d	3	Mouse anti-human IgG	<8

14. Construct a standard curve based on the concentrations of C4d in the standard solutions and their corresponding O.D. readings. Calculate the control and patient values from the standard curve to determine the concentration of C4d present in control and patient samples.

C. Assay validation: Duplicate wells should have O.D. within 10%. Both the positive and negative controls should be within established ranges to ensure that the results for patient samples are valid.

VI. IMMUNE COMPLEX ELISA ASSAYS

Assays that identify circulating immune complexes fall into three categories: (1) differential precipitation, (2) neoantigen identification, and (3) selective solid-phase immobilization. Immune complexes are readily detected by their differential precipitation under defined laboratory conditions. A reduction in temperature (test for cryoglobulins) and the addition of material that enhances hydrophobicity of the complexes (polyethylene glycol [PEG] precipitation assay) are two common strategies. The precipitation assays, however, lack sensitivity and precision. The second type of immune complex assay is based on the detection of neoantigenic determinants in the Fc region that develop after IgG complexes with antigen. Examples of this technique are conglutinin and monoclonal rheumatoid factor assays.

The third category is based on the ability of immune complexes to bind complement components. Purified C1q, which binds aggregated IgG, purified CR1 receptor, which binds C3b, C4b, and iC3b, and monoclonal antibodies with specificity for C1q, C3b, C3d, C3dg, or iC3b have been used to immobilize circulating immune complexes. The commercially available kits are ELISA-based assays that only differ in the capture protein coated to the microwells: C1q, CR1, or a monoclonal antibody (Table 4).[8] Except the C1q technique, the immune complex assays are relatively specific for IgG immune complex that has activated the complement cascade. The assay is performed by adding a dilution of patient serum to the microtiter well, which is then incubated for 30 to 60 min. Afterward, the wells are washed and an enzyme-conjugated anti-human IgG is added to bind IgG complexes that were retained by the capture reagent. After another 30- to 60-min incubation, the conjugate is washed away, the substrate solution is added, and the absorbance value is measured. The quantity of immune complexes present in the test specimen is determined by comparing its absorbance value to a standard curve generated with known quantities of aggregated IgG (in μg eq/ml). An "immune complex" standard is available from the Centers for Disease Control (CDC) ANA reference collection.

REFERENCES

1. **Wilson, J. G., Ratnoff, W. D., Shur, P. H., and Fearon, D. T.,** Decreased expression of the C3b/C4b receptor (CR1) and the C3d receptor (CR2) on B lymphocytes and of CR1 on neutrophils of patients with systemic lupus erythematosus, *Arthritis Rheum.*, 29, 739, 1986.
2. **Ross, G. D., Yount, W. J., Walport, M. J., Winfield, J. B., Parker, C. J., Fuller, C. R., Taylor, R. P., Myones, B. L., and Lachman, P. J.,** Disease-associated loss of erythrocyte complement receptors (CR1, C3b receptors) in patients with systemic lupus erythematosus and other diseases involving autoantibodies and/or complement, *J. Immunol.*, 135, 2005, 1985.

3. **Barnet, E. V.,** Circulating immune complexes: their biologic and clinical significance, *J. Allergy Clin. Immunol.*, 78, 1089, 1986.
4. **Myones, B. L.,** The measurement of complement fragments in clinical disease, *Clin. Immunol. Newslett.*, 11, 11, 1991.
5. **Mayer, M. M.,** Complement and complement fixation, in *Experimental Immunochemistry,* Kabat, E. A. and Mayer, M. M., Eds., Charles C Thomas, Springfield, IL, 1961, p. 133.
6. **Kent, J. F. and Fife, E. H.,** Precise standardization of reagents for complement fixation, *Am. J. Trop. Med.*, 12, 103, 1963.
7. **Platts-Mills, T. A., and Ishizaka, K.,** Activation of the alternative pathway of complement by rabbit cells, *J. Immunol.*, 113, 348, 1974.
8. **Cook, L. and Agnello, V. A.,** Detection of immune complexes, in *Manual of Clinical Immunology,* 4th ed., Rose, N. R., DeMacario, E. C., Fahey, J. L., Friedman, H., and Penn, G. M., Eds., American Society for Microbiology, Washington, D.C., 1992, 110.
9. **Mollnes, T. E.,** Antigenic changes of complement components: relevance for the analysis of complement activity, *Comp. Inflamm.*, 6, 134, 1989.
10. **Inoue, K.,** C5 neoepitopes appearing during activation, *Comp. Inflamm.*, 6, 219, 1989.
11. **Lund, E. D., Sorensen, L. S., and Brandslund, I.,** Specificities of monoclonal antibodies against the complement C3d split product, *Comp. Inflamm.*, 7, 18, 1990.
12. **Mollnes, T. E., Lea, T., and Tschopp, J.,** Activation-dependent epitopes in the terminal complement pathway, *Comp. Inflamm.*, 6, 223, 1986.
13. **Buyon, J. P., Tamerius, J., Belmont, M., and Abramson, S. B.,** Assessment of disease activity and impending flare in patients with systemic lupus erythematosus, *Arthritis Rheum.*, 35, 1028, 1992.
14. **Kolb, W. P., Morrow, P. R., and Tamerius, J. D.,** Ba and Bb fragments of factor B activation: fragment production, biological activities, neoepitope expression and quantitation in clinical samples, *Comp. Inflamm.*, 6, 175, 1989.
15. **Gawryl, M. S., Chudwin, D. S., Langlois, P. F., and Lint, T. F.,** The terminal complement complex, C5b-9, a marker of disease activity in patients with systemic lupus erythematosus, *Arthritis Rheum.*, 31, 188, 1988.
16. **Cooper, N. R.,** Assays for complement activation, *Clin. Lab. Med.*, 6, 139, 1986.
17. **Cook, L.,** unpublished data.

Chapter 10

Clinical Value of Testing for Complement Components and Immune Complexes

Linda Cook

CONTENTS

I. INTRODUCTION

Laboratory tests that measure the level of individual complement proteins, their multicomponent derivatives, and cleaved products provide information that may assist in the management of patients with immune-mediated disorders. These assays serve an integral role when evaluating complement immunodeficiency diseases. Testing may offer diagnostic as well as prognostic data for patients with systemic lupus erythematosus (SLE), vasculitis, and glomerulonephritis. On the other hand, immune complex testing is usually restricted to suspected diagnoses of glomerulonephritis and vasculitis. Assays for complement activation fragments and complexes may be particularly beneficial for monitoring disease activity in SLE, rheumatoid arthritis, vasculitis, glomerulonephritis, seronegative autoimmune disorders, allergic diatheses, and anaphylactic respiratory diseases.

II. FUNCTIONAL COMPLEMENT ASSAYS

Functional complement assays are designed primarily to provide a global assessment of complement activity. Disease states that are associated with complement activation lower the concentration of the complement proteins in the serum; therefore, serum CH50 and/or AP50 levels fall commensurately. Low CH50 levels correlate with the activity of systemic lupus erythematosus and with the clinical manifestations of other complement-fixing autoimmune diseases,[1] whereas normalization coincides with effective therapeutic intervention.

Since many variables influence the levels of individual complement components, results derived from functional assays should be interpreted cautiously. Synthesized by the liver, complement proteins are acute-phase reactants whose levels may increase

0-8493-5974-1/94/$0.00 + $.50

Table 1 **Levels of CH50, C3, C4, and Factor B in Various Clinical Situations**

CH50	C3	C4	Factor B	Clinical Condition
Normal	Normal	Normal	Normal	Normal
Low	Low	Low	Normal	Classical pathway activation
Low	Low	Normal	Low	Alternate pathway activation
Absent	Absent	Normal	Normal	C3 deficiency
Absent	Normal	Absent	Normal	C4 or C1INH deficiency
Low	Normal	Low	Normal	C2 or C1 deficiency, or cryoglobulinemia
Low	Low	Low	Low	Active immune complex disease, chronic liver disease, malnutrition
Absent	Normal	Normal	Normal	Complement deficiency other than C3, C4, or factor B
High	High	High	High	Acute or chronic inflammation

dramatically during an acute inflammatory response. Consequently, CH50 levels may be falsely normal or even elevated early in an infectious or inflammatory process. In addition, based on genetic differences, CH50 values vary widely among normal individuals. Inasmuch as CH50 represents an equilibrium between synthesis and catabolism activities of the entire system, any pathological process that preferentially decreases catabolism will increase CH50 test. Finally, the CH50 and AP50 assays measure the integrity of the entire pathway; therefore, alterations in the levels of individual components may not effect the results of CH50 or AP50.

CH50 and AP50 assays are best designed to detect complement deficiency states. The absence of a single component results in virtually no hemolytic activity. When complement deficiencies are suspected, mixing the patient's serum with a panel of sera deficient in a single component often identifies the deficient protein. The serum sample that lacks the same component as the patient's serum will not reconstitute hemolytic activity, whereas all other sera in the panel that contain the missing component will elevate the value of the CH50 result toward normal. A purified preparation of the missing protein can then be added to reconstitute the total hemolytic activity and confirm the identity of the missing protein. Specific complement deficiency for all components has been reported and generally manifests as an increased susceptibility to infection or as an autoimmune diathesis.[2]

Complement deficiencies are either secondary to the complete absence of the component or to the presence of a functionally inactive protein. For example, C1-esterase inhibitor (C1INH) deficiency may be caused by the presence of a functional protein that has been inactivated by a circulating inhibitor. Deficiencies characterized by absence of the protein are detected by quantitative measurements of the protein while functional deficiencies necessitate simultaneous performance of functional assays and tests that quantify the protein levels of individual components.

III. QUANTITATIVE TESTS FOR MEASURING CONCENTRATION OF COMPLEMENT COMPONENT

Measurement of the levels of complement components can be used to assess states of complement activation. Levels of C3, C4, and factor B are commonly determined by nephelometry in conjunction with the CH50 to detect complement activation (Table 1).

C3, C4, and factor B will be present in abnormally low quantities as the circulating proteins are degraded during active immune complex-mediated diseases. Nonfunctional complement proteins, however, will produce normal levels.

IV. IMMUNE COMPLEX ASSAYS

Inasmuch as circulating immune complexes have been identified in a broad variety of infectious, malignant, and autoimmune diseases, the measurement of immune complexes should intuitively have clinical value. However, correlation of the results derived from different assays is generally poor.[3,4] In a study done by the World Health Organization (WHO), many assays were shown to be sufficiently insensitive, imprecise, and technically demanding that the techniques would not be suitable for the clinical laboratory.[4] Such an observation may readily explain why numerous reports of immune complex assays are scattered throughout the scientific literature.

Therefore, the clinical value of immune complex assays remains controversial. The decision to implement such assays depends on the technical expertise of the clinical laboratory, on the nature of the patient population, and on the preferences of the requesting physicians.

V. ELISA ASSAYS FOR COMPLEMENT FRAGMENTS AND COMPLEXES

Enzyme-linked immunosorbent assays (ELISAs) that measure activation-induced epitopes on iC3b, C3dg, C4d, Ba, Bb, or C9(poly) have been shown to correlate with disease activity and to predict complement-mediated disease flares in systemic lupus erythematosus.[5-8] Since these assays are very sensitive and can measure nanogram quantities of activation products, they may be superior to the CH50 test and to nephelometric assays that measure levels of C3 and C4. The ELISA technique has detected elevated levels of complement fragments and complexes in adult respiratory distress syndrome, bronchial asthma, atopic dermatitis, idiopathic pulmonary fibrosis, rheumatoid arthritis, and during hemodialysis and cardiac bypass surgery.[9] The data from these studies, however, require independent corroboration before these ELISAs can be recommended for clinical use.

VI. MEASUREMENT OF COMPLEMENT IN FLUIDS

Compared to serum levels, the measurement of complement or immune complexes in synovial fluid, pericardial fluid, pleural fluid, or spinal fluid should provide a more sensitive indicator of inflammatory activity in the affected tissue. ''Normal levels'' of complement components in fluids vary considerably and usually are about 20% of the levels simultaneously measured in serum. Standard C3, C4, and B nephelometric assays and CH50 assays unfortunately do not accurately measure complement components present in these low levels. Complement activation is thus difficult to measure accurately and should never be done without simultaneously measuring serum levels. In most autoimmune disease states the detection of complement levels in body fluids is not clinically valuable.[10] Using ELISA to measure complement fragments in the synovial fluid of patients with rheumatoid, degenerative, and traumatic arthritis, the levels of C3a and Bb were found to be elevated in rheumatoid joints and the quantity of C3a correlated with disease activity.[11,12]

Table 2 **Case 1: A Patient with SLE**

Months	Disease Activity	ANA Titer	dsDNA (U/ml)	CH50 (Units)	C3 (mg/dl)	C4 (mg/dl)	SC5B-9 (μg/ml)
Normal	0	<1:40	<15	150–250	80–120	15–40	<0.5
Initial	4+	1:640 Homog	174	65	63	8	4.0
3	3+		58	71	46	8	5.2
5	2+	1:320 H	26	125	86	8	2.6
6	3+		115	78	85	8	41.0
7	2+		62	138	103	10	3.0
8	2+	1:160 H	74	119	77	5	4.1
9	3+		91	104	82	6	48.0
10	1+		55	139	82	5	4.3
11	1+	1:80 H	34	145	80	7	1.6

Data from Reference 13.

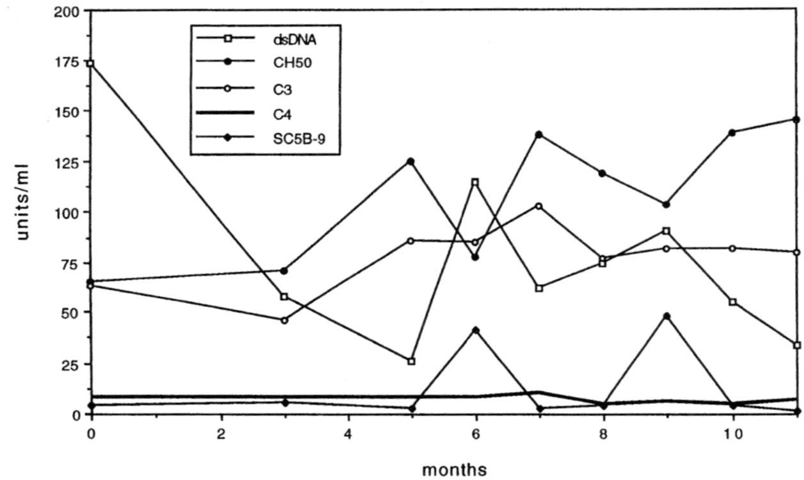

Figure 1 Relationship of complement components and activation products with anti-dsDNA antibody levels in a SLE patient who manifested various degrees of disease activity.

VII. CASE HISTORIES

Case 1: A patient with SLE[13] — The patient was a 29-year-old white woman who presented with Raynaud's phenomenon, malar rash, arthritis, leukopenia, and lymphopenia. Renal or central nervous system disease was not apparent. The lupus band test showed deposits of IgG and C3 at the dermal-epidermal basement membrane junction. Low-dose steroid therapy eliminated the rash but she continued to have active arthritis that finally abated 3 months later. She had two subsequent flares of arthritis at 6 and 9 months. After each episode her condition and symptoms improved. Laboratory studies over an 11-month period are found in Table 2 and Figure 1.

Table 3 **Case 2: A Patient with C4 Complement Deficiency**

Complement Protein	Patient	Sister	Mother	Father	Normal Range
Total CH50	125	46	104	201	150–250 Units
C2	0.4	0.5	2.5	0.9	1.5–3.5 mg/dl
C4	8	4	9	14	16–45 mg/dl
C3	72	59	69	108	77–135 mg/dl

Data from Reference 14.

Discussion: Laboratory data are consistent with SLE: (1) positive anti-nuclear antibody (ANA) (homogeneous), (2) elevated anti-dsDNA antibody, (3) low complement levels, and (4) positive SC5b-9 complex assay. As demonstrated in Figure 1, the level of anti-dsDNA correlated with flares of the patient's disease (see Chapter 7). When anti-dsDNA antibody is detectable in the patient's serum, assays that measure complement levels act as additional predictors for disease activity. C3 levels, C4 levels, and CH50 or AP50 tests decrease during active SLE. To reliably predict incipient flares, serial determinations are essential. Assays that measure cleavage fragments or complement complexes (e.g., SC5b-9) may supplant more traditional complement assays. As shown in Figure 1, the change in SC5b-9 levels rose 10- to 40-fold during disease flares at months 6 and 9, whereas the level of complement components changed by 50%.

Case 2: A patient with C4 complement deficiency (adapted from Reference 14) — An 18-year-old girl presented to her physician with an erythematous, scaly, and partially atrophic rash on her face and fingers. Skin biopsy was consistent with discoid lupus erythematosus. Tests for anti-nuclear antibodies and anti-dsDNA antibodies were negative. Results from complement testing are shown in Table 3. Testing revealed a 50% reduction in C4 level. Since a genetic deficiency in C4 was considered, her immediate family members were also studied. Both the sister and mother had significantly reduced C4 levels. The mother was asymptomatic but the sister also had lesions consistent with discoid lupus erythematosus.

Discussion: This case illustrates some of the rheumatologic manifestations of complement deficiencies. Complement deficiencies are classified as genetic (homozygous or heterozygous) and acquired. The most prevalent complement deficiency is acquired C1INH deficiency. The deficiency is caused by an anti-C1INH antibody that inactivates C1INH (also see Cases 5 and 6 below). Partial inherited C4 and C2 deficiencies also are common, whereas complete deficiencies of other components occur infrequently.

Individuals who inherit a complement deficiency are susceptible to infections and are prone to autoimmune diseases. Complete C3 deficiency or absence of terminal components (C5, C6, C7, or C8) is strongly associated with increased risk of recurrent gonococcal and meningococcal infections. Systemic lupus erythematosus, discoid lupus, atypical cutaneous lupus erythematosus, and glomerulonephritis are more prevalent among patients with complete C1q, C1r, C1s, C2, and C4 deficiencies. Approximately 50% of individuals with complete C2 deficiency develop autoimmune disease: SLE, 25%; SLE-like disease, 10%; and glomerulonephritis, 10%. For heterozygous C2 deficiency the prevalence of autoimmune disorders is approximately 3%.

C4 proteins are encoded by two similar genes on chromosome 6, the C4A and C4B loci. Six serologic alleles of C4A and two of C4B have been identified. At the DNA level, 35 different haplotypes have been described. C4 null alleles represent the absence

Table 4 **Case 3: A Patient with Factor D Deficiency**

	CH50	AP50	C3	C4	B	P	H	I	D
Normal	256–580	8–24	68–104	17–30	13–22	5–16	19–26	56–74	2–11
Patient	173	<1	114	27	19	14	21	72	0

Adapted from Reference 15.

of a C4A or C4B gene. C4 null genes are prevalent in the normal population: 64% have four C4 genes, 35% have three C4 genes, 10% have two C4 genes, and 1% has one C4 gene. The serum level of C4 reflects the number of functional gene products (e.g., two C4 genes produce a C4 level that is 50% of normal). Complete C4 deficiency is very rare (20 reports) and is strongly associated with SLE (75%). Partial deficiency of C4 significantly increases the risk for autoimmune disease. Approximately 15% of SLE patients have a complete absence of C4A genes. The complete absence of C4B genes has been associated with IgA nephropathy and glomerulonephritis. Discoid lupus erythematosus and urticaria may occur when one C4B gene is absent. An increased frequency of anti-SSA and anti-cardiolipin antibodies also have been reported with C4 deficiencies.

Case 3: A patient with factor D deficiency[15] — A 24-year-old male was admitted with generalized rash, spiking fever, arthralgias, and myalgia. History included two prior hospitalizations, the first at age 14 for meningococcal meningitis and another at age 19 for systemic infection with *Neisseria gonorrhoeae*. Routine serum and urine studies showed no significant abnormalities. Levels of IgG, IgA, and IgM, as well as IgG, subclasses were normal. The patient continued to spike fevers that were blood culture negative until the 32nd day, when cultures produced *Neisseria gonorrhoeae*. The patient was treated with penicillin G and cefotaxime. CH50 activity was slightly decreased but no alternate pathway activity was detectable (Table 4). Quantitative analyses demonstrated normal levels of C3, C4, factors B, P, H, and I. Factor D, however, was undetectable. AP50 was corrected by adding purified factor D.

Discussion: This case demonstrates that functional as well as quantitative assays are necessary to properly classify complement deficiency.

Case 4: A patient with C9 deficiency and coexistent SLE[16] — Based on the presence of generalized fatigue, polyarthralgias, Raynaud's phenomenon, and Coombs' positive hemolytic anemia, a 27-year-old Japanese woman was diagnosed with SLE. Prednisolone therapy produced remission. Her disease was quiescent until 8 years later when she again developed Raynaud's phenomenon. She had ulceration of one toe plus dry eyes and mouth. Laboratory studies showed anemia, a sedimentation rate of 29 mm/h, and an ANA-1:160 titer (homogeneous and speckled). A test for immune complexes was significantly elevated at 282 μG/ml (normal <30), anti-dsDNA antibody was 17.2 μG/ml (normal <10), anti-SSA was 1:16, and anti-SSB was negative. Although C3 and C4 levels were normal, CH50 was significantly decreased (Table 5). All complement protein levels were normal except for C9, which was undetectable. A functional assay for C9 corroborated the absence of functional C9 protein.

Discussion: This is the first report of a patient with C9 deficiency and SLE. Most cases of C9 deficiency occur in asymptomatic individuals of Japanese ancestry, whereas SLE has primarily been associated with complement deficiencies of components early in the pathway, especially C4 and C2.

Case 5: A patient with angioedema[17] — A 48-year-old woman was admitted to evaluate significant angioedema. Past history demonstrated juvenile rheumatoid arthritis

Table 5 **Case 4: A Patient with C9 Deficiency and Coexistent SLE**

Test	Patient Result	Normal Range
CH50	15.1	30–40 U/ml
C1q	14.6	8.7–14.6 mg/dl
C2	1.8	1.6–3.6 mg/dl
C3	76.0	71–138 mg/dl
C4	14.0	12–33 mg/dl
C5	12.7	8.0–15.0 mg/dl
C6	3.0	2.7–4.3 mg/dl
C7	3.5	1.9–5.3 mg/dl
C8	4.6	4.9–9.2 mg/dl
C9	<0.06	2.0–7.1 mg/dl

Data from Reference 16.

Table 6 **Case 5: A Patient with Angioedema**

Time (Months)	CH50 25–45	C3 60–130 (mg/dl)	C4 17–45 (mg/dl)	C1INH 12–23 (mg/dl)	C1q 9–15 (mg/dl)
0	5	53	2	2	2
2	4	74	3	3	1
4	5	75	1	3	1
6	5	70	3	3	2
8	3	53	4	2	1
10	6	50	3	3	1
12	5	69	3	22	1
14	6	82	4	8	2

Data from Reference 17.

at age 8. The disease resolved after 6 years. At age 22 a false-positive test for syphilis was noted. At age 35 she had a hysterectomy and was given estrogen replacement. About 1 month after surgery she began having recurrent bouts of nausea, vomiting, abdominal swelling, and pain. She underwent a cholecystectomy at age 42 wherein minimal splenomegaly was present. Her abdominal symptoms did not improve and she began to experience facial swelling. The abdominal pain and facial swelling continued to increase in frequency until they occurred every 2 to 3 weeks. She was then evaluated for rheumatologic disease. Laboratory tests for rheumatoid factor, anti-nuclear antibodies (ANAs), cryoglobulins, protein electrophoresis, and quantitation of immunoglobulin levels were normal. Serial levels of various complement components for the next 14 months are shown in Table 6. Laboratory studies revealed a significant decrease in CH50 activity and reductions in C4, C1q, and C1INH complement protein levels. Estrogen therapy was discontinued and the frequency of attacks decreased. Over the next 5 to 6 months she developed an autoimmune hemolytic anemia and frank splenomegaly. Prednisone therapy controlled the hemolysis. Due to progressive splenic enlargement, she underwent splenectomy 9 months after presentation. Post-splenectomy her hemolytic anemia resolved and she experienced no facial swelling or abdominal pain. Serial studies (Table 5) show that her complement levels, except C1INH, remained unaffected by the various therapies. C1INH rose to above normal post-splenectomy and then dropped to below normal in subsequent samples.

Discussion: Patient 5 is an example of an acquired complement deficiency. Acquired deficiencies are usually mediated by autoantibodies which bind complement proteins inhibiting the functional attributes of the cascade. The consequence is uncontrolled activation of C4 and C2 by C1qrs complexes and attendant triggering of the classical pathway. Since C3 inhibitory proteins block distal activation, serum levels of C3 and terminal components are usually normal. The autoantibodies also alter complement activity by enhancing clearance of the targeted protein. Furthermore, the antibody may cause a false-negative test by interfering with the assay designed to detect the protein. These autoantibodies are usually identified in patients with lymphoproliferative diseases and cancer.

Measurements of CH50, AP50, C3, C4, and other components are not useful to predict episodes of complement activation. In this patient, levels of complement components did not change significantly over the 14-month observation period. Complement fragments C4a and C3a mediate the clinical manifestation of C1INH deficiency; hence, during attacks of angioedema, serum levels of C4a and C3a should be significantly elevated. Indeed, technically demanding radioimmunoassays (RIA) have shown that levels of C4a, C3a, and their major breakdown products, C4a des-Arg and C3a des-Arg, increase during episodes of angioedema. Studies that measure these fragments by ELISAs are not available; however, the clinical utility of C4a and C3a testing is unclear.

Case 6: A patient with monoclonal gammopathy, panniculitis, and activated classical pathway[18] — A 59-year-old man was admitted with an acute febrile illness and found to have a subcutaneous nodule in the left groin. His temperature was 39.7°C, sedimentation rate was 125 mm/h, and liver function tests were slightly elevated. His serum contained an IgG_1 kappa monoclonal protein with the following immunoglobulin levels: IgG, 13.6 g/l; IgA, 0.95 g/l; and IgM, 1.04 g/l. Bone marrow biopsy failed to show increased plasma cell numbers. ANA, cryoglobulins, C3d-type immune complexes, direct antiglobulin, VDRL, and serological tests for hepatitis A and B were all negative. Table 7 illustrates that all early complement components of the classical pathway were significantly depressed while values were normal for components of the alternate pathway and for terminal complement components (data not shown). Biopsy of the subcutaneous nodule was consistent with lobular panniculitis. The patient did not improve with empiric antibiotic therapy or plasmapheresis. Alternate-day prednisone therapy, however, effectively normalized the temperature curve and reduced the nodule. Over the next 3 months, the patient had two additional flares of panniculitis. Results of complement testing remained similar to initial data presented in Table 7.

Discussion: This is the second report of panniculitis, hepatitis, and monoclonal gammopathy in association with depression of early complement component levels. The data are comparable to that described in case 5. The monoclonal IgG kappa protein in this patient may inactivate C1INH. The patient, however, had recurrent panniculitis and did not display symptoms usually associated with acquired C1INH deficiency.

Table 7 **Case 6: Patient with Monoclonal Gammopathy, Panniculitis, and Activated Classical Pathway**

Complement Component	Patient Level[a] (%)	Normal Range[a] (%)
C1q	10	54–146
C1INH	13	60–140
C4	5	48–151
C2	31	60–140
C3	165	68–132
CH50	10	80–120
AP50	100	60–140

[a]Expressed as the percent of functional component present compared to a pool of normal serum.
Data from Reference 18.

REFERENCES

1. **Estes, D. and Christian, C. L.,** The natural history of systemic lupus erythematosus by prospective analysis, *Medicine,* 50, 85, 1971.
2. **Cook, L. and Agnello, V. A.,** Complement deficiency and systemic lupus erythematosus, in *Systemic Lupus Erythematosus,* 2nd ed., Lahita, R. G., Ed., Churchill Livingstone, New York, 1992, 427.
3. **McDougal, J. S., Hubbard, M., McDuffie, F. C., Strobel, P. L., Smith, S. J., Bass, N., Goldman, J. A., Hartman, S., Myerson, G., Miller, S., Morales, R., and Wilson, C. H.,** Comparison of five assays for immune complexes in the rheumatic diseases, *Arthritis Rheum.,* 25, 1156, 1982.
4. **Lambert, P. H., Dixon, F. J., Zubler, R. H. et al.,** A WHO collaborative study for the evaluation of eighteen methods for detecting immune complexes in serum, *J. Clin. Lab. Immunol.,* 1, 1, 1978.
5. **Buyon, J. P., Tamerius, J., Belmont, H. M., and Abramson, S. B.,** Assessment of disease activity and impending flare in patients with systemic lupus erythematosus, *Arthritis Rheum.,* 35, 1028, 1992.
6. **Gawryl, M. S., Chudwin, D. S., Langlois, P. F., and Lint, T. F.,** The terminal complement complex, C5b-9, a marker of disease activity in patients with systemic lupus erythematosus, *Arthritis Rheum.,* 31, 188, 1988.
7. **Kolb, W. P., Morrow, P. R., and Tamerius, J. D.,** Ba and Bb fragments of factor B activation: fragment production, biological activities, neoepitope expression and quantitation in clinical samples, *Compl. Inflamm.,* 6, 175, 1989.
8. **Maillet, F., Fremeaux-Bacchi, V., and Kazatchkine, M. D.,** Limitations of ELISAs and RIAs for C3 and C4 cleavage fragments in the diagnosis of complement activation in vivo, *Compl. Inflamm.,* 7, 131, 1990.
9. **Myones, B. L.,** The measurement of complement fragments in clinical disease, *Clin. Immunol. Newslett.,* 11, 11, 1991.

10. **Hasselbacher, P.,** Arthrocentesis and synovial fluid analysis, in *Primer on the Rheumatic Diseases,* 9th ed., Schumacher, H. R., Ed., The Arthritis Foundation, Atlanta, GA, 1988, 55.
11. **Moxley, G. and Ruddy, S.,** Elevated C3 anaphylatoxin levels in synovial fluids from patients with rheumatoid arthritis, *Arthritis Rheum.,* 28, 1089, 1985.
12. **Ruddy, S.,** Unpublished studies, 1989.
13. **Gawryl, M. S., Chudwin, D. S., Langlois, P. F., and Lint, T. F.,** The terminal complement complex, C5b-9, a marker of disease activity in patients with systemic lupus erythematosus, *Arthritis Rheum.,* 31, 188, 1988.
14. **Voigtlander, V., Bahmer, F., and Hauptmann, G.,** Familial discoid lupus erythematosus associated with heterozygous C4 deficiency, *Acta. Dermatol. Venereol.,* 64, 552, 1984.
15. **Hiemstra, P. S., Langeler, E., Compier, B., Keepers, Y., Leijh, P. C. J., van den Barselaar, M., Overbosch, D., and Daha, M. R.,** Complete and partial deficiencies of complement factor D in a Dutch family, *J. Clin. Invest.,* 84, 1957, 1989.
16. **Kawai, T., Katoh, K., Narita, M., Tani, K., and Okubo, T.,** Deficiency of the 9th component of complement (C9) in a patient with systemic lupus erythematosus, *J. Rheumatol.,* 16, 542, 1989.
17. **Gelfand, J. A., Boss, G. R., Conley, C. L., Reinhart, R., and Frank, M. M.,** Acquired C1 esterase inhibitor deficiency and angioedema: a review, *Medicine,* 58, 321, 1979.
18. **Pascual, M., Widmann, J.-J., and Schifferli, J. A.,** Recurrent febrile panniculitis and hepatitis in two patients with acquired complement deficiency and paraproteinemia, *Am. J. Med.,* 83, 959, 1987.

V. Anti-Phospholipid Autoantibodies

Chapter 11

Anti-Phospholipid Antibodies: Nature and Mechanism of Action

E. Nigel Harris and Silvia S. Pierangeli

CONTENTS

I. INTRODUCTION

Phospholipid-binding antibodies are clinically important for a number of reasons. Historically, their occurrence in patients with syphilis was utilized to diagnose syphilis.[1-3] In the 1950s, investigators recognized the presence of these antibodies in some patients with systemic lupus erythematosus (SLE), and this became utilized as one of the laboratory tests in the diagnosis of SLE.[4,5] During the 1980s, a separate disorder of thrombosis and miscarriages in association with phospholipid-binding antibodies was recognized.[6-10] The central role of phospholipid-binding antibodies in diagnosing the disorder led to adoption of the name ''antiphospholipid syndrome''.[11] In addition to the above diseases, anti-phospholipid antibodies (aPL antibodies) can occur in other infectious,[10,12-15] drug-induced,[10,16,17] and autoimmune disorders.[10]

Although these antibodies appear primarily directed at negatively charged phospholipids, it is likely that they are heterogeneous.[10,18] Phospholipids are chemically such simple molecules that it is surprising that they can generate such an apparently diverse array of antibodies. However, when it is considered that phospholipids form large macromolecular configurations in aqueous solution (e.g., liposomes) and that the configuration of these structures can change depending on temperature, pH, phospholipid structure, and lipids with which they are mixed,[19] it is not surprising that such a variety of antibody specificities can be generated.

II. CLASSIFICATION OF ANTI-PHOSPHOLIPID ANTIBODIES

There is no satisfactory means of classifying these antibodies presently. The most popular method of classification is to use the test by which the antibody is identified.[10] Three tests are currently utilized: standard tests for syphilis, solid-phase anti-cardiolipin assays, and the so-called lupus anticoagulant test. A single patient may have any one, two, or all three tests positive. On the other hand, patients with quite different disease processes may have the same test positive. In the latter instance, it appears that although patients

0-8493-5974-1/94/$0.00 + $.50

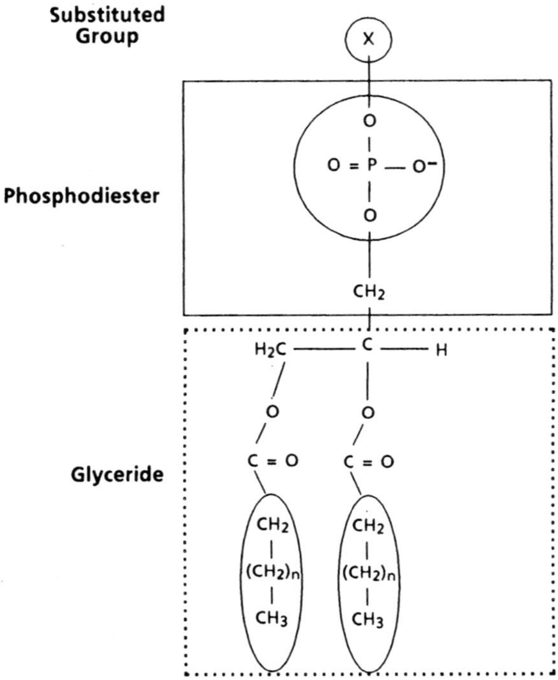

Figure 1 Diagrammatic representation of a phospholipid molecule. The phosphodiester group is negatively charged. When the substituted group (x) is uncharged (serine, inositol), the molecule has a net negative charge. When the substituted group is positively charged (choline, ethanolamine), the molecule is zwitterionic. Antibodies bind molecules with a net negative charge — perhaps the positively charged substituted group blocks antibody access to the phosphodiester. The glyceride portion of the molecule is not bound, but helps orient the molecule within liposomes to make them suitable for antibody binding.

with syphilis and patients with SLE may both have a positive test for syphilis, the antibodies that make this test positive differ, as discussed below. Although not proven satisfactorily, it is also likely that quite different antibodies may be responsible for positive solid-phase anti-cardiolipin and lupus anticoagulant tests. Hence, different subgroups of aPL antibodies may be recognized by different tests, but more than one subgroup may make the same test positive.

III. ANTIBODY SPECIFICITY

Wassermann and co-workers initially used infected liver tissue obtained from patients with syphilis as his source of antigen.[1] Shortly thereafter, alcoholic extracts of normal tissue were found to be a suitable source, and Landsteiner and colleagues demonstrated that the antigen with which these antibodies reacted was a lipid.[20] In 1942, Mary Pangborn demonstrated that this lipid was an acidic phospholipid,[2] which she later named cardiolipin[21] (since the lipid was extracted from beef heart). The structure of cardiolipin was elucidated by investigators such as MacFarlane and colleagues,[22,23] and by the late 1950s, synthetic analogues of cardiolipin[24,25] were being used for the Venereal Disease Research Laboratory (VDRL) test and related standard tests for syphilis. In the 1960s, by studying aPL antibodies induced by immunizing rabbits with phospholipid-protein conjugates, investigators reported that these antibodies did not bind cardiolipin alone, but cross reacted with negatively charged phospholipids.[26,27] Since the only region of the phospholipid molecule common to these different antigens was the phosphodiester group, these investigators concluded that the phosphodiester group was the epitope bound by the antibodies[26,27] (Figure 1). It was also noted, however, that the absence of fatty acid chains from the glyceride portion of the molecule affected antibody binding.[26,27] It is likely that the glyceride portion of the molecule with its long-chain fatty acids enables phospholipids to assume a liposomal conformation which the antibody recognizes.

Initial experiments to determine the binding specificities of aPL antibodies used agglutination reactions. To enable agglutination, the anionic phospholipid had to be mixed with phosphatidylcholine (PC) and cholesterol. PC and cholesterol do not appear to be part of the antigen for these antibodies, but may enhance the ''antigenicity'' of the anionic phospholipids, either by altering their configuration, or by promoting formation of liposomes which can be more easily agglutinated. PC and cholesterol came to be known as ''auxiliary phospholipids'' because they promoted agglutination of anionic phospholipids by aPL antibodies.[28]

When the anti-cardiolipin enzyme-linked immunosorbent assay (ELISA) was introduced in 1983,[29] a very different method of investigating the specificity of phospholipid-binding antibodies became available. It was now possible to coat plates with cardiolipin alone without the need for mixing with other auxiliary lipids. Three lines of evidence were developed to show that cardiolipin-binding antibodies cross reacted with negatively charged phospholipids. The first was that preincubation of anti-cardiolipin-positive sera with negatively charged phospholipid liposomes inhibited binding to cardiolipin-coated ELISA plates.[30] Second, binding to plates coated with negatively charged phospholids correlated to a high degree with binding to cardiolipin-coated plates.[31] Finally, antibodies purified with cardiolipin (or phosphatidylserine [PS]) liposomes exhibited comparable binding to plates coated with a variety of negatively charged phospholipids.[31] This cross-reactivity can only be explained by binding to the phosphodiester-glycerol portion of the molecule, since this is the only part of the molecule common to the negatively charged phospholipids (Figure 1).

If it is true that these antibodies bind phosphodiester groups, then one must explain why, in the experiments described above, there was no observed binding to zwitterionic phospholipids or to DNA, both of which have phosphodiester groups. Binding to zwitterionic phospholipids, such as PC, may not take place because the positively charged group (choline in phosphatidylcholine) interacts electrostatically with the phosphodiester and blocks antibody access (Figure 1). Indeed, removal of the choline by a phospholipase yields phosphatidic, which is avidly bound by these antibodies. On the other hand DNA has negatively charged phosphodiester groups, but preincubation of sera with single- or double-stranded DNA causes little or no inhibition of binding to cardiolipin,[30] and antibodies affinity purified with cardiolipin liposomes exhibited no binding to ELISA plates coated with DNA.[31] It is likely that the phosphodiester groups are bound by aPL antibodies only when arrayed on the surface of a liposome or similar structures. Hence, the glyceride portion of the molecule may be important in maintaining a liposomal or micellar configuration which can be recognized by these antibodies.

The simple chemical structure of phospholipids may not be the only determinant of binding by aPL antibodies. Phospholipids are insoluble and form large macromolecular suspensions in aqueous solutions.[19] Based on work by Rauch and colleagues, it has been postulated that anti-phospholipid specificity is also determined by the macromolecular configuration of the particular target antigen.[19,32] These workers have confined their work largely to egg phosphatidylethanolamine (EPE), which assumes a hexagonal configuration in aqueous solution at appropriate temperatures. Using both monoclonal and polyclonal antibody preparations, Rauch and colleagues report binding to EPE in hexagonal but not in bilayer configuration.[19,32] Indeed, hexagonal-phase EPE is now being marketed by one company in place of platelets to perform the ''platelet-neutralization test'', which is used to confirm the presence of the lupus anticoagulant. Phosphatidylethanolamine is not a negatively charged molecule but zwitterionic (i.e., it possesses both a negative and positive charge).

The exact configuration of negatively charged phospholipids and cardiolipin on a solid plastic plate is unknown, but they form bilayer structures in aqueous phase at *ambient* temperatures. The fact that cardiolipin or negatively charged phospholipids in aqueous solution can effectively inhibit binding of aPL antibodies to cardiolipin on a solid surface[30] suggests that the antigen structures recognized by these antibodies are the same on solid surfaces as in aqueous solution. Although Rauch and Janoff suggest that the lupus anticoagulant binds phosphatidylethanolamine, we have found that, with few exceptions,[33] most sera do not appear to recognize this molecule on solid surfaces. Negatively charged phospholipids have been shown by other groups to neutralize lupus anticoagulant activity,[34,35] and these phospholipids have been used to affinity purify antibodies with lupus anticoagulant activity.[31,34,35]

Hence, one group of investigators report that antibodies with lupus anticoagulant activity are specific for hexagonal-phase zwitterionic phospholipids,[32] whereas other investigators report that these antibodies bind negatively charged phospholipids in bilayer configuration.[31,34,35] This picture becomes all the more uncertain when one considers results which suggest that these antibodies may have a specificity other than for phospholipids. Some of this data are discussed below.

Recently, some investigators have reported a provocative observation suggesting that aPL antibodies do not bind phospholipids but a serum protein, identified as an apolipoprotein, β_2 glycoprotein 1 (β_2 GP1). At the center of this proposal is the observation by these groups that aPL binding to cardiolipin-ELISA plates is greater in the presence of bovine or human serum.[38-40] Indeed, these groups report that there is no cardiolipin binding in the absence of serum. The serum protein responsible for this phenomenon has been identified as β_2 GP1.[36,38] One group, based on work with only two antibodies, affinity purified with cardiolipin-phosphatidyl choline-cholesterol liposomes (as opposed to cardiolipin alone[31]), reported direct binding to β_2 GP1 by ELISA or by western blot.[36] Another group reported a similar observation with anti-cardiolipin-positive sera.[37] On the other hand, although McNeil and colleagues found no direct binding to β_2 GP1 alone, they reported that binding to cardiolipin did not take place in the absence of β_2 GP1.[38] This has led them to the alternative suggestion that aPL antibodies recognize epitopes shared by phospholipids and β_2 GP1.[38]

We have conducted several experiments to examine these observations. We have observed *no* direct binding of sera or whole immunoglobulins with anti-cardiolipin activity to ELISA plates coated with β_2 GP1 alone.[42] The same was true for affinity-purified anti-cardiolipin antibodies. In one experiment, where binding to cardiolipin-β_2 GP1 mixtures was examined by ELISA, binding was directly proportional to the concentration of cardiolipin only. There was enhanced binding of antibody to cardiolipin in the presence of β_2 GP1, as observed by other investigators,[38-40] but binding also took place in the absence of β_2 GP1.[42] We conclude that β_2 GP1 may alter the conformation of cardiolipin such that it is bound more avidly by anti-cardiolipin antibodies.[43] Alternatively, given that β_2 GP1 itself binds cardiolipin avidly, it may well be that this protein makes cardiolipin ''more available'' for binding on the ELISA plate, without necessarily altering cardiolipin configuration. It was noteworthy that when we compared inhibition of cardiolipin-binding activity by preincubation of antibodies with cardiolipin alone vs. cardiolipin + β_2 GP1, no difference in inhibition was observed.[44] Hence, the seeming enhancement of cardiolipin-binding activity by β_2 GP1 appears confined to solid-phase assays.[44]

Matsuura et al.[30] reported that β_2 GP1 enhanced the binding of sera from patients with the antiphospholipid syndrome to cardiolipin by ELISA, but reduced binding by syphilis sera. Although other groups have reported similar observations,[40] we found that in a preliminary study for five syphilis immunoglobulin preparations, there was either the same or slightly enhanced binding in the presence of β_2 GP1.

β_2 GP1 is reported to be a natural inhibitor of clotting by inhibiting adherence of clotting factors to phospholipids on platelet surfaces[45] or by preventing contact activation of the clotting cascade.[46] If aPL antibodies interfere with β_2 GP1-phospholipid interactions, it is conceivable that they may in this way exert a procoagulant effect.[28] This might explain the association of aPL antibodies with thrombosis.

An interesting observation made by Sammaritano and colleagues was that BALB/c mice immunized with human β_2 GP1 in Freund's adjuvant induced the formation of aPL antibodies.[47] Injection with bovine serum albumin (BSA) and Freund's adjuvant or Freund's adjuvant alone did not induce these antibodies. It is likely that on entering the circulation, β_2 GP1 complexes with negatively charged phospholipids and so induces aPL antibody formation. This finding (confirmed by Pierangeli and colleagues in our laboratory) suggests that aPL antibodies can be induced by exposure to phospholipids alone as well as by proteins that have an affinity for phospholipids. A similar mechanism may explain the induction of other autoantibodies specific for antigens that are poor immunogens. For example, proteins (or other substances) may induce anti-DNA antibodies because these proteins might have an avidity for DNA in the circulation.

In summary, it appears that aPL antibodies are specific for negatively charged phospholipids, but specificity is affected by the configuration of phospholipid aggregates, as well as by substances with which phospholipids are mixed (lipids, proteins) and the physical milieu (solid surface, aqueous solution, temperature) in which the aggregates are presented.

IV. MECHANISM OF ACTION IN THROMBOSIS

Why aPL antibodies are associated with thrombosis is unknown. One possibility is that these antibodies are merely markers of a syndrome, features of which are thrombosis and miscarriages. Alternatively, these antibodies may cause thrombosis and pregnancy loss. One is tempted to believe the latter possibility for many reasons. Both thrombosis and pregnancy loss are more frequent in patients with high compared to low antibody levels.[48-51] Two groups have reported that passive transfer of human aPL antibodies into pregnant mice has resulted in pregnancy loss in the recipient mice.[52,53] Lupus-prone MRL/lpr mice with anti-cardiolipin antibodies have been reported to get cerebral infarction,[54] pregnancy loss, and thrombocytopenia[55] in a manner similar to humans with these antibodies. Finally, phospholipids, whether on platelet membranes or endothelial cells, catalyze several steps of the clotting cascade (e.g., the conversion of prothrombin to thrombin or protein C activation), and it is possible that aPL antibodies may disrupt or alter coagulation protein-phospholipid interactions, so promoting thrombosis.

The first potential route by which these antibodies might cause thrombosis was proposed by Carreras and colleagues.[56,57] They reported that lupus anticoagulant-positive plasma inhibited prostacyclin production by endothelium or by human pregnant myometrium in culture.[56,57] Their experiments suggested that the lupus anticoagulant blocked arachidonic acid (the precursor of prostacyclin [PGI_2]) release from membrane phospholipids. PGI_2 is a potent inhibitor of platelet aggregation and a vasodilator; hence, interruption of its synthesis would result in platelet aggregation and clotting. Although some groups[58,59] supported the findings of Carreras and colleagues, several other groups have reported that lupus anticoagulant plasma either has no effect on, or even stimulates, PGI_2 production by human umbilical vein endothelial cells (HUVEC).[60-63] However, one investigative group has reported that these antibodies inhibit thrombin-induced PGI_2 release[64,65] — this report awaits substantiation. Because of conflicting results with respect to PGI_2, investigators have looked to other possible mechanisms of thrombosis by aPL antibodies.

An attractive possibility might be that these antibodies bind phospholipids in membranes of endothelial cells or platelets. In this way, endothelial or platelet function might be altered to exert a procoagulant effect. For those investigators who pursued this possibility, results have been disappointing thus far. Khamashta and colleagues reported that aPL antibodies bind disrupted but not intact platelet membranes.[65] Other investigators[66] and unpublished studies from our own laboratory have found that these antibodies have no effect on platelet function. Although Vismara and colleagues[67] found that antibodies in SLE sera can bind endothelial cells, there was no correlation with aPL antibodies. Similar results were found by other groups.[68,69] In a subsequent study, no significant binding to activated endothelial cells was found.[70]

One promising possibility may be that aPL antibodies may inhibit protein C activation. Although thrombin is central to fibrin formation, thrombin, once it is formed, sets in motion processes that turn off its own production. Thrombin binds thrombomodulin, a protein in the membrane of endothelial cells, and the thrombin-thrombomodulin complex activates protein C.[71] Activated protein C, in conjunction with another protein, termed protein S, degrades activated factors V and VIII. The breakdown of the latter factors will turn off thrombin generation. The process of protein C activation and subsequent factor Va and VIIIa degradation are believed to be catalyzed by endothelial membrane phospholipids. Three groups have presented data suggesting that aPL antibodies may inhibit protein C activation.[72-74] Marciniak and Romond have presented data in 15 patients with the lupus anticoagulant to show that these antibodies inhibit degradation of factor Va by protein Ca.[75] Whether these antibodies inhibit protein C activation or Va degradation, the net effect would be to favor thrombosis.

There has been much excitement recently about possible effects of aPL antibodies on the serum apo-lipoprotein β_2 glycoprotein 1 (β_2 GP1). Schousboe[46] first reported that β_2 GP1 might inhibit interaction of factor XII with negatively charged phospholipids, so delaying activation of the clotting cascade. Nimpf and co-workers reported that this protein might serve as a natural anticoagulant by inhibiting formation of the prothrombin activator complex, thus delaying thrombin formation.[45] In 1990, Galli and co-workers[36] reported that anti-cardiolipin antibodies bind β_2 GP1, and they speculated that these antibodies might neutralize the inhibitory action of β_2 GP1, so favoring thrombosis. Although several other groups have not found that these antibodies bind β_2 GP1 alone,[38,40,41] they do suggest that this protein enhances binding of aPL antibodies to cardiolipin presented on a solid surface. Oosting and colleagues[76] also report that β_2 GP1 is sometimes necessary for lupus anticoagulant activity, although data in our own laboratory show that these antibodies can inhibit thrombin generation *in the absence* of β_2 GP1.[77] The actual effect of aPL antibodies on β_2 GP1-phospholipid interactions is unsettled, but the possibility does exist that these antibodies may disrupt the hypothesized anticoagulant effects of β_2 GP1 and may so favor thrombosis.

Other mechanisms by which aPL antibodies may cause thrombosis might be by inhibition of fibrinolysis[78-82] or by inhibition of anti-thrombin III.[83,84] Both possibilities have been studied[78-84] and no evidence has been found to support either postulate thus far.

Although there is no one mechanism that has been presented to support the hypothesis that aPL antibodies are a direct cause of thrombosis, there are many promising leads to suggest that these antibodies may play a causative role.

V. THE LUPUS ANTICOAGULANT TEST

There are several methods published for performing the lupus anticoagulant test. All rely on the ability of antibodies with "lupus anticoagulant activity" to inhibit clotting. Inhibition is more marked in phospholipid-poor plasma, and abnormal prolongation of clotting tests is "corrected" by addition of phospholipids to the test system. These latter observations were the primary reasons why investigators first believed that the lupus anticoagulant reaction was caused by aPL antibodies. The detection of lupus anticoagulant is briefly reviewed here and that of anti-cardiolipin antibodies is reviewed in the following section.

Most patients with the lupus anticoagulant were first diagnosed because of the detection of a prolonged partial thromboplastin time (PTT). However, this test utilizes relatively "phospholipid-rich" reagents and is therefore not sensitive. The most sensitive test is the kaolin clotting time (KCT) performed with platelet-poor plasma.[85] In the KCT, only kaolin without phospholipids is added to the patient plasma to "start" the clotting cascade (factor XII activation) and the reduced phospholipid results in enhanced inhibition of clotting by the lupus anticoagulant. In the KCT test, phospholipid surfaces available to catalyze clotting are minimal, and inhibition by the lupus anticoagulant of clotting protein-phospholipid interactions more pronounced. Addition of relatively small quantities of phospholipids to this test system — in particular, phosphatidylserine/phospholipid mixtures — reduces the effect of these antibodies and results in normalization of the clotting time.[86]

The Russell viper venom time (RVVT) is preferred by some laboratories.[87] Essentially, Russell viper activates factor X to Xa, and Xa, with factors V and calcium catalyze prothrombin to thrombin conversion. The lupus anticoagulant antibodies inhibit conversion of prothrombin to thrombin, and can so prolong the RVVT. Other tests, such as the thromboplastin inhibition test, utilize dilute thromboplastin to magnify the effect of the lupus anticoagulant.[88] More details about the advantages and disadvantages of these tests in identifying the lupus anticoagulant are given elsewhere.[89]

Three criteria must be met for the lupus anticoagulant test: (1) the patient's PTT, RVVT, or KCT must be prolonged; (2) failure of the test to correct to normal if patient plasma is mixed with an equal volume of normal plasma (failure to correct suggests a clotting inhibitor is present. If the test did correct, it would indicate that the patient plasma was deficient in a clotting factor.); (3) correction of the prolonged clotting time by addition of phospholipids or platelets.[89]

VI. CONCLUSION

The subject of aPL antibodies and performance of tests for their detection continue to develop. If more is learned about the role of these antibodies in thrombosis and pregnancy loss, more predictive tests may be devised. Such tests may require that aPL antibodies be defined functionally, i.e., in terms of their ability to promote thrombosis as opposed to measurement of anticardiolipin concentration. The lupus anticoagulant assay, although a functional test, probably does not measure the "procoagulant" action of aPL antibodies. The continued interest of several laboratories in this subject promises much progress over the coming years.

REFERENCES

1. **Wasserman, A., Neisser, A., and Bruck, C.,** Eine serodiagnostische Reaktion bei Syphilis, *Dtsch. Med. Wochenschr.,* 32, 745, 1906.
2. **Pangborn, M. C.,** A new serologically active phospholipid from beef heart, *Proc. Soc. Exp. Biol. Med.,* 48, 484, 1941.
3. **DeBruijn, J. H.,** Chemical structure and serological activity of natural and synthetic cardiolipin and related compounds, *Br. J. Vener. Dis.,* 42, 125, 1966.
4. **Moore, J. E. and Mohr, G. F.,** Biologically false positive serologic tests for syphilis: type, incidence, and cause, *JAMA,* 150, 467, 1952.
5. **Moore, J. E. and Lutz, W. B.,** The natural history of systemic lupus erythematosus. An approach to its study through chronic biologic false positive reaction, *J. Chronic Dis.,* 1, 297, 1955.
6. **Johansson, E. A., Niemi, K. M., and Mustakallio, K. K.,** A peripheral vascular syndrome overlapping with systemic lupus erythematosus: recurrent venous thrombosis and hemorrhagic capillary proliferation with circulating anticoagulants and false-positive seroreactions for syphilis, *Dermatologia,* 155, 257, 1977.
7. **Soulier, R. P. and Boff, M. C.,** Avortement a repetition, thromboses et anticoagulant circulant antithromboplastine, *Nouv. Presse Med.,* 9, 859, 1980.
8. **Carreras, L. O. and Vermylen, J. G.,** "Lupus" inhibitor anticoagulant and thrombosis — possible role of inhibition of prostacyclin formation, *Thromb. Haemostas.,* 48, 28, 1982.
9. **Hughes, G. R. V.,** Thrombosis, abortion, cerebral disease and the lupus anticoagulant, *Br. Med. J.,* 287, 1088, 1983.
10. **Harris, E. N., Gharavi, A. E., and Hughes, G. R. V.,** Anti-phospholipid antibodies, *Clin. Rheum. Dis.,* 11, 591, 1985.
11. **Harris, E. N.,** Syndrome of the Black Swan, *Br. J. Rheumatol.,* 26, 324, 1987.
12. **Cohen, A. J., Phillips, T. M., and Kessler, G. M.,** Circulating coagulation inhibitors in the acquired immunodeficiency syndrome, *Ann. Intern. Med.,* 104, 175, 1986.
13. **Gold, J. E., Haubenstock, A., and Zalusky, A.,** Lupus anticoagulant and AIDS, *N. Engl. J. Med.,* 314, 1252, 1986.
14. **Canoso, T. R., Zon, L. I., and Groopman, J. E.,** Anticardiolipin antibodies associated with HTLV-III infection, *Br. J. Haematol.,* 65, 495, 1987.
15. **Vaarla, O., Palusuo, T., and Kleemola, M.,** Anticardiolipin response in acute infections, *Clin. Immunol. Immunopathol.,* 41, 8, 1986.
16. **Zarrabi, M. H., Zucker, S., Miller, F., and Derman, R. M.,** Immunologic and coagulation disorders in chlorpromazine-treated patients, *Ann. Intern. Med.,* 91, 195, 1979.
17. **Canoso, R. T. and Sise, H. S.,** Chlorpromazine-induced lupus anticoagulant and associated immunologic abnormalities, *Am. J. Hematol.,* 13, 121, 1982.

18. **Triplett, A. A. and Brandt, J. T.,** Lupus anticoagulants: misnomer, paradox, riddle, epiphenomena, *Hematol. Pathol.*, 2, 121, 1988.
19. **Janoff, A. S. and Rauch, J.,** The structural specificity of anti-phospholipid antibodies in autoimmune disease, *Chem. Phys. Lipids,* 40, 315, 1986.
20. **Landsteiner, K., Muller, R., and Plozl, O.,** Zur Frage der komplement bindungs reaktion bei syphilis, *Wien. Klin. Wochenschr.*, 20, 565, 1907.
21. **Pangborn, M. C.,** Acid cardiolipin and an improved method for the preparation of cardiolipin from beef heart, *J. Biol. Chem.*, 153, 343, 1944.
22. **MacFarlane, M. G. and Gray, G. M.,** Composition of cardiolipin, *Biochem. J.*, 67, 25, 1957.
23. **MacFarlane, M. G. and Wheeldon, L. W.,** Position of the fatty acids in cardiolipin, *Nature,* 183, 1808, 1958.
24. **DeBruijn, J. H.,** Chemical structure and serological activity of natural and synthetic cardiolipin and related compounds, *Br. J. Vener. Dis.*, 42, 121, 1966.
25. **DeHaas, G. H. and Van Deenan, L. L. M.,** Chemical structure and serological activity of synthetic and natural cardiolipin, *Nature,* 206, 935, 1965.
26. **Faure, M. and Coulon-Morelec, M.,** Entre la structure chimique du cardiolipide et son activite serologigue. Conservation du cardiolipide, *Ann. Inst. Pasteur (Paris),* 104, 246, 1963.
27. **Inoue, K. and Nojima, S.,** Immunochemical studies of phospholipids. IV. The reactivities of anti-sera against natural cardiolipin and synthetic cardiolipin analogues-containing antigens, *Chem. Phys. Lipids,* 3, 70, 1969.
28. **Kataoka, T. and Nojima, S.,** Immunochemical studies of phospholipids. VI. Haptenic activity of phosphatidylinositol and the role of lecithin as an auxiliary lipid, *J. Immunol.*, 105, 503, 1970.
29. **Harris, E. N., Gharavi, A. E., Boey, M. L. et al.,** Anticardiolipin antibodies: detection by radioimmunoassay and association with thrombosis in systemic lupus erythematosus, *Lancet,* ii, 1211, 1983.
30. **Harris, E. N., Gharavi, A. E., Loizou, S. et al.,** Cross reactivity of anti-phospholipid antibodies, *J. Clin. Lab. Immunol.*, 16, 1, 1985.
31. **Harris, E. N., Gharavi, A. E., Tincani, A. et al.,** Affinity purified anti-cardiolipin and anti-DNA antibodies, *J. Clin. Lab. Immunol.*, 17, 155, 1985.
32. **Rauch, J., Tannenbaum, M., Tannenbaum, H. et al.,** Human hybridoma lupus anticoagulants distinguish between lamellar and hexagonal phase lipid systems, *J. Biol. Chem.*, 261, 9672, 1986.
33. **Staub, H. L., Harris, E. N., Khamashta, M. L. et al.,** Antibody to phosphatidylethanolamine in a patient with lupus anticoagulant and thrombosis, *Ann. Rheum. Dis.*, 48, 166, 1989.
34. **Violi, F., Valesini, G., Ferro, D. et al.,** Anticoagulant activity of anticardiolipin antibodies, *Thromb. Res.*, 44, 543, 1986.
35. **Pengo, V., Thiagarajan, P., Shapiro, S. S., and Heine, J. J.,** Immunological specificity and mechanism of action of IgG lupus anticoagulants, *Blood,* 70, 69, 1987.
36. **Galli, M., Comfurius, P., Maasen, C. et al.,** Anticardiolipin antibodies directed not to cardiolipin but to a plasma protein co-factor, *Lancet,* 336, 1547, 1990.
37. **Arvieux, J., Roussel, B., Jacob, M. C., and Colomb, M. G.,** Measurement of anti-phospholipid antibodies by ELISA using b_2-glycoprotein 1 as an antigen, *J. Immunol. Meth.*, 143, 223, 1991.

38. **McNeil, H. P., Simpson, R. J., Chesterman, C. N., and Krilis, S. A.,** Antiphospholipid antibodies are directed against a complex antigen that includes a lipid-binding inhibitor of coagulation: β_2-glycoprotein 1 (apolipoprotein H), *Proc. Natl. Acad. Sci. U.S.A.,* 87, 4120, 1990.
39. **Matsuura, E., Igarashi, Y., Fujimoto, M. et al.,** Anticardiolipin antibodies directed not to cardiolipin but to a plasma protein co-factor, *Lancet,* 336, 1547, 1990.
40. **Sammaritano, L., Lockshin, M. D., and Gharavi, A. E.,** Antiphospholipid antibodies differ in aCL cofactor requirement, *Lupus,* 1, 51, 1992.
41. **Gharavi, A. E.,** Antiphospholipid cofactor, *Stroke,* 23(Suppl. I), I-7, 1992.
42. **Pierangeli, S., Davis, S., Ordi-Ros, J., and Harris, E. N.,** Do antiphospholipid (aPL) antibodies require b_2-glycoprotein 1 (b_2-GP1) for binding to target antigens?, *Arthritis Rheum. Suppl.,* 34 (Abstr.), S43, 1991.
43. **Harris, E. N. and Pierangeli, S.,** What is the "true" antigen for antiphospholipid antibodies?, *Lancet,* 336, 1505, 1990.
44. **Pierangeli, S., Harris, E. N., Davis, S. A., and DeLorenzo, G. J.,** β_2-Glycoprotein 1 (β_2GPI) enhances cardiolipin binding activity but is not the antigen for antiphospholipid antibodies, *Br. J. Haematol.,* 82:565–570.
45. **Nimpf, J., Bevers, E. M., Bomans, P. H. H., and Till, U.,** Prothrombinase activity of human platelets is influenced by b_2-glycoprotein 1, *Biochim. Biophys. Acta,* 884, 142, 1986.
46. **Schousboe, I.,** b_2-Glycoprotein 1: a plasma inhibitor of the contact activation of the intrinsic blood coagulation pathway, *Blood,* 66, 1086, 1985.
47. **Sammaritano, L. R., Wen, J., Elkon, K. B., and Gharavi, A. E.,** Induction of antiphospholipid antibodies by immunization with anticardiolipin cofactor, *Arthritis Rheum. Suppl.,* 34 (Abstr.), S43, 1991.
48. **Harris, E. N., Chan, J. K. H., Asherson, R. A. et al.,** Thrombosis, recurrent fetal loss, and thrombocytopenia: predictive value of the anti-cardiolipin test, *Arch. Intern. Med.,* 146, 2153, 1986.
49. **Lockshin, M. D., Druzin, M. L., and Qamar, T.,** Prednisone does not prevent recurrent fetal death in women with antiphospholipid antibody, *Am. J. Obstet. Gynecol.,* 160, 439, 1989.
50. **Loizou, S., Byron, M. A., Englert, H. R. et al.,** Association of quantitative anticardiolipin antibody levels with fetal loss and time of loss in systemic lupus erythematosus, *Q. J. Med.,* 68, 525, 1988.
51. **Alving, B. M., Barr, C. F., and Tang, B. D.,** Correlation between lupus anticoagulants and anticardiolipin antibodies in patients with prolonged activated partial thromboplastin times, *Am. J. Med.,* 88, 112, 1990.
52. **Branch, D. W., Dudley, D. J., Mitchell, M. D. et al.,** Immunoglobulin G fractions from patients with antiphospholipid antibodies cause fetal death in BALB/c mice: a model for autoimmune fetal loss, *Am. J. Obstet. Gynecol.,* 163, 120, 1990.
53. **Blank, M., Cohen, J., Toder, V., and Shoenfeld, Y.,** Induction of anti-phospholipid syndrome in naive mice with mouse lupus monoclonal and human polyclonal anti-cardiolipin antibodies, *Proc. Natl. Acad. Sci. U.S.A.,* 88, 3069, 1991.
54. **Smith, H. R., Hansen, C. L., Rose, R., and Canoso, R. I.,** Autoimmune MRL-lpr/lpr mice are an animal model for the secondary antiphospholipid syndrome, *J. Rheumatol.,* 17, 911, 1990.
55. **Gharavi, A. E.,** Anti-phospholipid syndrome in murine lupus, in *Phospholipid Binding Antibodies,* Harris, E. N., Exner, T., Hughes, G.R.V., and Asherson, R. A., Eds., CRC Press, Boca Raton, FL, 1991, 103.

56. **Carreras, L. O., Defreyn, G., Machin, S. J. et al.,** Arterial thrombosis, intrauterine death and lupus anticoagulant: detection of immunoglobulin interfering with prostacyclin formation, *Lancet,* 1, 214, 1981.
57. **Carreras, L. O. and Vermylen, J. G.,** "Lupus" anticoagulant and thrombosis — possible role of inhibition of prostacyclin formation, *Thromb. Haemostas.,* 48, 28, 1982.
58. **Marchesi, D., Parbtani, A., Frampton, G., Livio, et al.,** Thrombotic tendency in systemic lupus erythematosus, *Lancet,* 1, 719, 1981.

59a. **de Castellarnau, C., Vila, L., Sancho, M. J. et al.,** Lupus anticoagulant, recurrent abortion and prostacyclin production by cultured smooth muscle cells, *Lancet,* 2, 1137, 1983.

59b. **Hasselaar, P., Derksen, R. H. W. M., Blokzijl, L., and de Groot, P. G.,** Thrombosis associated with antiphospholipid antibodies cannot be explained by effects on endothelial and platelet prostanoid synthesis, *Thromb. Haemostas.,* 59, 80, 1988.

60. **Walker, T. S., Triplett, D. A., Javed, N., and Musgrave, K.,** Evaluation of lupus anticoagulants: antiphospholipid antibodies, endothelium associated immunoglobulin endothelial prostacyclin secretion, and antigenic protein S levels, *Thromb. Res.,* 51, 267, 1984.
61. **Rustin, M. H. A., Bull, H. A., Machin, S. J., and Isenberg, D. A.,** Effects of the lupus anticoagulant in patients with systemic lupus erythematosus on endothelial cell prostacyclin release and procoagulant activity, *J. Invest. Dermatol.,* 90, 744, 1988.
62. **Petrainolo, W., Bovill, E., and Hoak, J.,** The lupus anticoagulant stimulates the release of prostacyclin from human endothelial cells, *Thromb. Res.,* 50, 847, 1988.
63. **Schorer, A. E., Wickham, N. W. R., and Watson, K. V.,** Lupus anticoagulant induces a selective defect in thrombin-mediated endothelial prostacyclin release and platelet aggregation, *Br. J. Haematol.,* 71, 399, 1989.
64. **Watson, K. V. and Schorer, A. E.,** Lupus anticoagulant inhibition of *in vitro* prostacyclin release is associated with a thrombosis-prone subset of patients, *Am. J. Med.,* 90, 47, 1991.
65. **Khamashta, M. A., Harris, E. N., Gharavi, A. E., Derue, G., and Hughes, G. R. V.,** Immune mechanism for thrombosis: antiphospholipid antibody binding to platelet membranes, *Ann. Rheum. Dis.,* 47, 849, 1988.
66. **Out, H. J., de Groot, P. G., van Vliet, M. et al.,** Antibodies to platelets in patients with anti-phospholipid antibodies, *Blood,* 77, 2655, 1991.
67. **Vismara, A., Meroni, P. L., Tincani, A. et al.,** Relationship between anti-cardiolipin and anti-endothelial cell antibodies in systemic lupus erythematosus, *Clin. Exp. Immunol.,* 74, 247, 1988.
68. **Rosenbaum, J., Potter, B. E., Woo, P. et al.,** Measurement and characterization of circulating anti-endothelial cell IgG in connective tissue diseases, *Clin. Exp. Immunol.,* 72, 450, 1988.
69. **Le Roux, G., Wautier, M. P., Guillevin, L., and Wautier, J. L.,** IgG binding to endothelial cells in systemic lupus erythematosus, *Thromb. Haemostas.,* 56, 144, 1986.
70. **Del Papa, N., Meroni, P. L., Tincani, A. et al.,** Relationship between anti-phospholipid and anti-endothelial cell antibodies: further characterization of the reactivity on resting and cytokine-activated endothelial cells, *Clin. Exp. Rheumatol.,* 10, 37, 1992.

71. **Esmon, C. T.,** The roles of protein C and thrombomodulin in the regulation of blood coagulation, *J. Biol. Chem.,* 264, 4743, 1989.
72. **Comp, P. C., Debault, L. E., Esmon, N. L., and Esmon, C. T.,** Human thrombomodulin is inhibited by IgG from two patients with non-specific anticoagulants, *Blood,* 62 (Abstr.), 299a, 1983.
73. **Freyssinet, J. M., Wiesel, M. L., Gauchy, J., Boneu, B., and Cazenave, J. P.,** An IgM lupus anticoagulant that neutralizes the enhancing effect of phospholipid on purified thrombomodulin activity. A mechanism for thrombosis, *Thromb. Haemostas.,* 55, 309, 1986.
74. **Cariou, R., Tobelin, G., Bellucci, S., and Soria, J.,** Effect of lupus anticoagulant on antithrombogenic properties of endothelial cells — inhibition of thrombomodulin-dependent protein C activation, *Thromb. Haemostas.,* 60, 54, 198.
75. **Marciniak, E. and Romond, E. H.,** Impaired catalytic function of activated protein C: a new in vitro manifestation of lupus anticoagulant, *Blood,* 74, 2426, 1989.
76. **Oostin, J. D., Derksen, R. H. W. M., Entjes, H. T. I., Bouma, B. N., and de Groot, P. G.,** Lupus anticoagulant activity is frequently dependent on the presence of b_2GP1, *Thromb. Haemostas.,* 67, 499, 1992.
77. **Pierangeli, S., Goldsmith, G., Harris, E. N. et al.,** The mechanism of inhibition of thrombin generation by immunoglobulin with lupus anticoagulant activity, *Arthritis Rheum.,* 35:569.
78. **Angeles-Cano, E., Sultan, Y., and Clauvel, J. P.,** Predisposing factors to thrombosis in systemic lupus erythematosus: possible relation to endothelial damage, *J. Lab. Clin. Med.,* 94, 312, 1979.
79. **Francis, R. B., McGhee, W. G., and Feinstein, D. I.,** Endothelial-dependent fibrinolysis in subjects with the lupus anticoagulant and thrombosis, *Thromb. Haemostas.,* 59, 412, 1988.
80. **Tsakiris, D. A., Marbet, G. A., Markris, P. E., Settas, L., and Duckert, F.,** Impaired fibrinolysis as an essential contributor to thrombosis in patients with lupus anticoagulant, *Thromb. Haemostas.,* 61, 175, 1989.
81. **Sanfelippo, M. J. and Drayna, C. J.,** Prerkallikrein inhibition associated with the lupus anticoagulant: a mechanism of thrombosis, *Am. J. Clin. Pathol.,* 77, 275, 1982.
82. **Francis, R. B. and Neely, S.,** Effect of the lupus anticoagulant on endothelial fibrinolytic activity in vitro, *Thromb. Haemostas.,* 61, 314, 1989.
83. **Cosgriff, T. M. and Martin, B. A.,** Low functional and high antigenic antithrombin III level in a patient with the lupus anticoagulant, *Arthritis Rheum.,* 24, 94, 1981.
84. **Boey, M. L., Loizou, S., Colaco, C. B., Matkin, J. A., and Hughes, G. R. V.,** Antithrombin III in systemic lupus erythematosus, *Clin. Exp. Rheumatol.,* 2, 53, 1984.
85. **Exner, T., Rickard, K. A., and Kronenberg, H.,** A sensitive test demonstrating lupus anticoagulant and its behavioral patterns, *Br. J. Haematol.,* 40, 143, 1978.
86. **Kelsey, P. R., Stevenson, K. J., and Poller, L.,** The diagnosis of lupus anticoagulants by the activated partial thromboplastin time: the central role of phosphatidylserine, *Thromb. Haemostas.,* 52, 172, 1984.
87. **Thiagarajan, P., Pengo, V., and Shapiro, S. S.,** The use of the dilute Russell's viper venom time for the diagnosis of lupus anticoagulants, *Blood,* 68, 869, 1986.
88. **Schlieder, M. A., Nachman, R. L., Jaffe, E. A. et al.,** A clinical study of the lupus anticoagulant, *Blood,* 48, 499, 1976.

89. **Exner, T. and Triplett, D. A.,** Lupus anticoagulants: characteristics, methods of laboratory detection and some clinical associations, in *Phospholipid Binding Antibodies,* Harris, E. N., Exner, T., Hughes, G. R. V., and Asherson, R. A., Eds., CRC Press, Boca Raton, FL, 1991, chap. 8.

Chapter 12

Detection and Measurement of Anti-Phospholipid Antibodies

E. Nigel Harris, Silvia S. Pierangeli, and Marius Teodorescu

CONTENTS

I. PRINCIPLE OF REACTIONS

The test is based on the principle of indirect enzyme-linked immunosorbent assay (ELISA) (Chapter 1). The wells of polystyrene plates are coated with cardiolipin and the plastic is saturated with protein buffer, usually containing either fetal or adult bovine serum.[1,2] Blanks (reaction controls) are represented either by wells that are not coated with cardiolipin or by wells coated with cardiolipin and treated with specimen diluent buffer in lieu of the serum specimen. Diluted serum specimens or plasma along with the appropriate standards and controls are incubated in the wells. After incubation, the plates are washed with a buffer that lacks detergent and the wells are filled with either polyspecific or class-specific enzyme-labeled Ig antibody directed toward human immunoglobulins. After this incubation, unbound labeled antibody is removed by aspiration and washing with buffer. A specific substrate is added and the presence of autoantibodies is detected by a color change that is analyzed spectrophotometrically. The absorbance value for the blank well is subtracted from the value obtained for the well coated with cardiolipin. The blank is represented by a well in which cardiolipin is absent but the specimen is added or a well in which cardiolipin is present but the specimen is replaced by buffer. The level of anti-cardiolipin antibody then is calculated relative to a standard or interpolated from a standard curve.

II. SPECIMENS, SUPPLIES, AND EQUIPMENT

Plasma or serum are sufficient for testing. Lipemic sera should be avoided. The equipment and supplies are items that are available at any ELISA station (Chapter 1). Specific

0-8493-5974-1/94/$0.00 + $.50

supplies for anti-cardiolipin antibody testing are either prepared in the laboratory *(vide infra)* or obtained commercially (see the Appendix to this volume for sources).

III. STANDARDS AND CONTROLS

Anti-cardiolipin isotypes (IgG, IgM, IgA) may be measured separately or simultaneously on the same microtiter plate.[3] In general, the IgG isotype is most specific for the antiphospholipid syndrome (APS).[4-7] Nevertheless, sera from a few patients may have either IgM or IgA isotypes. A diagnosis of APS is more likely when more than one isotype is detectable (see Chapter 13).

Considerable inter-assay variation occurs if results are reported only as optical density (O.D.) readings (absorbance). To improve precision, a one-point calibrator may be used and results are calculated as a ratio of the O.D. reading of the unknown sample to that for the calibrator or may be converted to units. The validity of this calculation is predicted on two assumptions: (1) the relationship between O.D. readings and antibody concentration is linear, and (2) the O.D. readings for serum sample and calibrator fluctuate in the same direction when repeatedly tested. Neither assumption is entirely valid when ELISA is used to measure anti-cardiolipin (aCL) antibody as well as possibly antibodies directed against some proteins.[8] Hence, a single-point calibrator may not be suitable for precise aCL antibody testing.

To improve reproducibility, precision and inter-laboratory consensus of anti-cardiolipin testing, standards have been developed.[3,9] Nine standards currently exist; the IgG and IgM anti-cardiolipin standards have values that encompass the full range of the assay. Plotting O.D. readings of these standards vs. their concentration produces sigmoid curve.[3] To extend the linear portion of the sigmoidal curve, log-logit analysis of O.D. readings vs. their concentration is performed. The anti-cardiolipin concentration of an unknown sample can be interpolated from this curve. IgG anti-cardiolipin is reported as "GPL units", where 1 GPL unit = 1 mg/ml of an affinity-purified IgG aCL antibody.[9] IgM aCL activity, reported as "MPL units", was derived in a similar fashion. Recently, six IgA aCL standards, reported in APL units, have been introduced.

The Anticardiolipin Standardization Laboratory (Louisville, Kentucky) has prepared the standards discussed above by mixing varying proportions of a positive serum with pooled negative sera.[3] The standards were then aliquoted and lyophilized. Aliquots of the nine individual standards are available by request. These standards are reconstituted in distilled water prior to testing.

Although some investigators report differences in binding activity of APS sera to cardiolipin- and phosphatidylserine-coated wells,[12] we have not observed this phenomenon.[10,11] Thus, other negatively charged phospholipids may be substituted for cardiolipin and the same standards may be used.

IV. REAGENTS AND PROCEDURE WITH LAB-MADE ELISA REAGENTS

Coating the ELISA plate with antigen — Wells of ELISA plate are coated with cardiolipin or equivalent negatively charged phospholipid. Cardiolipin is diluted in ethanol at concentrations ranging from 25 to 75 mg/ml. Since other negatively charged phospholipids are not completely soluble in ethanol, a methanol-chloroform mixture is utilized. Because concentrated chloroform may damage the plastic used to manufacture the microwell plates, the negatively charged phospholipids should be dissolved in a methanol:chloroform mixture either at 4:1 or 5:1 (v/v).

The phospholipid solution (30 μg) is added to each well. Because these assays are subject to nonspecific binding, some investigators prefer to determine the binding of samples to phospholipid-coated as well as to uncoated wells.[2,13] If investigators choose this approach, alternating columns of wells of the ELISA plate are coated with either phospholipid suspension or with solvent. In this instance, each dilute serum sample is added to an antigen-coated and to an empty well. A net reading is then calculated as follows: O.D. reading (absorbance) of sample in coated well minus O.D. of sample in uncoated well. Some groups have preferred to use phosphatidylcholine (PC)-coated wells as their blanks because APS sera do not usually bind PC. This approach, however, has not been validated experimentally.

We have found that, under certain conditions, the uncoated well that serves as the blank gives falsely low reading for positive aCL samples. We speculate that empty wells have available sites to which immunoglobulins may stick nonspecifically. If the wells are coated with an "inert" antigen such as PC, many of the sites in the empty well become unavailable for nonspecific immunoglobulin attachment.

Several publications have reported differences in the reactivity of sera to different negatively charged phospholipids, e.g., phosphatidylserine vs. cardiolipin.[12,14] If such comparisons are planned, we advocate that binding studies be carried out on a single plate.[15] Duplicate columns of an ELISA plate are coated with each of the desired antigens, then each appropriately diluted sample is added to the various antigens across the plate. Using this method, we have found that most sera from patients with APS bind equally well to the different negatively charged phospholipids. On the other hand, syphilis sera bind to cardiolipin more avidly than to other negatively charged phospholipids.[15]

"Blocking" ELISA plates and dilution of serum samples — Immunoglobulins stick nonspecifically to the plastic of ELISA plates, even when appropriate blocking is performed. Hence, to reduce nonspecific binding, serum samples should be diluted in an appropriate buffer solution. Various protein-supplemented buffers have disparate impacts on anti-phospholipid (aPL) binding. As discussed (see Chapter 11), the apparent enhanced aPL reactivity that occurs in the presence of fetal calf serum (FCS) or adult bovine serum (ABS) is due to β_2 glycoprotein 1 (β_2 GP1).[16-18,24-29] The degree of enhancement of binding by β_2 GP1 varies from patient to patient.[18,30] Preliminary data in our laboratory suggest that other proteins may also influence binding. In this regard we found that the binding of samples diluted in 10% ABS/PBS (phosphate-buffered saline) was better than binding in 1% BSA/PBS + β_2 GP1, suggesting that, in addition to β_2 GP1 present in bovine serum, other serum proteins may have influenced binding.

Immediately prior to the aCL ELISA, the microwells are incubated with a protein/PBS buffer for least 1 h. After washing the plate, serum samples diluted with identical buffer are added to the wells. Consequently, nonspecific binding is minimized when the selected protein/PBS buffer is used both to block the plate and to dilute the serum samples.

The aCL ELISA first utilized 0.3% gelatin/PBS to block the wells and to dilute serum samples.[19] This diluent, however, was abandoned after it was found that nonspecific binding was considerable. Subsequently, 0.3% gelatin (w/v)/1% BSA (w/v) in PBS was adopted and results were more satisfactory.[10,11] In 1984 Koike and colleagues were the first to perform the assay with 10% FCS/PBS[21] and in 1985, Tincani and colleagues noted that 10% FCS/PBS (v/v) reduced nonspecific binding and appeared to increase the difference in O.D. readings between positive and negative samples.[20] In 1985, Loizou and colleagues also demonstrated that 10% FCS/PBS offered improved performance.[22] Shortly thereafter, Gharavi and colleagues showed that 10% ABS in PBS (v/v) yielded results comparable to 10% FCS and appeared to reduce nonspecific binding more effectively.[23] In the first "Anticardiolipin Standardization Workshop", valid assays were obtained with 10% ABS/PBS, 10% FCS/PBS, and 1% BSA/PBS, but not with 0.3% gelatin/PBS.[9] Currently, either 10% ABS/PBS or 10% FCS/PBS is recommended for blocking ELISA plates and diluting serum samples.[3]

The effect of temperature — The anticardiolipin ELISA should be performed at room temperature. Results from the first workshop indicate that assays performed at 37°C are unreliable,[9] an observation extensively documented by Lockshin and colleagues.[31] Although it has been speculated that 37°C may alter the conformation of the cardiolipin, available data are inconclusive. As a related issue, heating *normal* sera to 56°C produced false-positive test results.[32] In our hands, however, heating normal sera to 56°C for 30 min marginally influences O.D. readings.

Incubation times/washing plates — Standards and serum samples are diluted 1/50 in 10% ABS/PBS (v/v) or 10% FCS/PBS (v/v). This is best accomplished by adding 10 μl of the sample to 500 μl of diluent buffer in a test tube, and gently mixing in a vortex-type mixer to ensure good sample distribution in the diluent. The diluted standards and serum samples are added to ELISA plates in duplicate or triplicate (triplicate readings are recommended when a laboratory is first setting up the assay). A dilution of 1/50 is optimal because it minimizes nonspecific binding and enables sensitive determination of aCL concentration. However, different dilutions may be appropriate for different enzyme/substrate combinations.

After the serum samples are added to the wells, the plates are incubated for 1.5 to 3 h. Although binding of aCL antibodies to cardiolipin occurs rapidly, at least 1 h is needed to approach maximal readings. We have obtained the best results with a 3-h incubation period. Incubating sera for longer periods of time increases nonspecific binding. We suggest that the plate is incubated for at least 1 h after dispensing the *last* diluted serum sample.

Plate washing — After each step, plates are washed 2 or 3 times with PBS. A few laboratories have suggested PBS/Tween 20.[33] The first Anticardiolipin Standardization Workshop[3] and Gharavi and Lockshin[34] showed that Tween 20 reduced reproducibility.

Enzyme-labeled anti-human antibody — After washing, isotype-specific (IgG, IgM, or IgA), affinity-purified, enzyme-labeled anti-human antibodies diluted 1:1000 in 10% ABS (or 10% FCS/PBS) are added to the appropriate wells. In our experience alkaline phosphatase-labeled, isotype-specific anti-human antibodies yields optimal results, but other enzyme-substrate systems also are satisfactory if appropriately adjusted (see Chapter 1 and below for some commercial kits). Plates are incubated from 1 to 1.5 h after which the contents are discarded and the plates are washed.

Substrate and stopping the reaction — The enzyme substrate is then added. For alkaline phosphatase, the substrate, *p*-nitrophenyl phosphate (in tablet form), is dissolved in diethanolamine buffer immediately prior to use. To obtain reliable results the diethanolamine buffer (pH, 9.8) must be prepared carefully. The alkaline pH is essential for optimal enzyme reaction. Occasionally, the solution may be warmed to 37°C for 15 min to effect complete dissolution. After addition of the *p*-nitrophenyl phosphate solution to wells, the plate can be incubated at 37°C. Most laboratories have used a fixed incubation time. Alternatively, we read the plates when the highest positive IgG standard (90 GPL units), or highest positive IgM standard (92 MPL units), reaches an O.D.

reading of 0.9 to 1.0. In our hands, this approach ensures greater reproducibility. The use of a fixed incubation period may be unreliable because the enzyme-labeled antibody deteriorates with time. Furthermore, we do not stop the enzyme reaction with 3 *N* sodium hydroxide (NaOH). If the reaction is terminated, however, the time at which one of the highest positive standards reaches an O.D. of 0.8 should be chosen. This value is suggested because addition of NaOH appears to cause a slight increase in O.D. readings.

Calculating results and interpretation — The aCL concentration of a given antibody isotype is interpolated from a calibration curve. The log-logit curve of O.D. readings of the standards vs. their concentration is generated using software supplied by companies that sell ELISA readers.[35]

For comparative analysis, the unit value for each autoantibody can be reported numerically as units per milliliter and compared to the normal limits and the highest reported value. Normal limits and the highest reported value will vary with the system used for testing and the demographics of the sample population. As discussed above, results of IgG aCL concentrations are reported in GPL units. For the method described above, the following cut-offs are used: aCL negative, <10 GPL units; low positive, 10 to 20 GPL units; moderate positive, 20 to 80 GPL units; and high positive, >80 GPL units. Since the calibration curve plateaus at 80 GPL units, samples with higher concentrations of IgG aCL cannot determined. These samples should be sufficiently diluted so that the O.D. reading falls on the linear portion of the calibration curve (20 to 80 GPL units).[53] Readings in the low positive range of the assay (5 to 20 GPL) are prone to imprecision because log-logit curve fitting produces a slope with a low value. For IgM aCL the following cut-off values are used: negative, <10 MPL units; low positive, 10 to 20 MPL units; medium positive, 20 to 80 MPL; high positive, >80 MPL units. Ranges are being defined with the new APL standards for IgA. Cut-off values should be established for each laboratory whether the plates are made in the laboratory or commercial kits are used.

V. REAGENTS AND PROCEDURE WITH COMMERCIAL KITS (SEE APPENDIX)

Since commercially available aCL antibody kits vary in their design, enzyme/substrate used, and materials provided, each has its assets and pitfalls (see the Appendix). The kit described here can be used to screen for the presence of aCL antibody and also to measure specific antibody isotypes. The enzyme label is horseradish peroxidase (HRPO) and the substrate is tetramethyl benzidine (TMB) (see Chapter 1).

A. MATERIALS

- *Antigen-coated wells:* Detachable wells are provided in metalized pouches as pairs of strips along with frames. Half of the wells are coated with cardiolipin and saturated with bovine serum (fetal or adult) while the other half receive only bovine serum (blanks). Some commercial products do not supply blanks; the addition of specimen diluent to an antigen-coated well serves as a general blank for all specimens.
- *Specimen diluent:* Buffer containing bovine serum and 0.1% thimerosal.
- *Washing buffer:* Concentrate or powder.
- *Enzyme conjugate:*

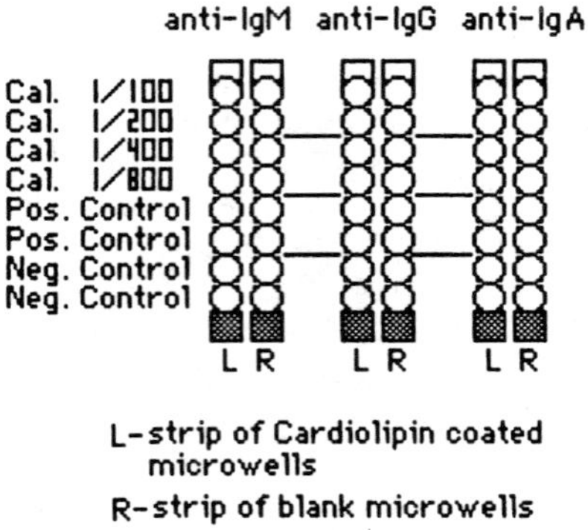

Figure 1 Example of a plate arrangement for calibrator, positive control, and negative control when determining class specificity and levels with standard curves.

1. Polyspecific (anti-IgM, IgG, and IgA) goat or rabbit antibody labeled with HRPO in stabilizer
2. Class-class specific antibody in the stabilizer (coloring is added to identify each specificity)

- *Substrate reagent and diluent:* 3,3′,5,5′-tetramethylbenzidine in an organic base that must be mixed with an equal volume of substrate diluent (citrate buffer containing hydrogen peroxide) immediately before each use. Ready-mixed substrate and buffer may also be available.
- *Stopping reagent:* 1 or 2 *M* phosphoric acid.
- *Calibrator and positive control:* Human serum that contains IgM, IgG, and IgA antibodies to cardiolipin and a preservative. As described above (see Section III), these sera are prepared by mixing appropriate proportions of serum from different patients. One serum mix may contain all isotypes or they may be offered separately.
- *Negative control:* Normal human serum containing a preservative.

B. PROCEDURE

Since less than 10% of specimens submitted to a specialized laboratory contain aCL antibodies, the incidence is relatively uncommon. Thus, for high-volume laboratories, it is cost-effective to initially screen for the presence of aCL antibody. The class specificities of the positive samples then are determined. A one-point calibrator offers sufficient precision for screening assay.

1. Dilute all sera (specimens, calibrator, positive and negative controls) 1/100 in specimen diluent. For screening, prepare the calibrator to be tested at the dilution of 1/100 in duplicate and for class specific prepare four or five twofold dilutions of the calibrator (Figure 1). The greatest precision is obtained if the most dilute calibrator has a value that falls in the normal range (e.g., 20, 10, 5, and 2.5 MPU for IgM with normal limit at 5 MPU).
2. Add diluted serum to a pair of wells, one antigen-coated and the other only protein-saturated. This is best accomplished by having two parallel strips of eight wells (Figure 1). The advantage of having a blank for each specimen is that immunoglobulin levels vary widely in patients with autoimmune diseases and so does the nonspecific binding.
3. After 30 min of incubation at room temperature, wash three to four times, blot very well on absorbent paper, and add 100 μl of conjugate solution to each well.

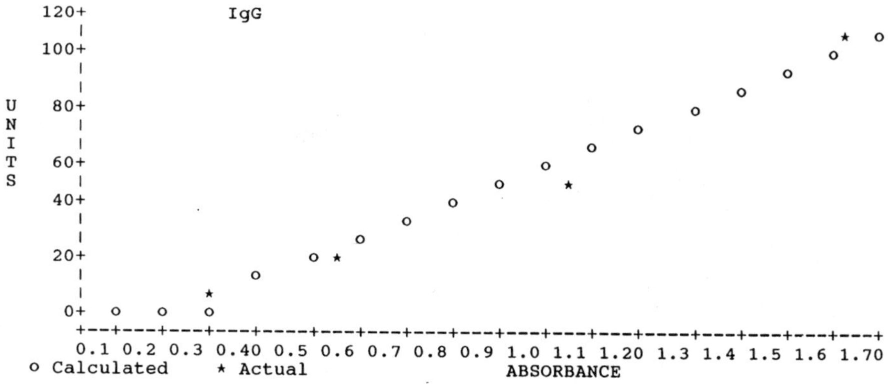

Figure 2 Example of a standard curve for IgG anti-cardiolipin antibody traced by computer based on four twofold dilutions with a commercial product. Specimen background absorbance values were subtracted. Note the area of linearity for best fit line.

4. Incubate the plate for 30 min at room temperature (18 to 30°C), wash and blot again.
5. Add 100 μl of the diluted substrate solution to each well; after 15 min at room temperature add stop solution and read in the ELISA reader.

C. CALCULATION OF RESULTS

The specific absorbance for each antigen is calculated by subtracting the absorbance of the blank well from the absorbance value of the well coated with cardiolipin. If the absorbance in the blank well is higher than in the cardiolipin well, the net absorbance is 0. The mean value is calculated from duplicate wells. Duplicate values should not differ by more than 30%. Larger differences are acceptable if the absorbance values are under 0.2.

Screening out negative specimens — The levels of aCL antibody in each specimen is calculated as a function of a calibrator. The calibrator for screening is assigned an arbitrary 100 units and the general calibration formula is applied:

$$\text{aCL level in specimen} = \frac{\text{anticardiolipin activity of calibrator}}{\text{net absorbance value of calibrator}} \times \text{net Abs. value of specimen}$$

A cut-off value is provided by the manufacturer and all values beyond a particular number of units (e.g., 7 units or 7% of the value of the calibrator) are ''suspect''. This value is designed to include all abnormal as well as most high normal specimens.

Determination of antibody class and levels — Units are calculated based on the standards issued by the Antiphospholipid Standardization Laboratory. These operational units have been defined by the Kingston Anti-Phospholipid Study (KAPS) (see Chapter 11). The one point calibrator (assayed in duplicate) or, to enhance increased precision, a 4-5 point standard curve (Figure 2) is used for the calculations. When highly sensitive enzyme systems are used, (e.g., HRPO and TMB), the curve may be calibrated such that the lower portion of the S shape falls within normal range. This allows the computer to place a best fit line between the points in the linear portion of the standard curve

```
Patient: DOE, JANE                                        Sample ID: 987
Physician: DR.XYZ  Inst: ABCD RHEUMOLOGY LABS
Drawn: 12/28/92    Reported: 12/28/92    Reported By: __________

Results expressed as Units/ml
```

Test (ELISA method)	Patient Result	Normal Max	High Value
ACA Quant (Curve) - IgM	8	5	130
ACA Quant (Curve) - IgG	52	15	200
ACA Quant (Curve) - IgA	3	6	200

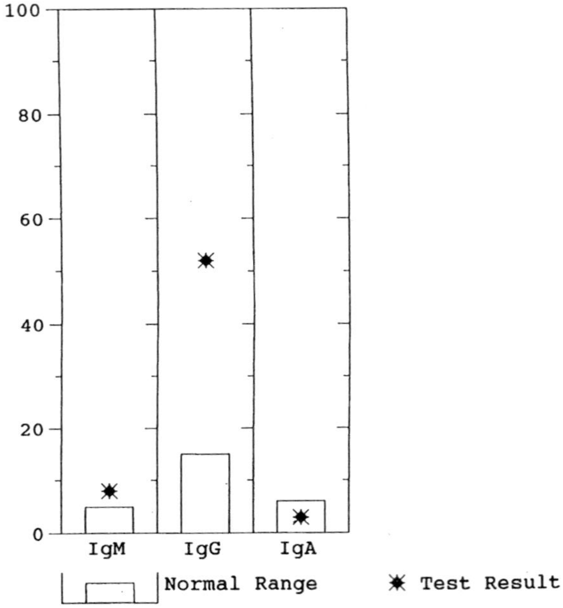

Figure 3 Example of a computer-generated report (TERIS™ Thera Test Laboratories, Inc., Chicago, IL) for anti-cardiolipin antibody in a patient with unexplained recurrent abortions.

(Figure 2). Also, since levels that fall on the upper portion of the curve are rare, repeating the test at a dilution that falls within the linear portion may offer the best precision. Certain manufacturers offer ELISA readers that contain the necessary software for data processing while others provide computer applications specially designed for aCL antibody (see also Chapter 1).

Reporting results within a range between normal maximum and a high abnormal value places a specimen into perspective. The results may be reported as negative or as low, moderate, or high positive, as shown above, and/or displayed graphically (Figure 3).

D. LIMITATION OF PROCEDURE

1. The aCL antibody test should not be performed on grossly hemolyzed, microbially contaminated, or lipemic samples.

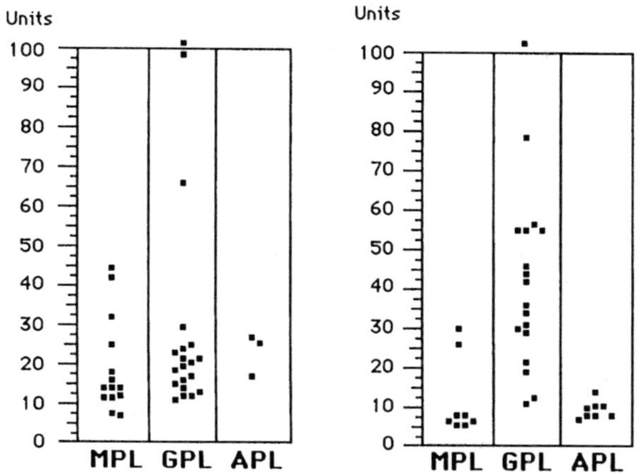

Figure 4 Distribution of abnormal values of IgG, IgM, and IgA anti-cardiolipin antibodies in 80 patients with unexplained recurrent abortions (left panel) and in 28 patients with systemic lupus erythematosus (right panel). (Normal values: 5 MPL, 10 GPL, and 6 APL.)

Table 1 **Percentages of Above-Normal Levels of IgG, IgM, and IgA aCL Antibodies in Patients with Recurrent Abortions and in Patients with SLE**

Abortions			Active SLE		
MPU	GPU	APU	MPU	GPU	APU
18	25	4	18	64	4

2. Diagnosis should not be made solely on the basis of a positive test result. The results must be interpreted in conjunction with all clinical information available to the physician (i.e., history, physical exam, and other diagnostic procedures).
3. A high percentage of confirmed active or seropositive syphilis patients will have elevated aCL levels. Confirmatory procedures should be performed to rule out syphilis in all positive individuals.

E. EXPECTED VALUES

Since the values may vary with age groups, normal values should be determined by the individual laboratory. Patients with SLE and recurrent unexplained spontaneous abortions have a relatively high frequency of aCL antibodies (Figure 4, Table 1).

F. CRITICAL LEVELS

Critical levels have not been defined for this antibody. Nevertheless, levels exceeding 100 GPL units should be reported as soon as possible to the clinician. The presence of IgG aCL antibody at moderate to high levels is considered to be positively associated with an increased risk of thromboembolic events or fetal loss (see Chapter 11). The presence of IgM aCL may precede the appearance of IgG isotype or may be nonspecific. The presence of IgA aCL antibody also may be associated with increased risk of fetal loss, but insufficient data exist at this time.

VI. QUALITY CONTROL

Materials used for quality controls (see also Chapter 1 for general procedures):

1. Positive and negative control sera provided with the kit by the manufacturer.
2. Internal positive controls (serum samples from known patients): three to five patients with variable levels of aCL antibody from low to high levels are measured, to be run with implementation of the test and at least every month. The values should fall within 30% of the expected original measurement expressed in units.

Special consideration should be given to ELISA for aCL antibody due to the lack of detergent in the washing solution. This may lead to artefacts in the form of false-positive results. Since, as mentioned above, this antibody is relatively rare, repeating the test on all positive specimens may offer superior value.

REFERENCES

1. **Harris, E. N., Gharavi, A. E., and Hughes, G. R. V.,** Antiphospholipid antibodies, *Clin. Rheum. Dis,* 11, 591, 1985.
2. **Biswas, R. M., Cronin, M. E., Bowerman, D. L. et al.,** A solid phase enzyme immunoassay (ELISA) for the detection and quantitation of anticardiolipin antibody, *Am. J. Clin. Pathol.,* 90, 591, 1988.
3. **Harris, E. N.,** Annotation. Antiphospholipid antibodies, *Br. J. Haematol.,* 74, 1, 1990.
4. **Harris, E. N., Chan, J. K. H., Asherson, R. A. et al.,** Thrombosis, recurrent fetal loss, and thrombocytopenia: predictive value of the anticardiolipin test, *Arch. Intern. Med.,* 146, 2153, 1986.
5. **Lockshin, M. D., Druzin, M. L., and Qamar, T.,** Prednisone does not prevent recurrent fetal death in women with antiphospholipid antibody, *Am. J. Obstet. Gynecol.,* 160, 439, 1989.
6. **Loizou, S., Byron, M. A., Englert, H. R. et al.,** Association of quantitative anticardiolipin antibody levels with fetal loss and time of loss in systemic lupus erythematosus, *Q. J. Med.,* 68, 525, 1988.
7. **Alving, B. M., Barr, C. F., and Tang, B. D.,** Correlation between lupus anticoagulants and anticardiolipin antibodies in patients with prolonged activated partial thromboplastin times, *Am. J. Med.,* 88, 112, 1990.
8. **Harris, E. N.,** The second international anti-cardiolipin standardization workshop/the Kingston Anti-Phospholipid Antibody Study (KAPS) group, *Am. J. Pathol.,* 94, 476, 1990.
9. **Harris, E. N., Gharavi, A. E., Patel, S. P., and Hughes, G. R. V.,** Evaluation of the anti-cardiolipin antibody test: report of a standardization workshop held April 4, 1986, *Clin. Exp. Immunol.,* 68, 215, 1987.
10. **Harris, E. N., Gharavi, A. E., Loizou, S. et al.,** Cross reactivity of antiphospholipid antibodies, *J. Clin. Lab. Immunol.,* 16, 1, 1985.
11. **Harris, E. N., Gharavi, A. E., Tincani, A. et al.,** Affinity purified anticardiolipin and anti-DNA antibodies, *J. Clin. Lab. Immunol.,* 17, 155, 1985.
12. **Triplett, D. A., Brandt, J. T., Musgrave, K. A., and Orr, C. A.,** The relationship between lupus anticoagulants and antibodies to phospholipid, *JAMA,* 259, 545, 1988.

13. **Cowchock, S., Fort, J., Manoz, S., Norberg, R., and Maddrey, W.,** False positive ELISA tests for anti-cardiolipin antibodies in sera from patients with repeated abortion, rheumatologic disorders and primary biliary cirrhosis: correlation with elevated polyclonal IgM and implications for patients with repeated abortion, *Clin. Exp. Immunol.,* 73, 289, 1988.
14. **Rote, N. S., Dostal-Johson, D., and Branch, W. D.,** Antiphospholipid antibodies and recurrent pregnancy loss: correlation between the activated partial thromboplastin time and antibodies against phosphatidylserine and cardiolipin, *Am. J. Obstet. Gyncol.,* 163, 575, 1990.
15. **Harris, E. N., Gharavi, A. E., Wasley, G. D., and Hughes, G. R. V.,** Use of an enzyme-linked immunosorbent assay and of inhibition studies to distinguish between antibodies to cardiolipin from patients with syphilis or autoimmune disorders, *J. Infect. Dis.,* 157, 23, 1988.
16. **McNeil, H. P., Simpson, R. J., Chesterman, C. N., and Krilis, S. A.,** Antiphospholipid antibodies are directed against a complex antigen that includes a lipid-binding inhibitor of coagulation: b2-glycoprotein 1(apolipoprotein H), *Proc. Natl. Acad. Sci. U.S.A.,* 87, 4120, 1990.
17. **Matsuura, E., Igarashi, Y., Fujimoto, M. et al.,** Anticardiolipin antibodies directed not to cardiolipin but to a plasma protein co-factor, *Lancet,* 336, 1547, 1990.
18. **Sammaritano, L., Lockshin, M. D., and Gharavi, A. E.,** Antiphospholipid antibodies differ in aCL cofactor requirement, *Lupus,* 1, 51, 1992.
19. **Harris, E. N., Gharavi, A. E., Boey, M. L. et al.,** Anticardiolipin antibodies: detection by radioimmunoassay and association with thrombosis in systemic lupus erythematosus, *Lancet,* 2, 1211, 1983.
20. **Tincani, A., Meroni, P. L., Brucato, A. et al.,** Anti-phospholipid and anti-mitochondrial type M5 antibodies in systemic lupus erythematosus, *Clin. Exp. Rheumatol.,* 3, 321, 1985.
21. **Koike, T., Seuishi, M., Funaki, M. E. et al.,** Anti-phospholipid antibodies and biological false positive serological test for syphilis in patients with systemic lupus erythematosus, *Clin. Exp. Immunol.,* 56, 193, 1984.
22. **Loizou, S., McCrea, J. D., Rudge, A. C., Reynolds, R., Boyle, C. C., and Harris, E. N.,** Measurement of anti-cardiolipin antibodies by an enzyme-linked immunosorbent assay (ELISA). Standardization and quantitation of results, *Clin. Exp. Immunol.,* 62, 738, 1985.
23. **Gharavi, A. E., Harris, E. N., Asherson, R. A., and Hughes, G. R. V.,** Anticardiolipin antibodies: isotype distribution and phospholipid specificity, *Ann. Rheum. Dis.,* 46, 1, 1987.
24. **Gharavi, A. E.,** Antiphospholipid cofactor, *Stroke,* 23(Suppl. I), I, 1992.
25. **Pierangeli, S., Davis, S., Ordi-Ros, J., and Harris, E. N.,** Do antiphospholipid (aPL) antibodies require, β2-glycoprotein 1 (β2-GPI) for binding to target antigens?, *Arthritis Rheum. Suppl.,* 34 (Abstr.), S43, 1991.
26. **Harris, E. N. and Pierangeli, S.,** What is the "true" antigen for antiphospholipid antibodies?, *Lancet,* 336, 1505, 1990.
27. **Pierangeli, S., Harris, E. N., Davis, S. A., and DeLorenzo, G. J.,** β2-glycoprotein 1 (β2-GPI 1) enhances cardiolipin binding activity but is not the antigen for antiphospholipid antibodies, *Br. J. Haematology,* 82, 565–570.
28. **Nimpf, J., Bevers, E. M., Bomans, P. H. H., and Till, U.,** Prothrombinase activity of human platelets is influenced by β2-glycoprotein 1, *Biochim. Biophys. Acta,* 884, 142, 1986.

29. **Schousboe, I.,** β2-glycoprotein 1: a plasma inhibitor of the contact activation of the intrinsic blood coagulation pathway, *Blood,* 66, 1086, 1985.
30. **Chamley, L. W., McKay, E. I., and Pattison, N. S.,** Cofactor dependent and cofactor independent anticardiolipin antibodies, *Thromb. Res.,* 61, 291, 1991.
31. **Lockshin, M. D., Qamar, T., Levy, R., and Best, M. D.,** lgG but not lgM antiphospholipid antibody binding is temperature-dependent, *J. Clin. Immunol.,* 8, 188, 1988.
32. **Hasselaar, P., Triplett, D. A., LaRue, A. et al.,** Heat treatment of serum and plasma induces false positive results in antiphospholipid antibody ELISA, *J. Rheumatol.,* 17, 186, 1990.
33. **Cheng, H. M. and Yap, S. F.,** Enhancement of anti-phospholipid antibody activity by Tween-20, *J. Immunol. Meth.,* 109, 253, 1988.
34. **Gharavi, A. E. and Lockshin, M. D.,** Enhancement of antiphospholipid activity by Tween 20, *J. Immunol. Meth.,* 114, 277, 1988.
35. **Pierangeli, A., Greenberg, R., and Harris, E. N.,** Determination of the calibration equation which achieves best accuracy and precision of the anti-cardiolipin assay, *Arthritis Rheum. Suppl.,* 32 (Abstr.), S123, 1989.

Chapter 13

Clinical Significance of the Anti-Phospholipid Antibodies

Ronald A. Asherson and Ricard Cervera

CONTENTS

I. INTRODUCTION

Vascular occlusive manifestations, spontaneous fetal losses, and thrombocytopenia are the main complications associated with the presence of anti-phospholipid antibodies (aPL). The term "antiphospholipid syndrome" (APS) was introduced as a means of categorizing those patients presenting with the above-mentioned manifestations. Although these antibodies are found predominantly in patients with systemic lupus erythematosus (SLE) — either defined according to the 1982 revised American Rheumatism Association criteria for the classification of SLE[1] or presenting with less than four of these criteria, termed "lupus-like" or "probable lupus"[2] — they are also being increasingly detected in the group of patients suffering from what has been termed a

0-8493-5974-1/94/$0.00 + $.50

"primary" APS,[3-7] as well as in a number of other specific conditions (Table 1), where they are usually unassociated with any features of the APS.[8] In addition, aPL may occur in up to 8% of normal populations, the frequency increasing with ageing,[9,10] and their production probably forms part of the "natural" repertoire of antibody production of the B cells in some individuals.

The value of aPL determination in a variety of thrombotic conditions has been the realization that:

1. Patients previously identified as suffering from so-called "idiopathic" vascular occlusions are now classifiable as suffering from the "primary" APS — thus, some patients with Sneddon's syndrome, Budd-Chiari syndrome, pregnancy-related or post-partum renal failure, and Addison's disease/hypoadrenalism are now clearly identifiable as belonging to this category.
2. A percentage of patients suffering from these conditions now have a basic identifiable coagulopathy which may require specific treatment.

II. CLINICAL ASSOCIATIONS

The clinical manifestations of aPL are dependent on vascular obstruction of both veins and arteries, as well as clot formation on the endocardium and its consequences. Single-vessel (large/medium) involvement or multiple vascular occlusions may give rise to a wide variety of presentations. Any combination of vascular occlusive events may occur in the same individual and the time interval between them also varies considerably from weeks to months or even years.

The identification and measurement of the aPL have resulted in the realization that many diverse syndromes may have a common etiopathogenic mechanism. As with other hypercoagulable states, the manifestations of the aPL-associated complications are often recurrent and tend to occur at times of hypercoagulability, e.g., prolonged bed rest, post-surgical procedures/biopsies, during late pregnancy, or in the puerperium. Additionally, patients may be difficult to anticoagulate or show resistance to anticoagulation.

A. OCCLUSIVE VASCULAR MANIFESTATIONS

The main occlusive vascular manifestations associated with aPL are summarized in Table 2.

1. Large and Medium-Sized Vessel Involvement

Venous — Deep vein thrombosis, often recurrent of the lower limbs, is the most common manifestation and, in approximately one third of patients, this may be accompanied by pulmonary embolism or even, less commonly, by thromboembolic pulmonary hypertension. Much less frequently, the venous occlusions result in occlusion of the inferior vena cava itself, sometimes extending into the renal or hepatic veins. Rarely, obstruction of the superior vena cava or cerebral venous sinuses may occur. Upper limb veins such as the subclavian are less commonly obstructed than the veins of the lower limbs. Venous occlusions are also liable to occur after intravenous procedures. Hypoadrenalism or, rarely, Addison's disease resulting from occlusion of adrenal veins with subsequent adrenal infarction occurring because of pressure on the adrenal arterial supply has recently been identified and reviewed[11] (case report no. 1). When large hepatic veins are occluded, typically a Budd-Chiari syndrome supervenes.

Table 1 **Diseases in which aPL Have Been Found**

Autoimmune diseases
Systemic lupus erythematosus
Rheumatoid arthritis
Scleroderma
Dermatomyositis-polymyositis
Mixed connective tissue disease
Sjögren's syndrome
Temporal arteritis/polymyalgia rheumatica
Takayasu's arteritis
Behçet's disease
Autoimmune hemolytic anemia
Idiopathic thrombocytopenic purpura
Hashimoto's thyroiditis
Myasthenia gravis
Drug-induced "lupus-like" syndromes
Chlorpromazine
Procainamide
Hydralazine
Quinidine
Phenytoin
Sulfonamides
Infectious diseases
Bacterial (tuberculosis, leprosy, syphilis, Lyme disease, infective endocarditis, *Klebsiella* infections)
Protozoan (*Pneumocystis carinii,* plasmodium)
Viral (acquired immunodeficiency syndrome [AIDS], mononucleosis, hepatitis, rubella, parvovirus)
Hematological diseases
Thrombotic thrombocytopenic purpura
Sickle cell disease
Polycythemia vera
Myelofibrosis
Monoclonal gammopathies
Von Willebrand's disease
Malignant diseases
Hairy cell leukemia
Malignant lymphoma
Waldenström's macroglobulinemia
Epithelial malignancies (lung, maxilla, prostate, esophagus, colon, cervix)
Hypernephroma
Other conditions
Renal failure undergoing dialysis
Degos' disease

Table 2 **Main Occlusive Vascular Manifestations Associated with aPL**

Vessel Involved	Clinical Manifestations
	Veins
Limbs	Deep vein thrombosis, thrombophlebitis
Brain	Cerebral venous sinuses thrombosis
Liver	
Large vessels	Budd-Chiari syndrome
Small vessels	Hepatomegaly, enzyme elevations
Adrenal glands	Addison's disease, hypoadrenalism
Lungs	Pulmonary embolism, thromboembolic pulmonary hypertension
Large veins	Superior vena caval syndrome
Skin	Livedo reticularis, skin nodules
Eyes	Retinal vein thrombosis
	Arteries
Limbs	Ischemia, gangrene
Brain	
Large vessels	Stroke, transient ischemic attacks, Sneddon's syndrome
Small vessels	Acute ischemic encephalopathy, multi-infarct dementia
Heart	
Large vessels	Myocardial infarction
Small vessels	
Acute	Circulatory collapse, cardiac arrest
Chronic	Cardiomyopathy, arrhythmia, bradycardia
Kidney	
Large vessels	Renal artery thrombosis, renal infarction
Small vessels	Renal thrombotic microangiopathy
Liver	Hepatic infarction, nodular regenerative hyperplasia
Aorta	
Arch vessels	Aortic arch syndrome
Abdominal	Claudication
Skin	Digital gangrene, superficial macules resembling vasculitis, chronic leg ulcers
Eyes	Retinal artery and arteriolar thrombosis

Arterial — These are less common than venous occlusions. Transient ischemic attacks, particularly amaurosis fugax, and strokes, often in younger people, are not infrequently a symptom of APS and testing of aPL in this group of patients is now mandatory.[12-17] The combination of cerebrovascular disease and livedo reticularis has become known as Sneddon's syndrome.[18] It is now clear that a proportion of these patients are, in reality, suffering from a "primary" antiphospholipid syndrome.[19-21] There is a high prevalence of valve lesions in patients with strokes and aPL and suggestions have been made that the cerebral infarctions are in fact mostly thromboembolic, stemming from thrombus superimposed on mitral or aortic valves. It should be emphasized that other risk factors, such as hypertension, hypercholesterolemia, excessive smoking, and oral contraceptives may also be present in these patients. Thus, aPL elevations may represent an additional risk factor for the development of cerebrovascular occlusive disease.

Other major arteries may also be involved; however, less frequently than the cerebral vessels. These include the coronary vessels,[22] large peripheral vessels,[23] or mesenteric arteries,[24] leading to myocardial infarctions, gangrene of the limbs, and bowel or splenic infarctions. Aortic arch occlusion or obstruction of axillary or subclavian arteries may cause an aortic arch syndrome.[25] Renal artery occlusions may mimic idiopathic renal artery stenosis and may result in renal infarction or hypertension. Several cases of this presentation have now been documented.[26-28] Hepatic infarction due to thrombosis of a major hepatic artery is rare, but has been described.[29] Splenic infarctions resulting in asplenia and its hematological manifestations may also occur.

2. Small-Sized Vessel Involvement

Not only may large or medium-sized vessels be affected, but small vessels may also be involved.

Brain — Small vessel occlusive vascular disease may give rise to two distinct syndromes:

- *Multiinfarct dementia:* This is no different to dementia arising because of degenerative states such as Alzheimer's disease or vascular dementia from any other cause. Cortical atrophy may or may not be demonstrable on computed tomographic (CT) scanning, while magnetic resonance imaging (MRI) may also either prove to be positive or negative. Cognitive tests should be performed on all patients in whom this condition is suspected and appropriate antithrombotic or anticoagulant therapy should be undertaken if progress of the condition is to be halted.[30,31]
- *Acute ischemic encephalopathy:* It is often difficult, in the absence of biopsy evidence, such as is possible in other more accessible organs, to determine how much of an acute organic brain syndrome in SLE patients is due to cerebral lupus, for which pulse steroid or immunosuppression is required, and how much is a result of small vessel occlusions, which require other treatments such as anticoagulation. The presence of typical MRI changes may assist in diagnosis. Moderate to high levels of IgG aPL in such patients should prompt the physician to consider antithrombotic or anticoagulant therapy, particularly if the desired response to steroids or immunosuppression is not obtained.[32]

Heart — Occlusion of multiple intramyocardial arterioles by fibrin thrombi, if acute, will result in circulatory collapse due to acute myocardial failure,[33] or if chronic, may present as either regional or global ventricular dysfunction.[34] Arrythmias theoretically could also occur if this vascular involvement affects the conducting apparatus.

Kidneys — Renal involvement with aPL may take several forms, all of which may be accompanied by hypertension. It is particularly important to identify these patients suffering from renal thrombotic microangiopathy during pregnancy and to distinguish this condition from eclampsia or glomerulonephritis, as plasmapheresis is often helpful in these patients.[35-38] Postpartum renal failure as a consequence of this condition may respond in a similar way. Patients with thrombotic microangiopathy may present with mild asymptomatic proteinuria, nephrotic level proteinuria, renal insufficiency, or complicating hypertension.

Table 3 **Manifestations Due to Direct Deposition of Clot on Endocardium**

Valves	
Acute	Vegetations, "pseudoinfective endocarditis"
Chronic	Valve dysfunction (regurgitation, stenosis), cerebral embolism, obstruction
Chambers	Thrombus, "pseudotumor", cerebral embolism

Liver — It appears that, in the liver most typically, complications associated with the aPL are particularly dependent on the size of the vessel involved, whether there is occlusion of arterioles or venules, and on the acuteness or chronicity of the process. This topic has recently been extensively reviewed[39] and diverse conditions, such as nodular regenerative hyperplasia or transaminitis only, may result.

Eye — Small vessel occlusions affecting the retinal vasculature will result in retinal ischemia and infarctions. Neovascularization may lead to secondary complicating vitreous hemorrhage, traction retinal detachments, or glaucoma.[40-42] Suggestions have been made that certain cases of optic neuritis may be vascular in origin and may be aPL-related.[43]

Skin — Involvement of small dermal vessels may give rise to a variety of skin manifestations, such as macules (resembling vasculitis), nodules, and superficial skin necrosis, apart from the more common livedo reticularis, skin ulcerations, and gangrene. This subject has also been extensively reviewed.[44]

B. MANIFESTATIONS DUE TO DIRECT DEPOSITION OF CLOT ON ORGAN SURFACES

The prime example of clot deposition on an organ surface is deposition on cardiac valves (Table 3), in particular the mitral valve (case report no. 2). There may be organization of clot leading to increasing mitral stenosis or incompetence. Clot may rarely extend into the atrium, mimicking an atrial myxoma, or may adhere to the ventricular surface of the valve projecting into, and partially obstructing, the ventricular cavity. Embolism, particularly to the brain, is a constant threat in such patients. Clot may also form on prosthetic valves and, if sufficiently large, may cause obstruction leading to death.[45-49] An increasing frequency of valve lesions themselves without obvious clot deposition, however, has been detected in patients with SLE,[50] as well as in patients with a "primary" APS.[51] The mechanism of production of these lesions is unclear in patients with the latter condition, as thus far no evidence of preceding valve damage by "valvulitis" has been demonstrable, due to obvious practical difficulties.

C. SPONTANEOUS FETAL LOSS

Recurrent fetal losses occur in patients with APS, whether in association with defined SLE, "lupus-like" disease ("probable" SLE), or in the context of the "primary" APS. They can occur in any trimester of pregnancy, although they are more common in the second and third trimesters (case report no. 3).

There are a number of mechanisms that have been proposed in order to explain how these fetal losses occur. The most accepted implies that fetal losses are associated with thrombosis of the placental vessels and subsequent infarction resulting in placental insufficiency, fetal growth retardation, and ultimately fetal loss.[60-62] Not all placentae examined, however, have shown areas of thrombosis or infarction and other mechanisms may be operative in these patients.

Table 4 **Manifestations Without any Clear Thrombotic Mechanisms**

Neurologic
Chorea
Transverse myelitis
Guillain-Barré syndrome
Psychosis
Bone
Avascular necrosis
Pulmonary
Nonthromboembolic pulmonary hypertension
Obstetric
Pre-eclamptic toxemia
Eclampsia

Table 5 **Hematological Manifestations**

Thrombocytopenia
Hemolytic anemia
Evans' syndrome[a]
Neutropenia

[a]Evans' syndrome is the association of autoimmune thrombocytopenic purpura and hemolytic anemia.

D. MANIFESTATIONS OCCURRING WITHOUT ANY CLEAR THROMBOTIC MECHANISMS

These include nonthromboembolic pulmonary hypertension,[52] chorea,[53] avascular necrosis of bone,[54] transverse myelitis,[55] Guillain-Barré syndrome,[56] migraine,[57] pre-eclamptic toxemia, and eclampsia[58] (Table 4).

Although small vessel occlusive disease may in fact be ultimately responsible for some of these conditions, lack of histopathological evidence of this mechanism makes any definitive statement regarding etiopathogenesis impossible. It has been suggested that a specific interaction with brain phospholipid in the basal ganglia may be responsible for the frequent occurrence of chorea in patients with APS.[53] CT and MRI scans in this group have been uniformly negative. Migraines seem to be frequent in aPL-positive patients. However, recent work from several institutions has demonstrated that there is no relationship of the aPL to migraine in SLE.[59]

E. HEMATOLOGICAL MANIFESTATIONS

These are summarized in Table 5. Several authors[63-67] have demonstrated a strong association between thrombocytopenia and the presence of aPL, mainly of the IgG isotype, in patients with SLE. It is usually mild (70 to 120 $\times$ 10^9 platelets/mm^3), benign, and does not require any active intervention. Extensive purpura of hemorrhage in the presence of aPL should lead one to suspect that the patient is in fact suffering from (1) a clotting factor deficiency, (2) idiopathic thrombocytopenic purpura, (3) uremia, (4)

Table 6 **Criteria for Classification of the Antiphospholipid Syndrome**

Clinical	Laboratory
Venous thrombosis	IgG aCL (moderate/high levels)
Arterial thrombosis	IgM aCL (moderate/high levels)
Recurrent fetal loss	Positive LA test
Thrombocytopenia	

Patients with the syndrome should have at least one clinical plus one laboratory finding during their disease; aPL test must be positive on at least two occasions more than 3 months apart.

overdosage with anticoagulation therapy, or (5) another cause, e.g., leukemia (particularly hairy cell) which may be accompanied by elevations of the aPL.

Hemolytic anemia, Evans' syndrome and neutropenia have also occasionally been found in association with the aPL.

III. THE ANTIPHOSPHOLIPID SYNDROME

This term was introduced as a means of categorizing and studying those patients with vascular occlusive manifestations, recurrent fetal losses, and/or thrombocytopenia associated with raised levels of aPL. The diagnosis of the APS should be based both on clinical and serological criteria (Table 6).

APS may be seen:

1. With defined SLE (four or more of the American Rheumatism Association criteria)
2. With "lupus-like" disease or "probable" SLE
3. As a "primary" syndrome
4. Rarely, with discoid lupus
5. In pediatric practice, with a preponderance of deep vein thrombosis, renovascular disease and hypertension, and chorea
6. In the "catastrophic" antiphospholipid syndrome
7. In patients with malignancies (carcinoma of lung, kidney, etc.)
8. With myeloproliferative disorders (Waldenström's macroglobulinemia, myeloma)
9. With lymphomas

In the nonlupus conditions, thrombocytopenia is often not a feature.

A. THE "PRIMARY" ANTIPHOSPHOLIPID SYNDROME

Since 1988, several series have been documented detailing the major clinical and serological characteristics of this syndrome. Essentially, these patients present features of any patient with APS, e.g., thrombosis (venous and/or arterial) and/or recurrent fetal losses, but without SLE or any other well-defined disease. A follow-up longer than 5 years is now considered necessary in order to rule out the development of SLE or any other autoimmune disorder.

Some of these patients may, however, have a few clinical manifestations resembling SLE or other connective tissue disorders. The clear separation of this group of patients and those with SLE and "lupus-like" disease is important. Patients with the "primary"

APS essentially do not have any of the "flares" (fever, arthralgias, myalgias), polyserositis, immune complex-type nephritis, or noncerebrovascular neurological disease seen in patients with SLE and lupus-like disease. They do not usually have other features closely associated with SLE, such as Raynaud's phenomenon, alopecia, mouth ulcers, or butterfly rashes, but they may demonstrate vasculitic skin rashes. Serologically, the anti-nuclear antibody level may be negative or low positive (<1:160). Antibodies to dsDNA, estimated by the *Crithidia* or Farr assays, are usually negative. However, in some patients, presumably in those more closely related to SLE, low-affinity anti-dsDNA antibodies may be demonstrable by enzyme-linked immunosorbent assay (ELISA). Antibodies to extractable nuclear antigens (ENA) are uniformly absent. Antibodies to ssDNA are usually present and of the IgM isotype. IgG antibodies to ssDNA of any significant level should lead one to suspect the development of lupus-like disease in these particular patients. Other immunological disturbances, such as rheumatoid factor, cryoglobulinemia, or immune complexes, may also be present. A number of patients may demonstrate a low C_4 level. In these cases, further studies are awaited in order to determine whether the low complement levels are due to complement activation or to a null allele at the C_{4a} or C_{4b} locus. A family history of SLE or other autoimmune disease may be elicitable.

B. THE "CATASTROPHIC" ANTIPHOSPHOLIPID SYNDROME

A minority of patients with aPL may develop an acute and catastrophic APS characterized by widespread vascular occlusions involving multiple organs. Ten such patients have been recently documented and reviewed in the literature.[68] These patients have in common:

1. Clinical evidence of multiple organ involvement (three or more): severe renal dysfunction often accompanied by accelerated or malignant hypertension; central nervous system symptomatology often heralded by behavior disturbances, but ending in disturbances of consciousness, such as stupor, and evidence of focal vascular disturbances, e.g., hemiparesis; respiratory difficulties such as the clinical and radiological picture of adult respiratory distress syndrome; skin manifestations such as livedo reticularis, acrocyanosis, or ischemic ulcerations and gangrene; or other organ failure due to multiple fibrin thrombi occluding small vessels, e.g., myocardial arteriolar thromboses, adrenal vessel occlusion, hepatic infarction, and, rarely, ischemic bowel ulceration.
2. Histopathological evidence of multiple large and small vessel occlusion.
3. Serological confirmation of the presence of aPL, usually in high titer. Other features of APS, such as thrombocytopenia, are also frequent. If the patient has SLE, activity of the disease is usually mild or absent, with low levels of antibodies to dsDNA.

This condition may superficially resemble other thrombotic conditions, such as thrombotic thrombocytopenic purpura (TTP), disseminated intravascular coagulation (DIC), cryoglobulinemia and other hypercoagulable states, or Raynaud's phenomenon with digital infarcts secondary to vascular pathology occurring particularly in patients with "overlap" syndromes. The presence of extensive purpura, fluctuating neurological signs, microangiopathic hemolytic anemia, and absence of aPL may assist in the differentiation of TTP. The diagnosis of DIC depends to a large extent on the presence of elevated fibrin split products as well as thrombocytopenia. DIC is very rarely associated with aPL, although several patients with SLE have developed this complication[68] and occult pulmonary embolism, common in patients with the antiphospholipid syndrome, may be the only manifestation of DIC.[69] The presence of cryoglobulins or the deficiency of protein C or S or antithrombin III will lead to the diagnosis of a specific hypercoagulable state. Finally, the diagnosis of Raynaud's phenomenon with digital infarcts will be made more in the setting of the typical clinical pattern of an "overlap" syndrome than on laboratory findings.

C. PEDIATRIC ANTIPHOSPHOLIPID SYNDROMES

Unlike the study of adults with APS, there are comparatively few reports on the frequency of aPL-associated conditions in the pediatric literature. Shergy et al.[70] have reported that up to 50% of children with SLE have aPL and that the clinical manifestations are similar to those encountered in adults, particularly recurrent deep vein thrombosis, strokes, chorea, renal artery thrombosis, or hypoadrenalism. These may be seen in infants as young as 9 months of age,[71] ranging through childhood to adolescence.[72,73]

Additionally, there have been several reports of aortic thrombosis in neonates due to maternal transfer of IgG aPL.[74,75]

IV. MANAGEMENT

A. GENERAL

There is no statistical documented evidence to date that elimination of the aPL may be achieved for any length of time, even with the use of energetic immunosuppression, e.g., "pulse" cyclophosphamide, plasmapheresis, or infusions of gammaglobulin. There is usually a rapid rebound to pretreatment levels within days to a week or two after discontinuation of therapy. In situations where such a short-term effect may be desirable, e.g., in pregnant patients with a particularly poor previous obstetric history, this form of treatment has been used. However, in long-term situations, e.g., in patients with recurrent thrombotic events, attempts to reduce elevated aPL levels are usually ineffective and are also difficult to monitor, as levels may fluctuate spontaneously, particularly with waxing and waning of lupus activity. In such at risk patients, therapy has been directed towards reducing the hypercoagulability present in this condition by the use of appropriate anticoagulant or antiaggregant compounds. The dosage and method of administration depends on the acuteness or chronicity of the situation, as well as the need to maintain the international normalization ratio (INR) at levels well above those recommended for the prophylaxis and treatment of idiopathic venous thrombosis or arterial occlusions. This is because of the essential hypercoagulability present in these patients, and resistance to anticoagulants present in some of them. Stroke and other arterial occlusions, e.g., myocardial infarction, is often due to primary vascular disease and, therefore, comparisons in therapy between patients suffering from the aPL coagulopathy and those with atherosclerotic disease cannot be made.

B. TREATMENT OF OTHER RISK FACTORS

Energetic efforts should be made to treat any associated risk factors, e.g., antihypertensives, cholesterol-lowering agents, treatment of active nephritis, avoidance of smoking or sedentarism, etc. Care should also be taken with the administration of oral contraceptives, particularly those with a high estrogen content, in patients with aPL.

There is evidence that their administration may result in complications such as vascular occlusions or chorea.[76] The administration of other drugs associated with drug-induced lupus, e.g., sulphonamides, may also on occasion result in thrombotic events, although this is unusual.

C. PROPHYLAXIS TO PREVENT OCCLUSIVE VASCULAR COMPLICATIONS IN ASYMPTOMATIC PATIENTS

Prophylaxis of arterial thrombosis in the general population is controversial, as it is in patients with aPL. In some trials within the general population and in patients with arteriosclerotic or hypertensive vascular disease,[77] the long-term use of aspirin has proven useful in the prevention of arterial occlusions, mainly of coronary vessels. Comparison between these groups of patients with overt vascular disease and those with aPL may be invalid. However, there may be a case for the prophylactic treatment of individuals with high levels of IgG aPL or persistent lupus anticoagulant (LA) activity using antiaggregants such as aspirin, specially in those with added risk factors. Hydroxychloroquine has also been shown to have an antiaggregant effect and its use may be considered.

On the other hand, prophylaxis of venous thrombosis is required for patients undergoing surgical procedures or who require a long stay in bed. In the general population, the use of low-dose subcutaneous heparin (10,000 to 15,000 units daily) is recommended in those circumstances. However, patients with aPL may show some resistance to these doses, as in other hypercoagulable states, and these doses may be insufficient for the prevention of recurrent thrombosis. It is therefore suggested that higher doses of subcutaneous heparin (25,000 units daily) or intravenous heparin (40,000 units daily) be administered to these patients.

D. TREATMENT OF OCCLUSIVE VASCULAR COMPLICATIONS

Experience in the treatment of patients with aPL and vascular complications is short and based mainly on retrospective studies. Until prospective and controlled studies are documented, the same procedures as apply to the general population should be followed. However, several special considerations should be emphasised:

1. Because of the tendency to recurrence, it is advised that patients should be anticoagulated on a long-term basis, and probably for life.
2. In the case of warfarin therapy, anticoagulation should ideally be controlled by the INR. In patients with aPL, the INR should be kept at levels of 3 to 4, rather than at 2 to 2.5. Recently, Rosove and Brewer[78] have reported the results of anticoagulation treatment after the first thrombotic event in 70 patients with APS. No recurrences were found during high-intensity warfarin treatment (INR >3.5). However, five patients developed bleeding which required interruption of warfarin therapy. There was poor protection by aspirin or low- to intermediate-intensity warfarin treatment (INR <3.5) in this study.
3. In the case of heparin, anticoagulation should be controlled by the recalcification test (Howell test) and not by the activated partial thromboplastin test (APTT), because of the interference of the LA with the latter. The principle of the recalcification test depends on the addition of calcium chloride to platelet-rich plasma which will initiate the coagulation process. The time taken for "soft" clot to form is compared with

normal standards from patients without heparin (5 to 7 min). Ideally, heparinized patients will take 10 to 15 min for clot formation. Heparin levels or the thrombin time may also be used for monitoring these patients.

4. Because of the not uncommon finding of fluctuating levels of the anticoagulation control tests, in some patients frequent and regular visits to anticoagulation clinics should be recommended. Instruction of patients as well as medical personnel as to the dangers of noncompliance is emphasized.
5. The use of steroids in the treatment of vascular occlusions is not recommended. In a recent 5-year follow-up study,[79] we found that those patients with thrombotic complications, usually a sicker group, were mostly all on steroid therapy as well as on immunosuppression at the time of the thrombotic event. Steroids do not seem to offer any protection and, therefore, are not indicated, unless required for the treatment of the underlying condition, e.g., SLE.

E. TREATMENT OF THE "CATASTROPHIC" ANTIPHOSPHOLIPID SYNDROME

Effective therapy depends on early recognition of this syndrome and the administration of anticoagulation and plasmapheresis. Pulse steroids and immunosuppression are generally ineffective. The use of streptokinase or other fibrinolytic agents in these resistant hypercoagulable patients needs to be considered. Concomitant hypertension and renal failure also requires effective treatment.[68]

F. PREVENTION OF FETAL LOSSES

The presence of aPL in pregnant women in the absence of a previous history of fetal loss is not an indication for treatment. In those with previous spontaneous fetal losses or miscarriages, several therapeutic approaches have been proposed, including subcutaneous heparin,[80,81] steroids,[82,83] azathioprine,[84] etc., but no controlled studies have as yet been performed.[85] However, low-dose (50 to 100 mg daily) aspirin administered from the beginning of pregnancy has proven useful and safe in an acceptable number of women with aPL.[86,87] However, because of the risk of hemorrhagic complications in both the newborn and the mother, aspirin should ideally be discontinued at least 48 to 72 h prior to delivery. Some authorities advocate the use of moderate doses of prednisone (15 to 20 mg/day) in the face of a rising titer of anti-cardiolipin antibody (aCL). In addition, close monitoring of pregnancy with doppler techniques, in order to detect placental vascular insufficiency, and early delivery by cesarian section with the first signs of fetal distress are mandatory. If the patient has been receiving warfarin because of previous thrombotic manifestations, this must be changed to subcutaneous heparin, certainly in the first trimester, as warfarin is teratogenic.

G. TREATMENT OF THROMBOCYTOPENIA

Thrombocytopenia associated to aPL is usually mild and does not require intervention. However, in a minority of cases it can be severe and refractory to prednisone therapy. Low-dose aspirin has proved useful in some cases,[88-90] but its administration may not be without risk, especially in patients with less than 20×10^9 platelets/mm^3. Immunosuppressive therapy, i.e., with azathioprine, may be effective in these situations. Intravenous gammaglobulin or danazol therapy may also be considered. In contrast, splenectomy should be recommended with caution in patients with aPL, due to an increased thromboembolic risk related to post-splenectomy thrombocytosis.[91]

V. CASE REPORTS

Case report no. 1 — A 43-year-old Greek man had a history of a right deep vein thrombosis (DVT) followed by a pulmonary embolism in 1970. He had been given anticoagulation therapy with warfarin for about 1 year. In 1981 he had a further right-sided DVT and was again given long-term anticoagulation with warfarin. This was complicated by the development of a hematoma of his right thigh in late 1986, which was associated with a fall in hemoglobin (9.3 g/dl) and elevation of the white cell count (15.2×10^9/l). He recovered after receiving treatment with intensive antibiotic therapy and transfusions. A false-positive serological test for syphilis was first noted in 1979 and had been found on repeated occasions since then. All immunological tests were repeatedly negative, including antibodies to dsDNA and extractable nuclear antigens. Anti-cardiolipin antibodies of the IgG isotype were first detected in 1987 and were repeatedly positive over the following year (18.8, 17.6, and 24.1 GPL units). The lupus anticoagulant was not measured until 1987 as the patient was taking anticoagulation therapy. However, this was found to be positive (kaolin cephalin thromboplastin time 18.4 s, normal $<$6.3 s). A diagnosis of "primary" antiphospholipid syndrome was made. Following his illness, he was found to have developed extensive bronze buccal and skin pigmentation. Addison's disease was suspected and diagnosed after determination of plasma cortisol levels and adrenocorticotropic hormone (ACTH) stimulation. Computerized tomography demonstrated bilateral small adrenal glands. He has been well since then and is taking replacement therapy and anticoagulation.

Case report no. 2 — A 27-year-old woman was admitted to hospital with a 3-week history of mild exertional shortness of breath. Three years previously she had suffered two episodes of DVT affecting both legs. At that time, laboratory investigations disclosed platelets 90×10^9 /l, lupus anticoagulant activity, and high levels of anti-cardiolipin antibodies of the IgG and IgM isotypes. A diagnosis of "primary" antiphospholipid syndrome was made and she was treated with heparin over 6 months. On admission, she was afebrile, there was a grade 3/6 pansystolic murmur at the apex radiating to the axilla, and crackles were heard throughout both lung fields. Lupus anticoagulant activity was detected according to a prolonged diluted Russell's viper venom time and platelet neutralization test. IgG and IgM anti-cardiolipin antibodies were found in high titers (140 GPL and 84 MPL, respectively). The anti-nuclear antibody test was positive at 1:100, whereas DNA binding and antibodies to extractable nuclear antigens were negative. Two-dimensional and Doppler echocardiography revealed mitral valve thickening and a nodular mass (52×40 mm) with vibratory movement attached to the anterior valve leaflet. Six blood cultures and serologies for *Mycoplasma, Legionella,* Q fever, *Clamydia,* and *Brucella* were repeatedly negative. Culture negative endocarditis was diagnosed and she was put on oral doxycycline and sulfamethoxazole-trimethoprim for 2 weeks, in addition to diuretic drugs and aspirin. Several follow-up examinations were performed over the next 6 months when she remained well.

Case report no. 3 — A 22-year-old woman was referred to our care because of eight spontaneous pregnancy losses at 8 to 18 weeks of gestation. Known causes of repeated abortion were excluded by evaluation of hysterosalpingography, karyotyping of woman and husband, toxoplasmosis serology, blood sugar levels, late luteal-phase endometrial biopsy and cultures, midluteal plasma progesterone, estradiol and prolactin, and thyroid function. Male factor as a cause of recurring abortion was also excluded. Lupus anticoagulant activity was detected according to a prolonged diluted Russell's viper venom time. IgG and IgM anti-cardiolipin antibodies were found in low titers.

Full immunological studies showed no abnormalities and a diagnosis of "primary" antiphospholid syndrome was made. In May 1988, she was put on aspirin (100 mg/daily). She became pregnant 2 months later. A sudden and pronounced rise in her lupus anticoagulant level was detected at 29 weeks gestational age. At that time, a chorioamnionitis and sepsis due to a group B streptococcus was diagnosed and fetal death ensued. Five months later, the patient became pregnant again while on aspirin therapy. At 24 weeks gestational age, she presented a pronounced rise in her lupus anticoagulant level and prednisone (15 mg/daily) was added to aspirin therapy. Pregnancy went to term, but a cesarean section was performed at 36 weeks of gestation due to an intrauterine growth retardation diagnosed by Doppler technique. A 2100-g small-for-gestational-age female baby was obtained. Postoperatively, the patient and her infant did well.

Case report no. 4 — A 43-year-old woman with a previous history of lupus nephritis and hypertension presented with a 18-month history of deteriorating mental function, personality change, and visual impairment. She had previously had two spontaneous first-trimester abortions, an episode of superficial thrombophlebitis, and frequent attacks of migraine. Her intellect and vision had continued to deteriorate despite good control of her blood pressure and there had been no improvement with prednisolone (20 mg daily) and azathioprine (100 mg daily) treatment. Formal psychometric testing confirmed an impairment of higher mental function. Serological investigations showed a positive anti-nuclear antibody (ANA) titer (1/80), but no antibodies to DNA. IgG anticardiolpin antibodies were present in high titer, while clotting tests were normal, and the Venereal Disease Research Laboratory (VDRL) test was negative. Circulating immune complexes were detected in low concentration and the C_4 level was reduced. Renal function tests showed a creatinine of 124 μmol/l and 24-h urinary protein loss of 0.7 g. Normal investigations included full blood count, erythrocyte sedimentation rate, thyroid function tests, serum vitamin B_{12} and red cells folate levels, chest X-ray, electrocardiogram, and examination of the cerebrospinal fluid. A computed tomographic brain scan showed bilateral lacunar infarcts (Figure 1). Under the diagnosis of multi-infarct dementia, a decision was made to start long-term anticoagulation, but before it was implemented the patient suffered a major stroke with a right lower quadrantanopia, dysphasia, and a monoplegia of her right upper limb.

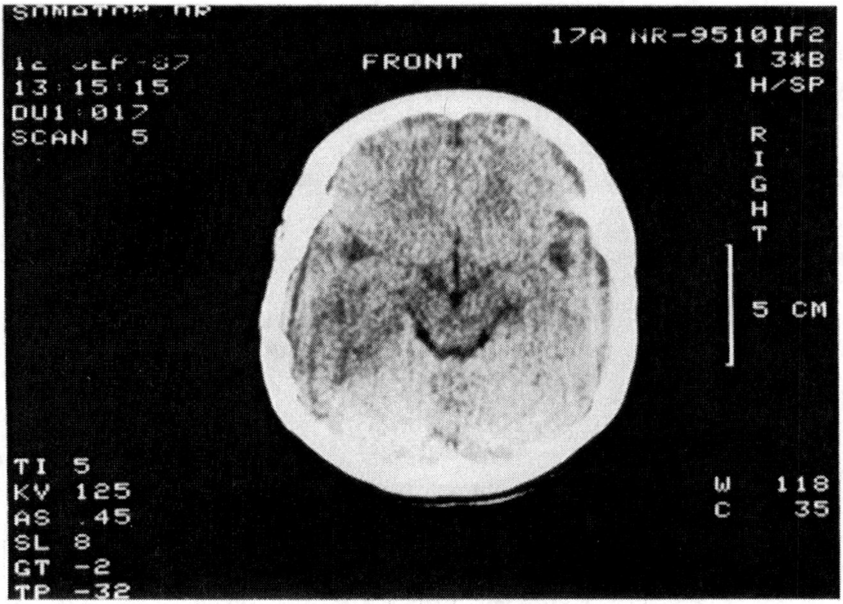

Figure 1 Computed tomographic brain scan showing bilateral lacunar infarcts.

REFERENCES

1. **Tan, E. M., Cohen, A. S., Fries, A. F., Masi, A. T., McShane, D. J., Rothfield, N. F., Schaller, J. G., Talal, N., and Winchester, R. J.,** The 1982 revised criteria for the classification of systemic lupus erythematosus, *Arthritis Rheum.*, 25, 1271, 1982.
2. **Asherson, R. A., Cervera, R., and Lahita, R.,** Latent, incomplete or lupus at all?, *J. Rheumatol.*, 18, 1783, 1991.
3. **Asherson, R. A.,** A 'primary' antiphospholipid syndrome?, *J. Rheumatol.*, 15, 1742, 1988.
4. **Asherson, R. A., Khamashta, M. A., Ordi-Ros, J., Derksen, R. H. W. M., Machin, S. J., Barquinero, J., Outt, H. H., Harris, E. N., Vilardell-Tarrés, M., and Hughes, G. R. V.,** The 'primary' antiphospholipid syndrome: major clinical and serological features, *Medicine (Baltimore)*, 68, 366, 1989.
5. **Alarcón-Segovia, D. and Sánchez-Guerrero, J.,** Primary antiphospholipid syndrome, *J. Rheumatol.*, 16, 482, 1989.
6. **Mackworth-Young, C. G., Loizou, S., and Walport, M. J.,** Primary antiphospholipid syndrome: features of patients with raised anticardiolipin antibodies and no other disorder, *Ann. Rheum. Dis.*, 48, 362, 1989.
7. **Font, J., López-Soto, A., Cervera, R., Balasch, J., Pallarés, L., Navarro, M., Bosch, X., and Ingelmo, M.,** The 'primary' antiphospholipid syndrome: antiphospholipid antibody pattern and clinical features of a series of 23 patients, *Autoimmunity*, 9, 69, 1991.

8. **Harris, E. N., Baguley, E., Asherson, R. A., and Hughes, G. R. V.,** Clinical and serological features of the antiphospholipid syndrome (APS), *Br. J. Rheumatol.*, 26 (Abstr.), 19, 1987.
9. **Manoussakis, M. N., Tzioufas, A. G., Silis, M. P., Pange, P. J. E., Goudevenos, J., and Moutsopoulos, H. M.,** High prevalence of anticardiolipin and other autoantibodies in a healthy elderly population, *Clin. Exp. Immunol.*, 69, 557, 1987.
10. **Font, J., Pallarés, L., Cervera, R., López-Soto, A., Navarro, M., Bosch, X., and Ingelmo, M.,** Systemic lupus erythematosus in the elderly. Clinical and serological characteristics, *Ann. Rheum. Dis.*, 50, 702, 1991.
11. **Asherson, R. A. and Hughes, G. R. V.,** Hypoadrenalism, Addison's disease and antiphospholipid antibodies, *J. Rheumatol.*, 18, 1, 1991.
12. **Landi, G., Calloni, M. V., Sabbadini, M. G., Mannucci, P. M., and Candelise, L.,** Recurrent ischaemic attacks in two young adults with lupus anticoagulant, *Stroke,* 14, 377, 1983.
13. **Levine, S. R. and Welch, K. M. A.,** The spectrum of neurologic disease associated with antiphospholipid antibodies, *Arch. Neurol.*, 44, 876, 1987.
14. **D'Alton, J. G., Preston, D. N., Bormanis, J., Green, M. S., and Kraag, G. R.,** Multiple transient ischaemic attacks, lupus anticoagulant and verrucous endocarditis, *Stroke,* 16, 512, 1985.
15. **Asherson, R. A., Khamashta, M. A., Gil, A., Vázquez, J. J., Chan, O., Baguley, E., and Hughes, G. R. V.,** Cerebrovascular disease and antiphospholipid antibodies in systemic lupus erythematosus, lupus-like disease, and the primary antiphospholipid syndrome, *Am. J. Med.*, 86, 391, 1989.
16. **Briley, D. P., Coull, B. M., and Goodnight, S. H.,** Neurological disease associated with antiphospholipid antibodies, *Ann. Neurol.*, 25, 221, 1989.
17. **Levine, S. R. and Welch, K. M. A.,** Cerebrovascular ischaemia associated with lupus anticoagulant, *Stroke,* 18, 257, 1987.
18. **Sneddon, J. E.,** Cerebrovascular lesions in livedo reticularis, *Br. J. Dermatol.*, 77, 180, 1965.
19. **Jonas, J., Kolble, K., Volcker, H. E., and Kalden, J. R.,** Central retinal artery occlusion in Sneddon's disease associated with antiphospholipid antibodies, *Am. J. Ophthalmol.*, 102, 37, 1986.
20. **Levine, S. R., Langer, S. L., Albers, J. W., and Welch, K. M. A.,** Sneddon's syndrome: an antiphospholipid syndrome?, *Neurology,* 38, 798, 1988.
21. **Asherson, R. A., Khamashta, M. A., and Hughes, G. R. V.,** Antiphospholipid antibodies and thrombosis, *Lancet,* ii, 272, 1988.
22. **Asherson, R. A., Khamashta, M. A., Baguley, E., Oakley, C. M., Rowell, N. R., and Hughes, G. R. V.,** Myocardial infarction and antiphospholipid antibodies in SLE and related disorders, *Q. J. Med.*, 73, 1103, 1989.
23. **Asherson, R. A., Derksen, R. H. W. M., Harris, E. N., Bingley, P. J., Hoffbrand, B. I., Gharavi, A. E., Kater, L., and Hughes, G. R. V.,** Large vessel occlusion and gangrene in systemic lupus erythematosus and 'lupus-like' disease: a report of six cases, *J. Rheumatol.*, 13, 740, 1986.
24. **Asherson, R. A., Mackworth-Young, C. G., Harris, E. N., Gharavi, A. E., and Hughes, G. R. V.,** Multiple venous and arterial thromboses associated with the lupus anticoagulant and antibodies to cardiolipin in the absence of SLE, *Rheumatol. Int.*, 5, 91, 1985.

25. **Asherson, R. A., Harris, E. N., and Gharavi, A. E.,** Aortic arch syndrome associated with anticardiolipin antibodies and the lupus anticoagulant, *Arthritis Rheum.,* 38, S94, 1985.
26. **Asherson, R. A., Derksen, R. H. W. M., and Hughes, G. R. V.,** Renal infarction associated with antiphospholipid antibodies in systemic lupus erythematosus and 'lupus-like' disease, *J. Urol.,* 140, 1028, 1988.
27. **Jouquan, J., Pennec, Y., Mottier, D., Youinou, P., Cledes, J., Leroy, J. P., and Le Menn, G.,** Accelerated hypertension associated with lupus anticoagulant and false positive VDRL in systemic lupus erythematosus, *Arthritis Rheum.,* 29, 147, 1986.
28. **Asherson, R. A., Noble, G. R., and Hughes, G. R. V.,** Hypertension, renal artery stenosis and the 'primary' antiphospholipid syndrome: a case report, *J. Rheumatol.,* 18, 1413, 1991.
29. **Mor, F., Beigel, Y., Inbal, A., Goren, M., and Wysenbeek, A. J.,** Hepatic infarction in a patient with the lupus anticoagulant, *Arthritis Rheum.,* 32, 491, 1989.
30. **Asherson, R. A., Mercy, D., Phillips, G., Sheehan, N., Gharavi, A. E., Harris, E. N., and Hughes, G. R. V.,** Recurrent stroke and multiinfarct dementia in systemic lupus erythematosus. Association with antiphospholipid antibodies, *Ann. Rheum. Dis.,* 46, 605, 1987.
31. **Coull, B. M., Bourdette, D. N., Goodnight, S. H., Jr., Briley, D. P., and Hart, R.,** Multiple cerebral infarctions and dementia associated with anticardiolipin antibodies, *Stroke,* 18, 1107, 1987.
32. **Fields, R. A., Sibbitt, W. L., Toubbeh, H., and Bankhurst, A. D.,** Neuropsychiatric lupus erythematosus, cerebral infarctions and anticardiolipin antibodies, *N. Rheum. Dis.,* 49, 114, 1990.
33. **Brown, J. H., Doherty, C. C., Alan, D. C., and Morton, P.,** Fatal cardiac failure due to myocardial microthrombi in systemic lupus erythematosus, *Br. Med. J.,* 296, 1505, 1988.
34. **Nihoyannopoulos, P., Gómez, P. M., Joshi, J., Loizou, S., Walport, M. J., and Oakley, C. M.,** Cardiac abnormalities in systemic lupus erythematosus: association with raised anticardiolipin antibodies, *Circulation,* 82, 369, 1990.
35. **Kant, K. S., Pollak, V. E., Weiss, M. A., Glueck, H. I., Miller, A. N., and Hess, E. V.,** Glomerular thrombosis in systemic lupus erythematosus: prevalence and significance, *Medicine (Baltimore),* 60, 71, 1981.
36. **Kincaid-Smith, P., Fairley, K. F., and Kloss, M.,** Lupus anticoagulant associated with renal thrombotic microangiopathy and pregnancy-related renal failure, *O. J. Med.,* 69, 795, 1988.
37. **Leaker, B., MacGregor, A. J., Isenberg, D. A., and Nield, G.,** Insidious loss of renal function in patients with anticardiolipin antibodies (ACLA) in absence of overt nephritis, *Br. J. Rheumatol.,* 19 (Suppl. 2), 108, 1990.
38. **D'Agati, V., Kunis, C., Williams, G., and Apple, G. B.,** Anticardiolipin antibody and renal disease: a report of three cases, *J. Am. Soc. Nephrol.,* 1, 777, 1990.
39. **Asherson, R. A., Khamashta, M. A., and Hughes, G. R. V.,** The hepatic complications of the antiphospholipid antibodies, *Clin. Exp. Rheumatol.,* 9, 341, 1991.
40. **Asherson, R. A., Merry, P., Acheson, J. F., Harris, E. N., and Hughes, G. R. V.,** Antiphospholipid antibodies: a risk factor for occlusive ocular vascular disease in systemic lupus erythematosus and the 'primary' antiphospholipid syndrome, *Ann. Rheum. Dis.,* 48, 358, 1989.
41. **Galepta, S. L., Plock, G. L., and Kushner, M. J.,** Ocular thrombosis associated with antiphospholipid antibodies, *Ann. Ophthalmol.,* 23, 207, 1991.

42. **Kleiner, R. C., Najarian, L. V., Schatten, S., Jabs, D. A., Patz, A., and Kaplan, H. J.,** Vasoocclusive retinopathy associated with antiphospholipid antibodies (lupus anticoagulant retinopathy), *Ophthalmology,* 96, 896, 1989.
43. **Openheimer, S. and Hoffbrand, B. I.,** Optic neuritis and myelopathy in systemic lupus erythematosus, *Can. J. Neurol. Sci.,* 13, 129, 1986.
44. **Alegre, V. A., Gastineau, D. A., and Winklemann, R. K.,** Skin lesions associated with circulating lupus anticoagulant, *Br. J. Dermatol.,* 120, 419, 1989.
45. **Anderson, D., Bell, D., Lodge, R., and Grant, E.,** Recurrent cerebral ischaemia and mitral valve vegetation in a patient with lupus anticoagulant, *J. Rheumatol.,* 14, 839, 1987.
46. **Asherson, R. A. and Lubbe, W. F.,** Cerebral and valve lesions in SLE: association with antiphospholipid antibodies, *J. Rheumatol.,* 15, 539, 1988.
47. **Lubbe, W. F. and Asherson, R. A.,** Intracardiac thrombus in systemic lupus erythematosus associated with lupus anticoagulant, *Arthritis Rheum.,* 31, 1453, 1988.
48. **Leventhal, L. J., Borofsky, M. A., Bergey, P. D., and Schumacher, H. R., Jr.,** Antiphospholipid antibody syndrome with atrial thrombosis mimicking an atrial mixoma, *Am. J. Med.,* 87, 111, 1989.
49. **Khamashta, M. A., Cervera, R., Asherson, R. A., Font, J., Gil, A., Coltart, D. J., Vázquez, J. J., Paré, C., Ingelmo, M., Oliver, J., and Hughes, G. R. V.,** Association of antibodies against phospholipids with heart valve disease in systemic lupus erythematosus, *Lancet,* 335, 1541, 1990.
50. **Asherson, R. A. and Cervera, R.,** Antiphospholipid antibodies and the heart: lessons and pitfalls for the cardiologist, *Circulation,* 84, 920, 1991.
51. **Cervera, R., Khamashta, M. A., Font, J., Reyes, P. A., Vianna, J. L., López-Soto, A., Amigo, M. C., Asherson, R. A., Azqueta, M., Paré, C., Vargas, J., Romero, A., Ingelmo, M., and Hughes, G. R. V.,** High prevalence of significant heart valve lesions in patients with the 'primary' antiphospholipid syndrome, *Lupus,* 1, 43, 1991.
52. **Asherson, R. A., Higenbottam, T. W., and Dihn Xuan, A. T.,** Pulmonary hypertension in a lupus clinic: experience with 24 patients, *J. Rheumatol.,* 17, 1292, 1990.
53. **Asherson, R. A., Derksen, R. H. W. M., Harris, E. N., Bouma, B. N., Gharavi, A. E., Kater, L., and Hughes, G. R. V.,** Chorea in systemic lupus erythematosus and lupus-like disease: association with antiphospholipid antibodies, *Semin. Arthritis Rheum.,* 16, 253, 1987.
54. **Asherson, R. A., Junghers, P., Liote, F., and Hughes, G. R. V.,** Ischaemic necrosis of bone associated with the "lupus anticoagulant" and antibodies to cardiolipin, *Proc. XVIth Int. Cong. Rheum.,* Sydney, Australia, 1983, 373.
55. **Lavalle, C., Pizarro, S., Drenkard, C., Sánchez-Guerrero, J., and Alarcón-Segovia, D.,** Transverse myelitis: a manifestation of systemic lupus erythematosus strongly associated with antiphospholipid antibodies, *J. Rheumatol.,* 17, 34, 1990.
56. **Frampton, G., Winer, J. P., Cameron, J. S., and Hughes, R. A. C.,** Severe Guillain-Barré syndrome in association with IgA anticardiolipin antibody in a series of 92 patients, *J. Neuro. Immunol.,* 19, 133, 1988.
57. **Hering, R., Couturier, E. G. H., Steiner, T. J., Asherson, R. A., and Clifford Rose, F.,** Anticardiolipin antibodies in migraine, *Cephalalgia,* 11, 19, 1991.
58. **Branch, D. W., Andres, R., and Digre, K. B.,** The association of antiphospholipid antibodies with severe pre-eclampsia, *Obstet, Gynaecol.,* 73, 541, 1989.

59. **Montalbán, J., Cervera, R., Font, J., Ordi, J., Vianna, J., Haga, H. J., Tintoré, M., Khamashta, M. A., and Hughes, G. R. V.,** Lack of association between anticardiolipin antibodies and migraine in systemic lupus erythematosus, *Neurology,* 42, 681, 1992.
60. **Lockshin, M. D., Druzin, M. L., Goei, S., Qamar, T., Magid, M. S., Jovanovic, L., and Ferenc, M.,** Antibody to cardiolipin as a predictor of fetal distress or death in pregnant patients with systemic lupus erythematosus, *N. Engl. J. Med.,* 313, 152, 1985.
61. **Lockshin, M. D., Qamar, T., Druzin, M. L., and Goei, S.,** Anticardiolipin antibody, lupus anticoagulant and fetal death, *J. Rheumatol.,* 14, 259, 1987.
62. **Walport, M. J.,** Pregnancy and antibodies to phospholipids, *Ann. Rheum. Dis.,* 48, 795, 1989.
63. **Cervera, R., Font, J., López-Soto, A., Casals, F., Pallarés, L., Bové, A., Ingelmo, M., and Urbano-Márquez, A.,** Isotype distribution of anticardiolipin antibodies in systemic lupus erythematosus: prospective analysis of a series of 100 patients, *Ann. Rheum. Dis.,* 49, 109, 1990.
64. **Delezé, M., Oria, C. M., and Alarcón-Segovia, D.,** Occurrence of both hemolytic anemia and thrombocytopenic purpura (Evans' syndrome) in systemic lupus erythematosus. Relationship to antiphospholipid antibodies, *J. Rheumatol.,* 15, 611, 1988.
65. **Delezé, M., Alarcón-Segovia, D., Oria, C. V., Sánchez-Guerrero, J., Fernández-Domínguez, L., Gómez-Pacheco, L., and Ponce de León, S.,** Hemocytopenia in systemic lupus erythematosus. Relationship to antiphospholipid antibodies, *J. Rheumatol.,* 16, 926, 1989.
66. **Harris, E. N., Asherson, R. A., Gharavi, A. E., Morgan, S. H., Derue, G., and Hughes, G. R. V.,** Thrombocytopenia in SLE and related autoimmune disorders: association with anticardiolipin antibody, *Br. J. Haematol.,* 59, 227, 1985.
67. **Harris, E. N., Chan, J. K. H., Asherson, R. A., Aber, V. R., Gharavi, A. E., and Hughes, G. R. V.,** Thrombosis, recurrent fetal loss, and thrombocytopenia. Predictive value of the anticardiolipin antibody test, *Arch. Intern. Med.,* 146, 2153, 1986.
68. **Asherson, R. A.,** The catastrophic antiphospholipid syndrome, *J. Rheumatol.,* 19, 508, 1992.
69. **Mustafa, M. H., Mispireta, L. A., and Pierce, L. E.,** Occult pulmonary embolism presenting with thrombocytopenia and elevated fibrin split products, *Am. J. Med.,* 86, 490, 1989.
70. **Shergy, W. J., Kredich, D. W., and Pisetsky, D. S.,** The relationship of anticardiolipin antibodies to disease manifestations in pediatric systemic lupus erythematosus, *J. Rheumatol.,* 15, 1389, 1988.
71. **Roddy, S. M. and Giang, D. W.,** Antiphospholipid antibodies and stroke in an infant, *Pediatrics,* 87, 933, 1991.
72. **Kelley, R. E. and Berger, J. R.,** Ischemic stroke in a girl with lupus anticoagulant, *Pediatr. Neurol.,* 3, 58, 1987.
73. **Pelkonen, P., Simell, O., Rasi, V., and Vaarala, O.,** Venous thrombosis associated with lupus anticoagulant and anticardiolipin antibodies, *Acta Paediatr. Scand.,* 77, 767, 1988.
74. **Finazzi, G., Cortelazzo, S., Viero, P., Galli, M., and Barbui, T.,** Maternal lupus anticoagulant and fatal neonatal thrombosis, *Thromb. Haemostas.,* 57, 238, 1987.

75. **Sheridan-Pereira, M., Porreco, R. P., Hays, T., and Burke, M. S.,** Neonatal aortic thrombosis associated with the lupus anticoagulant, *Obstet. Gynecol.,* 71, 1016, 1988.
76. **Asherson, R. A., Harris, E. N., and Hughes, G. R. V.,** Complications of oral contraceptives and antiphospholipid antibodies, *Arthritis Rheum.,* 31, 575, 1988.
77. **Antiplatelet Trialists' Collaboration,** Secondary prevention of vascular disease by prolonged antiplatelet treatment, *Br. Med. J.,* 296, 320, 1988.
78. **Rosove, M. H., and Brewer, P. M. C.,** Antiphospholipid thrombosis: results of treatment after the first thrombotic event in 70 patients, *Arthritis Rheum.,* 34 (Suppl.), S42, 1991.
79. **Asherson, R. A., Baguley, E., Pal, C., and Hughes, G. R. V.,** Antiphospholipid syndrome: five year follow up, *Ann. Rheum. Dis.,* 50, 805, 1991.
80. **Lubbe, W. F., Butler, W. S., Palmer, S. J., and Liggins, G. C.,** Lupus anticoagulant in pregnancy, *Br. J. Obstet. Gynaecol.,* 91, 357, 1984.
81. **Rosove, M. H., Tabsch, K., Howard, P., Wasserstrum, N., Howard, P., Hahn, B. H., and Kalunian, K. C.,** Heparin therapy for pregnant women with lupus anticoagulant or anticardiolipin antibodies, *Obstet. Gynecol.,* 75, 630, 1990.
82. **Ordi, J., Barquinero, J., Vilardell, M., Jordana, R., Tolosa, C., Selva, A., and Genover, E.,** Fetal loss treatment in patients with antiphospholipid antibodies, *Ann. Rheum. Dis.,* 48, 798, 1989.
83. **Prentice, R. L., Gatenby, P. A., Loblay, R. H., Shearman, R. P., Kronenberg, H., and Basten, A.,** Lupus anticoagulant in pregnancy, *Lancet,* ii, 464, 1984.
84. **Branch, D. W., Scott, J. R., Kochenour, N. K., and Hershgold, E.,** Obstetric complications associated with the lupus anticoagulant, *N. Engl. J. Med.,* 313, 1322, 1985.
85. **Walport, M. J.,** Pregnancy and antibodies to phospholipids, *Ann. Rheum. Dis.,* 48, 795, 1989.
86. **Balasch, J., Font, J., López-Soto, A., Cervera, R., Jové, I., Casals, F. J., and Vanrell, J. A.,** Antiphospholipid antibodies in unselected patients with repeated abortion, *Hum. Reprod.,* 5, 43, 1990.
87. **Elder, M. G., de Swiet, M., Robertson, A., Elder, M. A., Floyd, E., and Hawkins, D. F.,** Low-dose aspirin in pregnancy, *Lancet,* i, 410, 1988.
88. **Alarcón-Segovia, D. and Sánchez-Guerrero, J.,** Correction of thrombocytopenia with small dose aspirin in the primary antiphospholipid syndrome, *J. Rheumatol.,* 16, 1359, 1989.
89. **Dessein, P. H., Lamperelli, R. D., Phillips, S. A., Rubenchik, I. A., and Zwi, S.,** Severe immune thrombocytopenia and the development of skin infarctions in a patient with an overlap syndrome, *J. Rheumatol.,* 16, 1494, 1989.
90. **Iwahara, Y., Niiya, K., Yamato, K., and Myoshi, I.,** Thrombocytopenic purpura in a patient with lupus anticoagulant: requirement of both immunosuppressive and antithrombotic therapies, *Am. J. Haematol.,* 33, 75, 1990.
91. **Exner, T., Rickard, K. A., and Kronenberg, H.,** Studies on phospholipids in the action of a lupus coagulation inhibitor, *Pathology,* 7, 319, 1975.

VI. Cytokines in Autoimmune Diseases

Chapter 14

Classification, Description, and Activities of Cytokines and their Receptors

Mariana Linker-Israeli

CONTENTS

I. INTRODUCTION AND OVERVIEW

Cytokines are relatively small proteins or glycoproteins. They are essential for the regulation of normal immune reactions and inflammatory responses. Because of that, cytokines have become the object of intensive studies in rheumatic diseases.

As research on these molecules progresses, it is clear that their activity is associated with high specificity, but also with redundancy. Cytokines form a network where they may have additive, synergistic, or antagonistic activity: they can induce themselves and

0-8493-5974-1/94/$0.00 + $.50

other cytokines, but they can also downregulate cytokine production. Each cytokine can be produced by cells from different lineages, and can have multiple and overlapping effects on target cells of various types. On the other hand, each cytokine is encoded by a specific gene and, therefore, has specific amino acid sequences, and acts on cell targets by binding to unique receptors.

Normally, cytokines are under tight gene regulation, and are not expressed constitutively in resting cells. Cell activation transiently triggers the expression of most cytokines and their receptors. Therefore, persistent expression of the cytokines and receptors that are not constitutively expressed reflects aberrant endogenous cell activation, such as that found in autoimmune conditions. The effects that cytokines have on lymphocytes and monocytes suggest that they contribute to the aberrant antigen presentation and immune regulation in rheumatic diseases, and their inflammatory and tissue-damaging activities indicate that they have a direct pathogenic role in these diseases. Persistent inflammatory reactions become harmful to the host. Lymphocytes, macrophages, and polymorphonuclear cells all release the factors that mediate local inflammation and tissue damage. The molecules involved in these responses, such as corticoids, oxygen radicals, degrading enzymes, prostaglandins, and leukotrienes, are produced as a result of cytokine activity, and, in turn, modulate cytokine production/activity. Therefore, anticytokine therapy may offer a logical alternative treatment in rheumatic diseases.

Following cell activation, soluble forms of cytokine receptors are also induced and secreted. These are truncated molecules, lacking the transmembrane and/or cytoplasmic domains. They may inhibit cytokine activity on target cells by interfering with binding of the free cytokine to its membrane-bound receptors. On the other hand, they may provide transportation for cytokines and delivery to target cells bearing high-affinity membrane-bound receptors. The availability of cytokine-binding nonblocking proteins that can protect and transport, and the high affinity of the membrane-bound cytokine receptors enable cytokines to deliver signals even when produced in low quantities at relatively long distances from the involved site.

The interaction cytokine receptor involves specific binding and signal transduction. In many cases, these two activities reside in different subunits of the respective receptor. The signal is transduced after initial cytokine-receptor binding, by interaction of the complex with a GTP-binding protein, and activation of pathways that yield second messengers. Common activation pathways include the proteinase kinase C (PKC), intracellular Ca^{2+} fluxes, and phosphotidylinositol (PI) turnover. Nuclear-binding factors are induced that recognize regulatory sequences of responding genes, and deliver positive or negative signals.

The development of recombinant cytokines, specific antibodies, and sensitive assays has made possible the study of cytokines *in vitro*. However, a major concern is the relevance of these studies to *in vivo* processes. First, cytokine measurements in body fluids express only the balance between levels of cytokines and those of inhibitory or amplifying molecules, such as soluble receptors, anti-cytokine antibodies, or other cytokine-or receptor-binding molecules. Therefore, even slightly aberrant levels of cytokines may be indicative of disease. Further, *in vitro* studies of individual cytokines also pose problems, since, in the natural environment, a single stimulus may elicit multiple cytokines that interact with the cytokine under study.

In the last 15 years, many new cytokine activities have been investigated. The cytokines and the proteins they bind have been purified, cloned, sequenced, and mapped to respective chromosomes. In this chapter, discussion will be confined to the cytokines that, to date, have been consistently associated with rheumatic diseases.

II. INFLAMMATORY CYTOKINES AND THEIR RECEPTORS

A. IL-1

Interleukin-1 (IL-1) evolved probably more than 400 million years ago, preceding immunoglobulins, and is present, in addition to mammals, in starfish, amphibians, fish, and birds. IL-1 is rarely expressed constitutively, and may be induced by mitogens, antigens, and cytokines, including IL-1. Generally, it originates as a 31-kDa precursor molecule that produces, upon cleavage from the carboxy terminal, the mature, 17-kDa form. Two species of IL-1 have been sequenced and cloned: IL-1α and IL-1β. Both are encoded by genes mapped to chromosome 2, and consist of 7 exons. IL-1α is detected mainly in association with the cell membrane, and is active in interactions where direct cell-to-cell contact is needed. Most of the IL-1 detected in culture supernatants or in body fluids is IL-1β, which is thought to act as a soluble mediator. Possibly, the two IL-1 forms are under separate transcriptional control.[1-6]

1. Effects of IL-1

IL-1 was originally described as endogenous pyrogen, EP, later as lymphocyte activating factor, LAF, and has many other biological effects. It is an important factor in rheumatic disease because of its immunoregulatory potential, and its systemic and local effects in inflammation and tissue damage.

Immunoregulatory effects — IL-1 supplies co-mitogenic and differentiation signals for lymphocytes (T, B, and natural killer [NK]) at different stages of maturation, by inducing the expression of growth/differentiation factors, including IL-2, tumor necrosis factor (TNF)-α, IL-6, and IL-1 itself, of cytokine receptors (i.e., IL-2R), adhesion molecules, and the IgG kappa light chain.

Effects on nonimmune tissue, inflammation, and tissue damage — Il-1 affects the central nervous system by inducing fever, slow-wave sleep, and the release of neuropeptides, and may be a cofactor in synaptic transmission. IL-1 acts on hepatocytes by upregulating synthesis of selected acute-phase proteins and downregulating synthesis of albumin. IL-1 injections into the joint space are followed by tissue destruction, bone resorption, and proteoglycan degradation. These are mediated by induction of the collagenase and cyclooxygenase genes in synovial cells, the latter followed by prostaglandin (PGE_2) production, enhancement of proteoglycanase production in chondrocytes, in synergy with TNF-α, proliferation of osteoblasts producing PGE_2 and plasminogen activating factor, and activation of endothelial cells as evidenced by expression of adhesion molecules and the release of PGE_2, PGI_2, and platelet activating factor (PAF). IL-1 also indirectly increases fibroblast proliferation, possibly synergizing with other growth factors, such as platelet-derived growth factor (PDGF). IL-1 may have a direct role in lupus nephritis, as it induces mesangial cell proliferation and superoxide production. Very little amounts of IL-1 are sufficient for delivering signals to target cells. When as little as 10 ng/ml IL-1 was injected into animals, it induced other cytokines, such as IL-6 (increasing synthesis of acute-phase proteins), colony stimulating factors (possibly related to its radioprotective effect), and other typical acute-phase responses. In fact, several effects that had been previously attributed to IL-1 are directly mediated by cytokines that are induced by IL-1. Thus, IL-1 is co-mitogenic for thymocytes by induction of IL-2. IL-1 triggers acute-phase proteins, probably by induction of IL-6, and causes neutrophilia by induction of IL-8. Besides inducing these cytokines, IL-1 also synergizes with IL-2, TNF-α, IL-6, and IL-8, *in vitro* and *in vivo*.[1-2,7-8]

2. IL-1 Receptors (IL-1R)

Although different in their primary structures and biophysical properties, IL-1α and IL-1β bind to the same receptors. IL-1R are constitutively expressed. Two types of IL-1R have been described. Both are transmembrane molecules that belong to the Ig supergene family. IL-1R type I, (IL-1RtI), is an 80-kDa molecule that fully transduces the IL-1 signal, and is found on T, B, and NK lymphocytes, macrophages, fibroblasts, endothelial cells, hepatocytes, and keratinocytes. The type II receptor (IL-1RtII), is a 68-kDa molecule having a very short cytoplasmic domain, associated mainly with B cells, neutrophils, and bone marrow cells. There is recent evidence that cellular expression of the two receptors is not mutually exclusive. The two types differ in kinetics of ligand internalization and, although both species of IL-1 bind to either receptor, the affinity of binding may differ, with IL-1α binding more efficiently to IL-1RtI, and IL-1β binding preferentially to IL-1RtII. A soluble form of the IL-1RtII was found in spent media of Raji cells. Soluble IL-1 receptors may act as immuno suppressants, since injection of recombinant IL-1RtI to mice delayed allograft rejection. However, neither type of receptor has been detected yet in human plasma or urine.[9-13]

3. Regulation of IL-1 Expression

IL-1 production is triggered by endotoxin and other microbial products that stimulate both IL-1 and TNF-α production. Viruses, synthetic adjuvants, complement components, thrombin, bile salts, androgen metabolites, and cytokines such as TNF-α, all induce IL-1 expression. IL-1 expression is downregulated by α2-macroglobulin and lipids that inhibit several other cytokines. Further, specific IL-1 inhibitory activities have been found in human urine and plasma. The IL-1 receptor antagonist, IL-1ra, could be of particular clinical relevance. This inhibitor acts at the level of the IL-1/receptor interaction. It is an 18- to 22-kDa molecule that has some degree of homology with IL-1, competes with it for receptor occupancy, yet does not provide the cells with an IL-1 signal. Since IL-1 affects inflammation, tissue remodeling, and bone resorption, the IL-1ra may prove to be an efficient drug for the treatment of rheumatic diseases.[1,15-17]

B. TNF-α

At the end of the 19th century, Coley reported that spent medium derived from cultures of *Streptococcus* or *Serratia* induced hemorrhagic necrosis of human tumors. Studies on this factor were abandoned because of toxicity, but were revived in the course of studies on the hemorrhagic necrosis of tumors that may occur in the context of acute bacterial infections, and when serum of endotoxin-treated mice passively transferred tumor-necrotizing properties. TNF-α was isolated and characterized. This molecule is identical to the cachectin that was described by other groups studying the pathogenesis of wasting in chronic disease. TNF-α and the related cytokine lymphotoxin (TNF-β) are encoded by closely linked genes contained within the MHC on chromosome 6, proximal to the D locus. Both cytokines bind to the same receptors. The immature form of TNF-α contains a 76-amino acid pro-segment that is cleaved, and the mature form is a 17 kDa protein. The carboxy terminal of the molecule is particularly important for bioactivity. TNF-α is produced primarily by macrophages stimulated with LPS or by monocytes primed with Interferon-γ. It is also induced in T cells stimulated with Phorbol Myristic Acetate (PMA) and the calcium Ionophore A 23187, or viruses.[18-21]

1. TNF-α Effects

Upon injection into rats, TNF-α induces hypotension, metabolic acidosis, transient hyperglycemia followed by hypoglycemia, hemorrhagic infarction of the gastrointestinal tract, adrenal and pancreatic hemorrhages, acute renal tubular necrosis, severe interstitial pneumonitis leading to occasional respiratory arrest. TNF-α is a potent endogenous pyrogen. It is involved in the pathogenesis of malaria and graft-versus-host disease, and of Gram-negative septic shock. TNF-α downregulates adipocyte differentiation and lipo protein lipase (LPL) levels, inhibits expression of adipose tissue-specific proteins, and antagonizes lipogenic effects of insulin. It also downregulates erythropoiesis by directly affecting hemopoietic stem cells. TNF-α induces in endothelial cells production of a procoagulant factor and inhibits thrombomodulin. The TNF-triggered hemorrhagic necrosis of tumors may be mediated by these effects, as well as by the IL-1 that TNF-α induces in endothelial cells. Although TNF-α may directly affect hypothalamic neurons, its pyrogenic activity is due in part also to a TNF-triggered, IL-1-mediated effect. Another indirect effect of TNF is induction of acute-phase proteins in hepatocytes, probably mediated by TNF-induced IL-6.

Since immune stimulation induces in T cells both TNF and its receptor, TNF may modulate, in autocrine and/or paracrine fashion, immune responses. Indeed, TNF-α may determine cell activation, differentiation, and cell-to-cell interaction, as it enhances, in lymphocytes, expression of activation molecules such as MHC class II and IL-2 receptors, and in dermal fibroblasts and vascular endothelial cells, MHC class I expression. Important in local inflammation may be the TNF-α modulation of phagocytic and cytotoxic activity of neutrophils, possibly by increasing production of superoxide anions and hydrogen peroxide. TNF-α stimulates degranulation and stops neutrophil migration while inducing neutrophil adhesion to endothelial cells. *In vitro,* TNF accelerates neutrophil-mediated destruction of endothelial cells. The effects of TNF-α on connective tissue also suggest a role for this cytokine in the inflammation occurring in rheumatic bones and joints: like IL-1, albeit 1000-fold less potent, TNF stimulates bone resorption; it triggers proteoglycan degradation in cartilage, and suppresses its synthesis *in vitro;* finally, TNF induces production of PGE-2 and collagenase by synovial cells and skin fibroblasts. Besides the soluble TNF-α, the membrane-anchored cytokine also functions in cytotoxic and other cell-to-cell interactions.[22-35]

2. TNF Receptors (TNF-R)

All tissues, except red blood cells, can express TNF-R; therefore, it is not surprising that TNF-α acts on a variety of target cells. Constitutive expression of TNF-R was observed on various resting cells, except lymphocytes, that express the receptor only following activation. By studying binding of radio-labeled TNF to various cell lines, two types of TNF-binding molecules have been detected: the 75- to 80-kDa type A (TNF-RI), that has been associated primarily with activated T and B lymphocytes, and the 55- to 60-kDa type B (TNF-RII) receptor. Both bind to TNF with high affinity. Soluble forms of both types of TNF receptor, resulting from enzymatic cleavage of the membrane-bound molecule, have been detected in urine of normal individuals and in supernatants of activated cells. Soluble TNF receptors compete with the membrane-bound receptor, as they bind cytokine with equal affinity. Therefore, they may be used in the treatment of conditions in which TNF is the major pathogenic factor, such as sepsis.[36-39]

3. Regulation of TNF-α Expression

Deregulated expression of TNF has been associated with autoimmunity. As with other cytokines, TNF-α synthesis is modulated by positive and negative signals: IL-1, gamma-interferon, and granulocyte macrophage colony-stimulating factor (GM-CSF) increase TNF-α expression; glucocorticoids strongly inhibit it.[30,40]

C. IL-6

IL-6 was initially assigned different names, depending on the biological activities and target cells under investigation, and the groups that independently performed the respective studies. To name several, it was referred to as B cell stimulatory factor-2 (BSF-2), interferon β-2, hybridoma/plasmacytoma growth factor (HPGF), hepatocyte stimulating factor (HSF), monocyte granulocyte inducer type-2 (MGI-2), and 26-kDa factor. IL-6 may be induced in a variety of cells, including monocytes, endothelial cells, and mesangial kidney cells. It was originally described as secreted by T helper clones, but a recent report has shown that CD8 T cells constituted the major source of IL-6 in the serum of tumor-bearing mice.

IL-6 can be constitutively expressed in some myelomas and plasma cell leukemias, and the content of IL-6 in the sera of patients with multiple myeloma or plasma cell leukemia correlated with disease activity, suggesting an autocrine role for IL-6. Non-neoplastic, activated T and B cells can produce IL-6, and, indeed, infiltrating T and B cells in rheumatoid arthritis (RA) synovium, and systemic lupus erythematosus (SLE)-derived peripheral blood monocytes and lymphocytes express this cytokine.[41-43]

1. IL-6 Effects

As suggested by the many names under which it has been described, IL-6 has pleiotropic effects. IL-6 is important in the regulation of immune responses by supplying growth and differentiation signals. IL-6 also enhances cytotoxic activity of natural killer cells (NK) and lymphokine-activated killer cells (LAK); it therefore has potential use in immunotherapy of selected tumors. In early stages of activation of T cells, IL-6 is a competence factor, inducing, with IL-1 or IFN-γ, IL-2 and IL-2R expression in IL-2-activated CD4 T cells, and directly affecting differentiation of cytotoxic CD8 T cells. In late stages of activation, it is essential for the differentiation of activated B lymphocytes into Ig secreting cells. It is a growth factor for EBV-transformed B cells and some mature T cells from thymus and periphery. Thus, a relative abundance of endogenous IL-6 may support the growth, proliferation, and differentiation of autoreactive T and B clones. In fact, endogenous IL-6 is essential for spontaneous autoantibody production by SLE-derived peripheral blood mono-nuclear cells (PBMC), and deregulated IL-6 expression has been detected in autoimmunity. Along with its immunoregulatory effects, IL-6 is the principal inducer of acute phase proteins by hepatocytes, and supports mesangial cell proliferation *in vitro* and *in vivo*. Therefore, it may have a local role in lupic mesangial glomerulonephritis. In essence, many IL-6 activities overlap with those of IL-1 and TNF-α. It regulates osteoclast activity and bone resorption, and this may be one pathogenic effect of this cytokine in rheumatic diseases. However, IL-6 does not induce expression of the cyclooxygenase gene and does not modulate expression of adhesion molecules by endothelial cells.[44-62]

2. IL-6 Receptors (IL-6R)

IL-6R are expressed on activated B cells and on resting T cells. Unlike the receptors for IL-1, which were found mostly on CD4 cells, IL-6R are expressed by both CD4 and CD8 T cell subsets. The IL-6R consists of two molecules. The α chain is an 80-kDa glycoprotein with an Ig-like domain structurally homologous to other human cytokine receptors, such as the receptors for IL-1 and PDGF. It belongs to the cytokine receptor family, along with the IL-2R (p55) and the GM-CSF receptor. The α chain specifically binds IL-6, but its cytoplasmic domain lacks tyrosine kinase activity; therefore, signal transduction is mediated by another molecule. This is a 130-kDa glycoprotein that is induced upon cell activation, and associates with the 80-kDa chain. The two chains form a high-affinity functional receptor, as they each bind noncompetitively to its specific site on the IL-6 molecule. A soluble form of the IL-6R has been detected in the urine of normal individuals.[63,64]

3. Regulation of IL-6 Expression

Many factors that modulate IL-1 and TNF will also act on IL-6 expression. Induction of IL-6 expression may be achieved by bacterial derivatives such as lipopolysaccharide (LPS), and viruses such as human immunodeficiency virus (HIV). Further, the inflammatory cytokines IL-1 and TNF-α, as well as cross-linking Fc receptors on monocytes, can induce IL-6, explaining, in part, the relative abundance of this cytokine in the body fluids of patients with rheumatic diseases. Dexamethasone, IL-4, and TGF-β have downregulating effects.[41-43,65]

D. IL-8

IL-8 was also assigned several names, including neutrophil-activating factor, NAF, or peptide, NAP. Generally, IL-8 is not expressed constitutively. It is a 10-kDa product of monocytes induced with mitogens or cytokines (IL-1 and TNF-α). Cytokines, but not LPS, induce IL-8 also in non-monocytic cells: endothelial and epithelial cells, fibroblasts, and chondrocytes.

1. IL-8 Effects

IL-8 effects resemble those of other chemotactic factors, such as PAF, C5a, and FMLP, as it has strong chemotactic activity on neutrophils and induces, in these cells, expression of adhesion molecules, exocytosis, and a rapid and transient respiratory burst. The IL-8-induced chemotaxis can persist for a long time, possibly due to the unusual resistance of IL-8 to inactivation by plasma peptidases, and its low rate of degradation by proteases. Unlike other chemoattractants that affect various polymorphonuclear cells and monocytes, IL-8 specifically attracts neutrophils, and has only marginal effects on eosinophils and basophils.

Since IL-8 is resistant to degradation by serum and exudate peptidases, it may accumulate in areas of acute inflammation and, thus, play an important role in the RA joint. Indeed, IL-1-stimulated synovial cells produce IL-8-like, neutrophil-activating factors. Further, there is a concentration of neutrophils within the inflamed rheumatic joint. The infiltrating neutrophils may be triggered into secreting cartilage-degrading enzymes. Indeed, *in vitro,* in cocultures of neutrophils with ^{35}S-sulfate-labeled cartilage, even a 10^{-7} *M* concentration of rIL-8 could cause cartilage degradation.

On the other hand, IL-8 may also have anti-inflammatory activity: it inhibited polymorphonuclear cell adhesion to IL-1- or TNF-activated endothelial cells *in vitro,* and the migration of polymorphonuclear cells to acute inflammatory sites *in vivo.*[66-71]

2. IL-8 Receptors (IL-8R)

As mentioned previously, the effects of IL-8 on neutrophils are similar to those of other chemotactic factors (PAF, C5a, and FMLP). Although an IL-8 pulse desensitizes neu-

Table 1 **Inflammatory Cytokines**

Cytokine	Immune Regulation	Inflammation
IL-1α IL-1β	Cofactors for proliferation/ differentiation of lymphocytes. ↑ Cytokines and their receptors and adhesion molecules.	↑ TNF-α, IL-6, IL-8, CSFs, APPs, PGE_2, fever, O_2-. ↑ Fibroblast proliferation, bone resorption, cartilage destruction. Endothelial cell activation.
TNF-α TNF-β	Growth/differentiation of lymphocytes. ↑ IL-2R, adhesion molecules, and MHC class I.	Similar to IL-1 and IL-6.
IL-6	Proliferation/differentiation of T, B, and NK cells.	↑ APP. ↑ bone resorption, mesangial proliferation. Unlike IL-1, CO, PLA_2 genes, endothelial activation, fibroblast proliferation are not ↑. ↓ IL-1-induced response.
IL-8		Attracts, activates neutrophils, cartilage

trophils to further stimulation with IL-8, it does not cross-desensitize these cells to C5a or PAF stimulation. Therefore, it was concluded that IL-8 delivers signals through its own receptor. The majority (3 to 4 × 10^4 sites/cell) of IL-8R on neutrophils are low affinity binding. Approximately 5 × 10^3 high-affinity receptors/cell are also expressed by neutrophils[72] (Table 1).

III. GROWTH/TRANSFORMING GROWTH FACTORS AND THEIR RECEPTORS

A. IL-2

In the late 1970s, it was reported that activated T cells of murine and human origin could be maintained *in vitro* for long periods of time, when grown in "conditioned medium", i.e., cell-free spent medium of phytohemagglutinin (PHA)-stimulated lymphocytes. Eventually, the growth factor that was responsible for the continuous proliferation of these T cell clones was identified as T cell growth factor (TCGF) or interleukin-2. Since then, the vast amount of research conducted on IL-2 and its receptors pioneered methods and concepts applied for the research of the other interleukins. Even the original IL-2-dependent cytotoxic T lymphocytic line (CTLL) is still used as an exquisitely sensitive indicator cell in biological assays for IL-2 activity. Unlike the cytokines discussed in the previous section, which can be synthesized by a multitude of cells, IL-2 is mainly a product of activated T lymphocytes. In response to various stimuli, and depending on the mode of activation, both CD4 and CD8 T cell subsets can produce it. IL-2 is a 15.5-kDa glycoprotein that has been cloned and sequenced. Its general genomic organization is similar to IL-4 and GM-CSF, suggesting they all belong to a family of molecules that have evolved from a common gene.

1. IL-2 Effects

IL-2 is pivotal to the initiation and maintenance of immune responses. It is considered a true progression factor, conferring competence upon activated cells that have entered G_1 from the G_0 resting phase, to continue into subsequent phases of the cell cycle. The IL-2 proliferative and differentiating effects have been used in immunotherapy of tumors for inducing and expanding LAK and cytotoxic T cells. IL-2 alone or with IL-1, IL-6, TNF-α, and IFN-γ provide activation, growth, and differentiation signals to B cells. IL-2 directly triggers in B cells expression of the secretory form of the μ and the J chain. Therefore, deregulated endogenous IL-2 expression that has been reported in rheumatic diseases may contribute to the characteristic B cell hyperactivity, either by direct effects on B cells, or by maintaining the growth of aberrant autoimmune T helper clones.[73-80]

2. IL-2 Receptors (IL-2R)

The stimulus that triggers production of IL-2 may also trigger expression of its receptor. There are at least two molecules that bind to IL-2: the low-affinity p55 α chain (Tac), and the signal-transducing, intermediate-affinity p75 β chain. The p75 chain is expressed constitutively on T lymphocytes and on NK cells. Activation of cells with lectin/antigen induces the low-affinity p55 chain, and formation of a heterodimeric α-β complex that functions as a high-affinity receptor, efficiently transducing signals, even in the presence of very low amounts of cytokine. Following disappearance of the original activating stimulus (*in vivo* antigen clearance, for example), and internalization of the receptor-IL-2 complex, the decreasing amounts of membrane-bound p75 chains and the preferential activation of p55 transcription by IL-2 rapidly decrease the expression of high-affinity receptors, precluding further usage of the cytokine, and returning the cells to a resting stage.

Cell activation, *in vitro* or *in vivo*, also triggers the secretion/shedding of the p55 chain. Aberrantly high levels of soluble IL-2R may explain the hyporesponsiveness to exogenous stimuli in rheumatic diseases, since, in spite of relative low affinity, soluble IL-2 receptors can inhibit IL-2 activity, and thus constitute a natural immunosuppressant.[73,80-83]

B. TGF-β

The term designates a family of closely related proteins (β1, β2, β1.2, β3, and β5), well conserved in various species. Of these, only TGF-β1 has been consistently detected in humans. TGF-β was found in high levels in human platelets and in bone, but it may be produced by other cell types also. TGF-β is probably active in the early stages of embryonic development, coordinating morphogenesis and the remodeling of tissues of mesenchymal origin. It stimulates osteoblasts and inhibits osteoclasts, possibly coordinating bone remodeling. Like other cytokines, it supplies either positive or negative signals to its target cells, depending on their lineage and degree of differentiation. Thus, while TGF-β acts as a differentiating factor by upregulating cytokine secretion by macrophages and secretion of IgA by activated B lymphocytes in the presence of IL-2 and IL-5, it also inhibits proliferation of T and B cells and macrophages, and the secretion of IgG and IgM by activated B cells. These immunoregulatory activities may suggest its use for therapy in rheumatic diseases. TGF-β has even more direct effects in inflammation and tissue destruction, as it both stimulates production and inhibits degradation of extracellular matrix. TGF-β may also play a role in glomerulonephritis.[84-86]

Table 2 **Growth Factors**

Factor	Immune Regulation	Inflammation
IL-2	Growth, proliferation, and differentiation of T, B, and NK cells.	
TGF-β	↓ Proliferation and ↑ differentiation of monocytes and lymphocytes.	Modulates collagen; bone remodeling. ↑ Chemotaxis inflammatory cells. ↓ LPS-induced IL-1, TNF.

1. TGF-β Receptors (TGF-βR)

TGF-βR are constitutively expressed, with most cells expressing three distinct types. Type I (53 kDa), type II (70-85 kDa), and type III (230-350 kDa), the latter being a heparan sulfate proteoglycan that can be detected also in soluble form. Signal transduction is done via types I and II[84] (Table 2).

IV. INTERFERONS AND THEIR RECEPTORS

The term interferons was coined in the late 1950s, to describe factors that were produced by cells following infection with virus, and protecting other cells from subsequent infection. Three major classes of interferons have been detected in all mammalian species that have been studied to date: IFN-α and IFN-β, known also as type I IFNs, and IFN-γ, known also as immune IFN, because of its role in the regulation of immune responses. At least 23 loci have been associated with the human IFN-α family, 14 of them containing coding sequences for functional proteins. The human IFN-α genes do not contain introns, and are all clustered on chromosome 9, proximal to the IFN-β gene. Duplicated IFN-β genes have been found in some individuals. In contrast, IFN-γ is encoded by a unique gene containing four exons and three introns, and located on chromosome 12. There is virtually no homology between IFN-γ and IFN-α and -β, which seem to have derived from a common gene, 300 million years ago, before the divergence of mammals, reptiles, and birds from fish and amphibia. IFN-α proteins have apparent molecular weights of 16 to 27 kDa, and are found as monomers. Recombinant IFN-γ has a molecular weight of 17 kDa and migrates as a dimer, but the functional unit is a tetramer. IFN-α is predominantly induced in peripheral blood cells and IFN-β in fibroblasts and epithelial cells. IFN-γ (immune IFN) is mainly induced in T and NK cells by lectins/antigens.[87-89]

A. INTERFERON EFFECTS

Negative signals — Initial studies documented the antiviral activity of IFNs. *In vitro,* even fentomolar concentrations of IFNs can confer resistance to subsequent infection with RNA and DNA viruses by interfering with various stages in the viral life cycle. The IFN-induced resistance of cells to viral or parasitic infection has been associated with induction of two double-stranded RNA (viral)-dependent enzymes: [2,5-A_n] synthetase and a protein kinase, that can inhibit protein synthesis *in vitro. In vivo,* prophylactic treatment of household contacts of infected individuals reduced by 78% the risk of contracting rhinovirus colds. Interferon treatment was approved also for non-A, non-B type viral hepatitis. Interferons markedly inhibit proliferation of neoplastic cells, possibly due to the induction of reactive oxygen radicals. Based on studies in experimental models, the Food and Drug Administration (FDA) approved IFN treatment for hairy cell leukemia and Kaposi's sarcoma in acquired immune deficiency syndrome (AIDS). Further, encouraging clinical results were reported in IFN treatment of basal cell carcinoma and laryngeal stimuli. The IFN-induced cell arrest in the G_1 phase of the cell cycle coincides with downregulation of proto-oncogenes c-*myc,* c-ha-*ras,* and c-*fos* whose expression is associated with early proliferative events. Interferons inhibit synthesis of collagens types I and II by dermal and synovial fibroblasts and articular and costal chondrocytes. This inhibition is associated with decrease in levels of mRNA for procollagen types I and II. Further, cytokines such as IL-1, which have an important role in rheumatic diseases, are transcriptionally suppressed by IFNs. However, IFN treatment in rheumatic diseases may be complicated by the positive signals that IFNs supply to the immune system.

Positive signals — In contrast to their antiproliferative effects, IFNs upregulate a number of other proteins, besides the dsRNA-dependent enzymes mentioned above, that are important in differentiation and in cell-to-cell immune interactions: binding and adhesion, antigen presentation and recognition, migration and homing, and response to other cytokines. Interferons modulate expression of molecules encoded by the major histocompatibility locus (MHC). All interferons increase expression of MHC class I (HLA-A, -B, and -C) and the associated β2-microglobulin. This increase is due, at least in part, to stimulation of the rate of transcription. On the other hand, only IFN-γ modulates expression of MHC class II molecules (DR, DP, DQ), and MHC class III molecules, mostly C2 and factor B. IFN-γ induces MHC class II expression in cells from various lineages. IFN-γ transcriptionally regulates MHC class I by induction of nuclear-binding factors to interferon response sequences (IRS) in the MHC gene promoter region. Intrinsic differences in inducibility of MHC class I genes are determined by the nucleotides present in the IRS. Interference with the constitutive attenuation of MHC gene transcription may constitute an additional mechanism by which IFN-γ upregulates MHC gene expression. Deregulated expression of MHC can modulate antigen presentation and promote autoreactivity. Indeed, in one study, IFN-γ treatment enhanced the rate of relapse for patients with multiple sclerosis. Interferons facilitate interaction of cytokines and growth factors with their target cells by inducing expression of specific receptors and of specific cytokines. IFN-α and -β enhanced the content of glucocorticoid receptors on HL-60 cells, and IFN-γ enhanced expression of receptors for TNF-α and IL-2 on T lymphocytes and monocytes. Further, IFN-γ increased the transcription rate of TNF-α. The expression of adhesion molecules, such as ICAM-1 and ELAM-1, that play an important role in immune responses and inflammation is enhanced by IFN-γ. Cell-mediated responses, NK- and T cell (CTL)-mediated cytotoxic activities are both enhanced by IFN-γ. Also, IFN-γ induces expression of FC gamma receptors on macrophages and eosinophils, possibly augmenting also in this way cytotoxic reactions in local sites of inflammation.[90-105]

B. INTERFERON RECEPTORS

There is a high degree of structural homology between the various IFN-α subtypes and IFN-β, and their effects, both *in vitro* and *in vivo,* are overlapping. It is therefore not surprising that they share a common receptor. The α/β receptor is a 110- to 130-kDa molecule encoded by a gene mapped to chromosome 21. The IFN-γR has also been cloned. It is an approximately 54-kDa glycoprotein, and its gene is located on chromosome 6. Soluble IFN-γ receptors have been found in human urine.[87,88]

Table 3 **Interferons**

Interferon	Immune Regulation	Inflammation
IFN-α, IFN-β	Cytotoxic. MHC-class I induction. ↑ GC receptors.	Antiviral.
IFN-γ	Cytotoxic. ↑ MHC-class I, II, III, IL-2R, Fc-γR, TNF, and adhesion molecules.	Antiviral. Mϕ and eosinophil act. ↓ IL-1-induced cytokines

C. REGULATION OF IFN EXPRESSION

Interferons are directly induced by viruses, bacteria, and dsRNA. IL-1, TNF-α, and IL-2 can also induce or upregulate interferons. An inner network seems to exist between type I and type II IFNs. Thus, IFN-α- and IFN-β-incubated human monocytes secrete a 15-kDa protein that induces secretion of IFN-γ from CD3+ cells. In contrast, interleukin-4 (IL-4) can have downregulating effects[87-89] (Table 3).

REFERENCES

1. **Dinarello, C. A.,** Interleukin-1 and interleukin-1 antagonism, *Blood,* 77, 1627, 1991.
2. **Dinarello, C. A.,** Interleukin-1 and biologically related cytokines, *Adv. Immunol.,* 44, 153, 1989.
3. **Bailly, S., Ferrua, B., Fay, M., and Gougerot-Pocidalo, M. A.,** Paraformaldehyde fixation of LPS-stimulated human monocytes. Technical parameters permitting the study of membrane IL-1 activity, *Eur. Cytokine Net.,* 1, 147, 1990.
4. **Sipe, J. D.,** The molecular biology of Interleukin-1 and the acute-phase response, *Adv. Intern. Med.,* 34, 1, 1990.
5. **Clark, B. D., Collins, K. L., Gandy, M. S., Webb, A. C., and Auron, P. E.,** Genomic sequence for human prointerleukin-1 β: possible evolution from a reverse transcribed prointerleukin-1 α gene, *Nucleic Acids,* 14, 7897, 1986.
6. **Turner, M., Chantry, D., Buchan, G., Barrett, K., and Feldmann, M.,** Regulation of expression of human IL-1 α and IL-1 β genes, *J. Immunol.,* 143, 3556, 1989.
7. **Bevilaqua, M. P., Pober, M. S., Wheeler, M. E., Coran, R. S., and Gibron, M. A.,** IL-1 acts on human cultured human vascular endothelium to increase the adhesion of polymorphonuclear cells, monocytes, and related leukocyte lines, *J. Clin. Invest.,* 76, 2003, 1985.
8. **Okusawa, S., Gelfand, J. A., Kejima, T., Connoly, R. J., and Dinarello, C. A.,** Interleukin-1 induces a shock-like state in rabbits. Synergism with TNF and the effect of cyclooxygenase inhibition, *J. Clin. Invest.,* 81, 1162, 1988.
9. **Chizzonite, R., Truitt, T., Kilian, P. L., Stern, A. S., Nunes, P., Parker, K. P., Kaffka, K. L., Chua, A. D., Lugg, D. K., and Gubler, U.,** Two high-affinity IL-1 receptors represent separate gene products, *Proc. Natl. Acad. Sci. U.S.A.,* 86, 8029, 1989.
10. **Scapigliatti, G., Ghiara, P., Bartalini, A., and Boraschi, D.,** Differential binding of IL-1 α and IL-1 β to receptors on B and T cells, *FEBS Lett.,* 243, 394, 1989.

11. **Sims, J. E., March, C. J., Cosman, D., Widmer, M. B., McDonald, H. R., McMahan, C. J., Grubin, C. E., Wignall, J. M., Jackson, J. L., Call, S. M., Gillis, S., and Dower, S. K.,** cDNA expression and cloning of the IL-1 receptor, a member of the immunoglobulin superfamily, *Science,* 241, 5875, 1988.
12. **Giri, J., Newton, R. C., and Horuk, R.,** Identification of IL-1-binding protein in cell-free supernatants: evidence for IL-1 receptor, *J. Biol. Chem.,* 265, 17416, 1990.
13. **Fanslow, W. C., Sims, J. E., Sassenfeld, H., Morissey, P. J., Gillis, S., Dower, S. K., and Widmer, M. B.,** Regulation of alloreactivity in vivo by a soluble form of the IL-1 receptor, *Science,* 248, 739, 1990.
14. **Liao, Z., Grinshaw, R. S., and Rosenstreich, D. L.,** Identification of a specific IL-1 inhibitor in the urine of febrile patients, *J. Exp. Med.,* 159, 126, 1984.
15. **Barak, V., Treves, A. J., Yanai, P., Halpein, M., Wasserman, D., Biran, S., and Braun, S.,** IL-1 inhibitory activity secreted by a human myelomonocytic cell line (M 20), *Eur. J. Immunol.,* 16, 1449, 1986.
16. **Arend, W. P., Welgus, H. G., Thompson, R. C., and Eisenberg, S. P.,** Biological properties of recombinant human monocyte-derived IL-1 receptor antagonist, *J. Clin. Invest.,* 85, 1694, 1990.
17. **Seckinger, P., Klei-Nulen, J., Alander, C., Thompson, R. C., Dayer, J. M., and Raisz, L. G.,** Natural and recombinant IL-1 receptor antagonists block the effects of IL-1 on bone resorption and prostaglandin production, *J. Immunol.,* 145, 4181, 1990.
18. **Aggarwal, B. B., Kohr, V. J., Hass, P. E. et al.,** Human tumor necrosis factor: production, purification, and characterization, *J. Biol. Chem.,* 260, 2345, 1985.
19. **Beutler, B., Milsark, J. W., and Cerami, A.,** Passive immunization against cachectin/tumor necrosis factor protects mice from lethal effects of endotoxin, *Science,* 229, 869, 1985.
20. **Aderka, D., Holtman, H., Toker, L., Hahn, T., and Wallach, D.,** Tumor necrosis factor induction by Sendai virus, *J. Immunol.,* 136, 2938, 1986.
21. **Tracey, K. J., Beutler, B., Lowry, S. F. et al.,** Shock and tissue injury induced by recombinant human cachectin. *Science,* 234, 470, 1986.
22. **Tracey, K., Fong, Y., Hesse, D. G., Manogue, K. R., Lee, A. T., Kuo, G. C., Lowry, S. F., and Cerami, A.,** Anti-cachectin/TNF monoclonal antibodies prevent septic shock during lethal bacteremia, *Nature,* 330, 265, 1989.
23. **Torti, F. M., Dieckman, B., Beutler, B., Cerami, A., and Ringold, G. M.,** A macrophage factor inhibits adipocyte gene expression: an in vitro model of cachexia, *Science,* 229, 867, 1985.
24. **Cuturi, M. C., Murphy, M., Costa-Giomi, M. P. et al.,** Independent regulation of tumor necrosis factor and lymphotoxin production by human peripheral blood lymphocytes, *J. Exp. Med.,* 165, 1581, 1987.
25. **Grau, G. E., Fajarels, L. F., Piguet, P. F. et al.,** TNF (cachectin) as an essential mediator in murine cerebral malaria, *Science,* 237, 1210, 1987.
26. **Waage, A., Halstensen, A., and Espevick, T.,** Association between TNF in serum and fatal outcome in patients with meningococcal disease, *Lancet,* 1[8529], 355, 1987.
27. **Perlmutter, D. H., Dinarello, C. A., Punsal, P. I., and Colten, H. R.,** Cachectin/TNF regulates hepatic acute-phase gene expression, *J. Clin. Invest.,* 78, 1349, 1986.

28. **Scheurich, P., Thoma, B., Ucer, U., and Pfizenmaier, K.,** Immunoregulatory activity of recombinant human tumor necrosis factor (TNF)-α induction of the TNF receptors on human T cells and TNF-α mediated enhancement of T cell responses, *J. Immunol.,* 138, 1786, 1987.
29. **Sung, S. J., Bjorndhal, J. M., Wang, C. Y., Kao, H. T., and Fu, S. M.,** Production of tumor necrosis factor/cachectin by human T cell lines and peripheral blood lymphocytes stimulated by phorbol myristate acetate and anti-CD3 antibody, *J. Exp. Med.,* 167, 937, 1988.
30. **Stashenko, P., Dewhirst, F. E., Peros, W. J., Kent, R. L., and Ago, J. M.,** Synergistic interactions between IL-1, TNF, and LT in bone resorption, *J. Immunol.,* 138, 1464, 1987.
31. **Collins, T., Lapierre, L. A., Fiers, W., Strominger, J. L., and Pober, J. S.,** Recombinant TNF-α increases mRNA levels and surface expression of HLA-A, B antigens in vascular endothelial cells and dermal fibroblasts in vitro, *Proc. Natl. Acad. Sci. U.S.A.,* 83, 446, 1986.
32. **Saklatvala, J.,** TNF-α stimulates resorption and inhibits synthesis of proteoglycan in cartilage, *Nature,* 322, 547, 1986.
33. **Dayer, J. M., Beutler, B., and Cerami, A.,** Cachectin/TNF stimulated collagenase and prostaglandin E_2 production by human synovial cells, *J. Exp. Med.,* 162, 2163, 1985.
34. **Decker, T., Lohman-Mathes, M. L., and Gifford, G. E.,** Cell-associated TNF as a killing mechanism of activated cytotoxic monocytes, *J. Immunol.,* 138, 957, 1987.
35. **Luettig, B., Decker, T., and Lohmann-Matthes, M. L.,** Evidence for the existence of two forms of membrane tumor necrosis factor: an integral protein and a molecule attached to its receptor, *J. Immunol.,* 143, 4034, 1989.
36. **Aggarwal, B. B., Eessalu, T. E., and Hass, P. E.,** Characterization of receptors for human tumor necrosis factor and their regulation by γ-interferons, *Nature,* 318, 665, 1985.
37. **Hohmann, H. P., Remy, R., Brockhaus, M., and van Loon, A. P.,** Two different cell types have different major receptors for human tumor receptor factor, *J. Biol. Chem.,* 264, 14927, 1989.
38. **Andrews, J. S., Berger, A. E., and Ware, C. E.,** Characterization of the receptor for TNF and LT on human T lymphocytes, *J. Immunol.,* 144, 2582, 1990.
39. **Engelmann, H. D., Aderka, M., Rubinstein, M., Rotman, D., and Wallach, D.,** TNF-binding protein purified to homogeneity from human urine protects from TNF toxicity, *J. Biol. Chem.,* 264, 11974, 1989.
40. **Cannistra, S. A., Rambaldi, A., Spriggs, D. R. et al.,** Human GM-CSF induces expression of the TNF gene by the U937 cell line and by normal human monocytes, *J. Clin. Invest.,* 79, 172, 1987.
41. **Hirano, T., Akira, S., Taga, T., and Kishimoto, T.,** Biological and clinical aspects of interleukin-6, *Immunol. Today,* 11, 443, 1990.
42. **Van Snick, J.,** Interleukin-6, an overview, *Annu. Rev. Immunol.,* 8, 253, 1990.
43. **Hirano, T., Taga, T., Nakano, N., et al.,** Purification to homogeneity and characterization of human B cell differentiation factor (BCDF or BSF p.2), *Proc. Natl. Acad. Sci. U.S.A.,* 82, 5490, 1985.
44. **May, L. T., Helfgott, D. C., and Sehgal, PBB.,** Anti-β-interferon antibodies inhibit the increased expression of HLA B7 mRNA in TNF-treated human fibroblasts: structural studies of the β_2 interferon involved, *Proc. Natl. Acad. Sci. U.S.A.,* 83, 8957, 1986.

45. **Van Damme, J., Opdenakker, G., Simpson, R. J. et al.,** Identification of the human 26-kD protein, interferon β_2, as a B cell hybridoma/plasmacytoma growth factor induced by interleukin-1 and TNF, *J. Exp. Med.*, 165, 914, 1987.
46. **Gauldie, J., Richards, C., Harnish, D., Landsorp, P., and Bauman, H.,** Interferon β_2/B cell stimulatory factor type 2 shares identity with monocyte-derived hepatocyte-stimulating factor and regulates the major acute-phase protein response in liver cells, *Proc. Natl. Acad. Sci. U.S.A.*, 84, 7251, 1987.
47. **Shabo, Y., Lotem, J., Rubinstein, M. et al.,** The myeloid blood cell differentiation inducing protein MG1-2A is interleukin-6, *Blood,* 72, 2070, 1988.
48. **Haegeman, G., Content, J., Volkaert, G. et al.,** *Eur. J. Biochem.*, 159, 625, 1986.
49. **Utsumi, K., Takai, Y., Ohzeki, S., Fujiwara, H., and Hamaoka, T.,** Enhanced production of IL-6 in tumor-bearing mice and determination of cells responsible for its augmented production, *J. Immunol.*, 145, 397, 1990.
50. **Freeman, G. J., Freedman, A. S., Rabinowe, S. N. et al.,** IL-6 gene expression in normal and neoplastic B cells, *J. Clin. Invest.*, 83, 1512, 1989.
51. **Bataille, R., Jourdan, M., Zhang, X. G., and Klein, B.,** Serum levels of IL-6, a potent myeloma growth factor, as a reflection of disease severity in plasma cell dyscrasias, *J. Clin. Invest.*, 84, 2008, 1989.
52. **Hirano, T., Matsuda, T., Turner, M., Miyasaka, N., Buchan, G., Tang, B., Sato, K., Shimizu, M., Maini, R., Feldman, M., and Kishimoto, T.,** Excessive production of IL-6/BSF-2 in rheumatoid arthritis, *Eur. J. Immunol.*, 18, 1797, 1988.
53. **Linker-Israeli, M., Dean, R. J., Wallace, D. J., Prehn, J., Ozeri-Chen, T., and Klinenberg, J. R.,** Elevated levels of endogenous IL-6 in systemic lupus erythematosus: a putative role in pathogenesis, *J. Immunol.*, 147, 117, 1991.
54. **Horii, Y., Muraguchi, A., Iwano, M., Matsuda, T., Hirayama, T., Yamada, H., Fujii, Y., Dohi, K., Ishikawa, H., Omoto, Y., Yoshizaki, K., Hirano, T., and Kishimoto, T.,** Involvement of IL-6 in mesangial proliferative glomerulonephritis, *J. Immunol.*, 143, 3949, 1989.
55. **Yoshizaki, K., Matsuda, T., Nishimoto, N., Kuritani, T., Taeho, L., Aozasa, K., Nakahata, T., Kawai, H., Tagoh, H., Komori, T., Kishimoto, S., Hirano, S., and Kishimoto, T.,** Pathogenic significance of interleukin-6 (IL-6/BSF-2) in Castleman's disease, *Blood,* 74, 1360, 1989.
56. **Breen, E. C., Rezai, A. R., Nakajima, K., Beall, G. N., Mitsuyasu, R. T., Hirano, T., Kishimoto, T., and Martinez-Maza, O.,** Infection with HIV is associated with elevated IL-6 levels, *J. Immunol.*, 144, 480, 1990.
57. **Jablons, D. M., Mule, J. J., McIntosh, J. K., Sehgal, P. B., May, L. T., Huang, C. M., Rosenberg, S. A., and Lotze, M. T.,** IL-6/IFN-β2 as a circulating hormone: induction by cytokine administration in humans, *J. Immunol.*, 142, 1542, 1989.
58. **Bronckaert, P. D., Spriggs, R., Demetri, G., Kuffe, D. W., and Fiers, W.,** Circulating IL-6 during continuous infusion of TNF-α and IFN-γ, *J. Exp. Med.*, 169, 2257, 1989.
59. **Krutmann, J., Kirnbauer, R., Jock, A., Schwartz, T., Schopf, E., May, L. T., Sehgal, P. B., and Luger, T. A.,** Cross-linking Fc_r receptors on monocytes triggers IL-6 production: role in anti-CD3-induced cell activation, *J. Immunol.*, 145, 1342, 1990.

60. **Luger, T. A., Krutman, J., Kirnbauer, R., Urbanski, A., Schwartz, T., Klapcher, G., Kock, A., Micksche, M., Malejczyck, J., Schauer, E., May, L. T., and Sehgal, P. B.,** IL-6/IFN-β augments the activity of human natural killer cells, *J. Immunol.,* 143, 1206, 1989.
61. **Gallagher, G., Stimson, W. W., Findlay, J., and Al-Azzawi, F.,** IL-6 enhances the induction of human lymphokine-activated killer cells, *Cancer Immunol. Immunother.,* 31, 49, 1990.
62. **Mule, J. J., Custer, M. C., Travis, W. D., and Rosenberg, S. A.,** Cellular mechanisms of the anti-tumor activity of recombinant IL-6 in mice, *J. Immunol.,* 148, 2622, 1992.
63. **Yamasaki, K., Taga, T., Hirata, Y. et al.,** Cloning and expression of the human IL-6 (BSF-2/IFNβ_2) receptor, *Science,* 241, 825, 1988.
64. **Novick, D., Engelman, H., Wallach, D., and Rubinstein, M.,** Soluble cytokine receptors are present in normal urine, *J. Exp. Med.,* 170, 1409, 1989.
65. **Schindler, R., Mancilla, J., Endres, S., Ghorbani, R., Clark, S. C., and Dinarello, C. A.,** Correlations and interactions in the production of IL-6, IL-1, and TNF in human blood mononuclear cells: IL-6 suppresses IL-1 and TNF, *Blood,* 75, 40, 1990.
66. **Yoshimura, T., Matsushima, K., Oppenheim, J., and Leonard, E. J.,** Neutrophil chemotactic factor produced by LPS-stimulated human blood leukocytes: partial characterization and separation from IL-1, *J. Immunol.,* 139, 788, 1987.
67. **Van Damme, J., Van Beeumen, J., Opdenakker, G., and Billiau, A.,** A novel, NH_2-terminal sequence characterized human monokine possessing neutrophil chemotactic, skin reactive, and granulocytosis-promoting activity, *J. Exp. Med.,* 167, 1364, 1988.
68. **Peveri, P., Waltz, A., Dewald, B., and Baggiolini, M.,** A novel neutrophil-activating factor produced by human mononucleolar phagocytes, *J. Exp. Med.,* 167, 1547, 1988.
69. **Watson, M. L., Westwick, J., Fincham, N. J., and Camp, R. D.,** Elevation of PMN cytosolic free calcium and locomotion stimulated by novel peptides from IL-1-treated human synovial cell cultures, *Biochem. Biophys. Res. Commun.,* 155, 1154, 1988.
70. **Mohr, W. and Wessinghage, D.,** The relationship between polymorphonuclear granulocytes and cartilage destruction in RA, *J. Rheumatol.,* 37, 81, 1978.
71. **Elford, P. R. and Cooper, P. H.,** Induction of neutrophil-mediated cartilage degradation by IL-8, *Arthritis Rheum.,* 34, 325, 1991.
72. **Bessemer, J., Hujber, A., and Khun, B.,** Specific binding, internalization and degradation of human neutrophil activating factor by human polymorphonuclear leukocytes, *J. Biol. Chem.,* 264, 17409, 1989.
73. **Smith, K. A.,** Cytokines in the nineties, *Eur. Cytokine Net.,* 1, 7, 1990.
74. **Gillis, S., Mochizuki, D. Y., Conlon, P. J. et al.,** Molecular characterization of interleukin-2, *Immunol. Rev.,* 63, 167, 1982.
75. **Fujita, T., Takaoka, C., Matsui, H., and Taniguchi, T.,** Structure of the human interleukin-2 gene, *Proc. Natl. Acad. Sci. U.S.A.,* 80, 7437, 1983.
76. **Blakman, M., Tiggs, M. A., Minie, M. E., and Koshland, M. E.,** A model system for peptide hormone action in differentiation: Interleukin-2 induces a β lymphoma to transcribe the J-chain gene. *Cell,* 47, 609, 1986.
77. **Jelinek, D. F. and Lipsky, P. E.,** The roles of IL-2 and IFN-γ in human B cell activation, growth and differentiation, *Eur. J. Immunol.,* 16, 825, 1986.

78. **Alcocer-Varela, J. and Alarcon-Segovia, D.,** Decreased production of and response to interleukin-2 by cultured lymphocytes from patients with systemic lupus erythematosus, *J. Clin. Invest.,* 69, 1388, 1982.
79. **Linker-Israeli, M., Bakke, A. C., Kitridou, R. C., Gendler, S., Gillis, S., and Horwitz, D. A.,** Defective production of interleukin-1 and interleukin-2 in patients with systemic lupus erythematosus (SLE), *J. Immunol.,* 130, 2651, 1983.
80. **Kahaleh, M. B. and LeRoy, E. C.,** Interleukin-2 in scleroderma. Correlation of serum level with extent of skin involvement and disease duration, *Ann. Intern. Med.,* 110, 446, 1989.
81. **Robb, R. J., Greene, W. C., and Rusk, C. M.,** Low and high affinity cellular receptors for IL-2: implications for the level of Tac antigen, *J. Exp. Med.,* 160, 1126, 1984.
82. **Rubin, L. A., Kurman, C. C., Fritz, M. E., Biddison, W. E., Boutin, B., Yarchoan, R., and Nelson, D. E.,** Soluble IL-2 receptors are released from activated human lymphoid cells in vitro, *J. Immunol.,* 135, 3172, 1985.
83. **Kondo, N., Kondo, S., Shimizu, A., Honjo, T., and Hamuro, J.,** A soluble anchor minus IL-2 receptor suppresses in vitro IL-2 mediated immune responses, *Immunol. Lett.,* 19, 299, 1988.
84. **Sporn, M. B. and Roberts, A. B.,** The transforming growth factors β, in *Peptide Growth Factors and their Receptors,* Sporn, M. B. and Roberts, A. B., Eds., Springer-Verlag, New York, 1990, 419.
85. **Lebman, D. A., Lee, F. D., and Coffman, R. L.,** Mechanism for TGF-β and IL-2-enhancement of IgA expression in lipopolysaccharide-stimulated B cell cultures, *J. Immunol.,* 144, 952, 1980.
86. **Border, W. A., Okuda, S., Languino, L. R., Sporn, M. B., and Ruoslahti, E.,** Suppression of experimental glomerulonephritis by antiserum against transforming growth factor β_1, *Nature,* 346, 371, 1990.
87. **Petska, S., Langer, J. A., Zoon, K. A., and Samuel, C. E.,** Interferons and their actions, *Annu. Rev. Biochem.,* 56, 727, 1987.
88. **Blackwill, F. R.,** Peptide regulatory factors/interferons, *Lancet,* 5.13, 1060, 1989.
89. **Ohlson, M., Feder, J., Cavalli-Sforza, L. L., and von Gabain, A.,** Close linkage of α and β interferons and infrequent duplication of β interferon in humans, *Proc. Natl. Acad. Sci. U.S.A.,* 82, 4473, 1985.
90. **Gray, P. W., Leung, D. W., Pennica, D. et al.,** Expression of human immune interferon cDNA in E. coli and monkey cells, *Nature,* 295, 503, 1982.
91. **Recht, M., Borden, E. C., and Knight, E., Jr.,** A human 15 kDa interferon-induced protein induces the secretion of interferon gamma, *J. Immunol.,* 147, 2617, 1991.
92. **Auget, M., Dembic, Z., and Merlin, G.,** Molecular cloning and expression of the human interferon-γ receptor, *Cell,* 55, 273, 1988.
93. **Gordon, D. R.,** The common cold — relief at last?, *N. Engl. J. Med.,* 314, 114, 1986.
94. **Talpaz, M., Kantarjian, H. M., McCredie, K. B., Keating, M. J., Trujillo, J., and Gutterman, J.,** Clinical investigation of human alpha interferon in chronic myelogenous leukemia, *Blood,* 65, 1280, 1987.
95. **Kimchi, A.,** Autocrine interferon and the suppression of the c-myc nuclear oncogene, *Interferon,* 8, 86, 1987.
96. **Dani, C., Mechti, N., Piechaczyk, M. et al.,** Increased rate of degradation of c-myc mRNA in interferon-treated Daudi cells, *Proc. Natl. Acad. Sci. U.S.A.,* 82, 4896, 1985.

97. **Strunk, R. C., Cole, F. S., Perlmutter, D. H., and Colten, H. R.,** Interferon increases expression of class III complement genes C_2 and factor B in human monocytes and in murine fibroblasts transfected with human C_2 and factor B genes, *J. Biol. Chem.,* 260, 15280, 1985.
98. **Hakem, R., Le Boutellier, P., Jezo-Bremond, A., Harper, K.,** Differential regulation of HLA-A3 and HLA-B7 MHC class I gene by IFN is due to two nucleotide differences in their IFN response sequences, *J. Immunol.,* 147, 2384, 1991.
99. **Radford, J. F., Jr., Chen, E., Hromas, R., and Ginder, G. D.,** Cell-type specificity of interferon-gamma mediated HLA class I gene transcription in human hematopoietic tumor cells, *Blood,* 77, 2008, 1991.
100. **Panitch, H. S., Hirsh, R. L., Haley, A. S., and Johnson, K. P.,** Exacerbation of multiple sclerosis in patients treated with gamma interferon, *Lancet,* i, 893, 1987.
101. **Fridman, W. H., Gresser, I., Bandu, M. T., Aguet, M., and Neauport-Sautes, C.,** Interferon enhances the expression of Fc_γ receptors, *J. Immunol.,* 124, 2436, 1980.
102. **Valerius, T., Repp, R., Kaiden, J. R., and Platzer, E.,** Effects of IFN on human eosinophils in comparison with other cytokines. A novel class of eosinophil activators with delayed onset of action, *J. Immunol.,* 145, 2950, 1990.
103. **Cotran, R. S. and Prober, S.,** Cytokine-endothelial interactions in inflammation, immunity, and vascular injury, *J. Am. Soc. Nephrol.,* i, 225, 1990.
104. **Sica, G., Lama, G., Tartaglione, R., Pierelli, L., Frati, L., della Cuna, G. R., and Marchetti, P.,** Effects of natural beta interferons and recombinant alpha 2-b interferon on proliferation, glucocorticoid receptor content, and antigen expression in cultured HL-60 cells, *Cancer,* 65, 920, 1990.
105. **Beutler, B., Krochin, N., Milsark, I. W., Goldberg, A., and Cerami, A.,** Induction of cachetin (Tumor Vecrosis Factor) synthesis by Influenza virus: deficient production by endotoxin resistant (C-3H/HEJ) macrophages. *Clin. Res.,* 34, 491A, 1986.

Chapter 15

Measurement of Cytokines and their Receptors by Immunoassay

Mona L. Hall and Elizabeth G. Posillico

CONTENTS

I. INTRODUCTION

Cytokines are intercellular signalling molecules that play a central role in activating and sustaining the immune response. Moreover, cytokines are sensitive markers of immune activation and elevated levels are present in numerous disease states, including rheumatoid arthritis. Additionally, the ability of target cells to shed cytokine receptors as a means of downregulating the response to the cytokine ligand permits soluble receptor levels to also serve as barometers of immune system activity. Consequently, the measurement of cytokines and cytokine receptor levels is warranted in order to understand their role in the pathophysiology of a disease and to assess their clinical value as indicators of the onset and/or prognosis of a disease.

Within the arthritic joint, resident fibroblast and synovial cells are joined by infiltrating mononuclear and polynuclear leukocytes. Since these cells are all capable of secreting and responding to cytokines, it is not surprising that the synovial fluid of rheumatoid arthritis patients contains a variety of cytokines. Cytokines implicated in the pathophysiology of rheumatoid arthritis include interleukin (IL)-1, IL-6, IL-8, tumor necrosis factor (TNF) and transforming growth factor (TGF)-β.[1-7] These cytokines, as well as the soluble IL-2 receptor,[8-9] have been measured in synovial fluid, serum, plasma, or in the supernatants of mononuclear cell cultures. To date, only the concentrations of IL-6 and IL-2R have demonstrated a correlation with prognosis and disease severity.

0-8493-5974-1/94/$0.00 + $.50

IL-6 levels exceeded those of IL-1 or TNF-α and were correlated with leukocyte counts, erythrocyte sedimentation rate, the presence of acute-phase proteins, and the parameters of local inflammation — joint temperature, swelling, and pain.[2-4] Also, a strong positive correlation was observed between disease activity and IL-2 receptor levels.[8,9] The prognostic value of IL-2 receptor levels was also noted, since IL-2 receptor levels rapidly declined upon treatment. Further studies are required to evaluate the diagnostic value of IL-6 and IL-2R in rheumatoid arthritis.

II. METHODS FOR CYTOKINE AND CYTOKINE RECEPTOR MEASUREMENT

A. BIOASSAYS

Cytokines were initially identified based on their bioactivity on target cells. Therefore, bioassays which measure effects of cytokines (i.e., cell proliferation) *in vitro* became the traditional method for the determination of cytokine levels (Table 1). However, bioassays have several disadvantages which are problematic for routine use in the clinical and research laboratory. First, bioassays lack specificity, since a number of other cytokines or immunomodulators may modulate the response of the indicator cell line. Second, considerable assay-to-assay variability is inherent to bioassays due to inconsistencies in the target cell response, and varying aptitude of the technician who must perform the labor-intensive procedure. Lastly, bioassays cannot be applied to measure levels of soluble cytokine receptors.

B. IMMUNOASSAYS

With the advent of cytokine-specific antibodies, two alternatives to the bioassay were developed — the radioimmunoassay (RIA) and enzyme-linked immunoassay (EIA). These immunoassays employ antibodies to recognize unique antigenic regions on the cytokine and thereby ensure specificity despite the presence of other immunomodulators. The RIA procedure is based on the competition of unlabeled antigen (cytokine) with radiolabeled cytokine for a specific antibody. The amount of radiolabeled cytokine bound by the antibody is inversely related to the cytokine concentration in the sample. The principles of RIA methodologies have been expertly reviewed.[23]

More recently, the enzyme-linked immunoassay (EIA) has gained predominance due to the assay speed (hours vs. days), long shelf life (months vs. weeks), and lack of radioactive waste. Quantitation of cytokine levels by EIA is achieved with the use of two antibodies which form an immune complex, followed by an enzyme-based detection system. The cost of separately purchased reagents and the time required for optimization of assay performance and quality control has dissuaded laboratories from use of in-house EIAs, in favor of the convenience provided by commercially available cytokine EIAs. Differences between commercial EIAs do exist, however, and a careful review of the performance claims is recommended. The criteria for evaluation of the various commercial EIA kits are provided in this chapter. The performance characteristics (i.e., precision, accuracy, sensitivity, and specificity) and inclusion of positive controls should serve as the basis for choosing between the available commercial EIA kits.

III. ENZYME-LINKED IMMUNOASSAY

A. PRINCIPLES OF THE PROCEDURE

The antibody sandwich EIA is the assay format typically used to detect cytokines and cytokine receptors in the well of a microtiter plate coated with a specific capture antibody.

Table 1 **Bioassays for Human Cytokines**

Cytokine	Indicator Cells	Biological Effect	Ref.
IL-1	D10.G4.1 murine TH2 cell line	Co-stimulation of cell proliferation	10
IL-2	CTLL-2 murine T cell line	Cell proliferation	10–13
IL-3	TF-1 human erythroleukemic cell line	Cell proliferation	14
IL-4	Human peripheral T cells	Co-stimulation of cell proliferation	11, 12, 15
IL-5	TF-1 human erythroleukemic cell line	Cell proliferation	12, 14
IL-6	Murine B9 hybridoma cells	Cell proliferation	11, 16
IL-7	Pre-B cell lines	Stimulation of cell proliferation	10–12
IL-8	Human neutrophils	Chemotaxis	10–12
IL-9	Human MO7E megakaryoblastic leukemia cells	Cell proliferation	10, 17
IL-10	Murine MC/9 mast cell line	Co-stimulation of cell proliferation	18
IL-11	T10 murine plasmacytoma cell line	Cell proliferation	10
IL-12	Human peripheral T cells	Co-stimulation of cell proliferation	19
IFN-γ	Fibroblastoid L929 cells	Virus yield reduction	10, 11
LIF	Murine leukemia M1 cells	Cell differentiation	12, 20
MCAF	Human monocytes	Chemotaxis	11, 21
SCF	Human MO7E megakaryoblastic leukemia cells	Cell proliferation	22
TGF-β	Mv1Lu mink lung epithelial cells	Cell proliferation	11, 12
TNF-α, β	Fibroblastoid L929 cells	Cytotoxicity	11, 12

Abbreviations: IL (Interleukin); IFN (Interferon); LIF (Leukemia Inhibitory Factor); MCAF (Monocyte Chemotactic and Activating Factor); SCF (Stem Cell Factor); TGF (Transforming Growth Factor); TNF (Tumor Necrosis Factor).

Following incubation with the antigen, unbound substances (serum proteins, other cytokines, inflammatory mediators, rheumatoid factors, etc.) are washed out. A second antibody is added to complete the formation of the antibody-antigen-antibody "sandwich" (Figure 1).

Subsequent reactions are required to permit spectrophotometric detection of the immune complex. An enzyme-catalyzed color change serves as the basis for the detection system. The second antibody may be directly conjugated to the enzyme responsible for

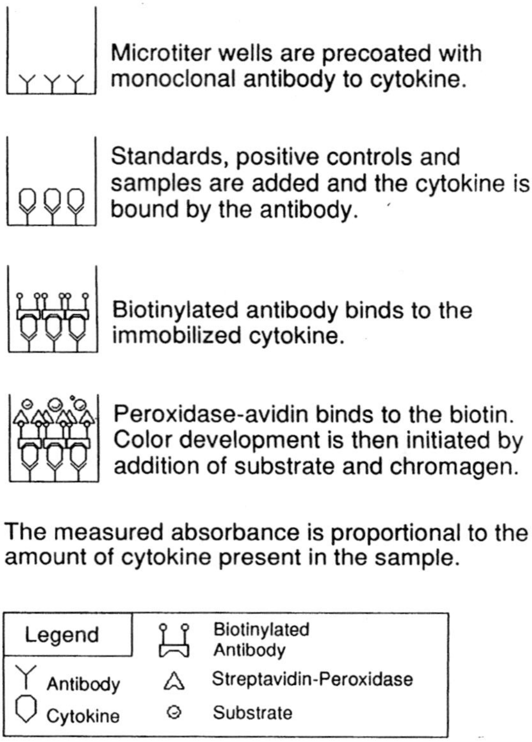

Figure 1 The principle of an enzyme-linked immunoassay (EIA).

color development. Alternatively, a step using the signal amplification of the biotin-avidin system may be employed. In this case, the second antibody is conjugated to biotin, which then forms a high-affinity complex with the avidin-conjugated enzyme.

The enzyme-catalyzed color change is initiated by the addition of a substrate/chromogen solution and acidification terminates the reaction. The absorbance values are read on a microplate spectrophotometer (EIA reader). The absorbance values of the standards are plotted and the values of the experimental samples are determined from the standard curve.

B. REAGENTS, SUPPLIES, AND EQUIPMENT

EIA kits for the measurement of cytokines or soluble cytokine receptors normally contain sufficient reagents and materials for performing a standard curve and sample determinations for a total of 96 wells. The kit contents include the cytokine or cytokine receptor standard, a primary and secondary antibody, an enzyme-based detection system, appropriate buffers, substrate, chromogen, and stop solution. Positive controls are supplied in only a few commercial kits. Otherwise, a positive control pool should be prepared by the user to evaluate assay performance. Also, the convenience of performing multiple assay runs is afforded only by those kits which provide a stripwell plate, and adequate reagent supply. A complete listing of all materials required for cytokine measurement is provided below:

1. EIA kit validated for serum, plasma, and culture supernatants
2. Precision pipettes with disposable tips
3. Multichannel pipette
4. Disposable reagent troughs
5. Disposable 10-ml pipettes
6. Distilled or deionized water for wash buffer
7. Plastic wash bottle for dispensing wash buffer
8. Absorbent towels for blotting plate dry
9. Disposable plastic tubes for reagent dilutions
10. EIA reader with A_{450} and A_{492} filters
11. 37°C incubator (high humidity)
12. Timer
13. Graph paper or graphing program

C. PREPARATION OF STANDARDS

Highly purified cytokine or cytokine receptor standards are provided with each kit. The mass value of the standards must be related to a reference standard, which is carefully calibrated on a mass basis (i.e., amino acid analyzed material). It must be emphasized that reference standards offered by the Biologic Response Modifiers Program are calibrated in terms of activity units for use in a bioassay and, therefore, do not necessarily qualify as a standard for an immunoassay.

Standards should represent a clinically relevant range that is useful, considering the anticipated values in the unknown test samples. A standard curve range spanning several log concentrations and a sensitivity less than or equal to 25 pg/ml is achievable by EIA methodology. Therefore, the standard curve range of an EIA will generally span from 10–25 pg/ml to 1–2 ng/ml, a range relevant to detection of cytokine and cytokine receptor levels in rheumatoid arthritis. Second, the standard curve should form a steep linear slope in order to ensure accuracy and permit linear regression analysis. Positive controls will assist in establishing the validity of the standard curve for the determination of unknown samples. If positive controls are not provided with the EIA kit then a laboratory positive control pool should be prepared to evaluate assay performance.

The standards and the positive control(s) should be formulated in a diluent which appropriately reflects the matrix of the samples. No shift in the standard curve should occur between standards in the diluent and standards in the sample milieu (i.e., culture medium, control serum, or control plasma). Second, the diluent should provide adequate stability of the reconstituted standards to allow for multiple assay runs with one kit. Batching samples to complete a 96-well plate is not always convenient, particularly in clinical settings. Assay flexibility is determined by the amount of reagents provided and stability of the reconstituted standard. Therefore, stabilities of the reconstituted standards should optimally exceed one month.

D. SAMPLE COLLECTION AND STORAGE

1. Biological Samples

Cytokine production can be the result of any number of stimuli, extreme care must be taken during sample collection to avoid false positives. Endotoxin, a product of Gram-negative bacteria, is a worrisome contaminant, since it stimulates production of IL-1, TNF, IL-6, and IL-8 by monocytes. The use of ethylene diamine tetraacetate (EDTA) as an anticoagulant and stabilizer during plasma and synovial fluid collection can cir-

Table 2 **Sample Collection and Storage**

Important notes

1. The EIA kit should be qualified for the measurement of serum, plasma, or culture supernatants.
2. A standardized collection procedure should be used for all samples within a study.
3. For correlation analysis, other parameters of disease activity should be performed (e.g., clinical index rating, synovial fluid leukocyte count).
4. Record use of anti-inflammatory drugs and consider pre- and post-treatment samples in the study.

Sample type

1. Plasma collection
   a. Aseptic
   b. EDTA anticoagulant (purple-top tube)
   c. Centrifuge within 10 min at 4°C
   d. Collect clear supernatant
2. Serum collection
   a. Aseptic
   b. Red-top tube
   c. Clot at room temperature 45–60 min
   d. Centrifuge immediately at 4°C
   e. Collect clear supernatant
3. Synovial fluid collection
   a. Aseptic
   b. EDTA stabilized (purple top tube)
   c. Centrifuge at 1800 *g* for 30 min at 4°C
   d. Collect clear supernatant

Sample appearance

1. Specimens should be clear.
2. Hemolyzed or lipemic samples should not be used in the study.

Storage of samples

1. Aliquot 200-μl samples in microfuge tubes.
2. Freeze and store aliquots at −70°C; Storage at −20°C is a suitable alternative.
3. Each sample should undergo only one freeze/thaw cycle; aliquot accordingly.

cumvent this problem, since it apparently inhibits endotoxin-induced cytokine production.[24] Also, rapid separation of serum, plasma, and synovial fluid from cells is critical. Otherwise, cells resting within a test tube may recapture circulating cytokine and cause artificially low or negative values.[25] A sample collection and storage procedure relevant for the measurement of cytokine or cytokine receptor levels has been summarized in outline format (Table 2).

2. Special Considerations

Most EIA kits require a dilution of the serum and plasma samples, since matrix constituents can otherwise interfere with accurate cytokine or cytokine receptor measurement. Studies on the effects of synovial fluid, however, have not been conducted and dilution recommendations are not provided by the EIA kit manufacturer. Synovial fluid consists of a plasma dialysate, formed by the passage of blood though the capillary endothelium, to which highly polymerized hyaluronate is added by synovial cells. Although qualification of an EIA kit for use with plasma can serve as a preliminary requirement, the EIA kit should be validated for accurate measurement in synovial fluid using the following protocol:

1. Spike a known amount of cytokine or cytokine receptor standard into synovial fluid
2. Perform a dilution series of the sample (e.g., undiluted, 1:2, 1:3, 1:4)
3. Determine the cytokine or cytokine receptor levels with the EIA kit, remembering to multiply by the dilution factor
4. Adopt the dilution factor which affords the best percent recovery of cytokine or cytokine receptor.

3. Mononuclear Cell Culture Supernatants

Alternatively, an *in vitro* approach can be employed which assesses the cytokine or cytokine receptor levels released from mononuclear cells isolated from the peripheral blood (PBMC) or from the synovial fluid (SFMC). These mononuclear cells are readily obtained from the blood or synovial fluid after centrifugation over Ficoll-Hypaque (density = 1.077). The buffy coat remaining at the interface contains the mononuclear cell population. Cytokine or cytokine receptor levels in the culture supernatants may be measured as the result of constitutive release or stimulus-induced release. Phytohemagglutinin (PHA) is often chosen as the stimulus, since it will stimulate monocyte and lymphocyte populations, resulting in the production of the entire array of cytokines and the release of soluble receptors. In contrast, lipopolysaccharides (LPS) will stimulate only the monocyte population, limiting determinations to the monocyte-derived cytokines (e.g., IL-1, TNF, interferon [IFN]-γ, IL-6, and IL-8). A protocol involving the stimulation of approximately 1×10^6 mononuclear cells/ml should yield cytokine and cytokine receptor levels detectable by immunoassay. In order to optimize the measurement of all cytokines and cytokine receptors of interest, a dose-response with the cell stimulus and the kinetics of cytokine and cytokine receptor accumulation in the culture medium after stimulation should first be determined.

E. CALCULATION AND REPORTING OF RESULTS

Data can be analyzed either by manually graphing the standards or by entering the data into a program capable of linear regression analysis (Figure 2). Linear regression analysis is commonly implemented due to the availability of computer programs and built-in capabilities of advanced EIA readers. The mass concentration of the standards are entered as the independent variable (the x-axis) and the corresponding absorbance values are entered as the dependent variable (y-axis). The data are then fit with a line equation:

$$\begin{aligned} \text{Absorbance} &= \text{slope(pg/ml)} + \text{y-intercept} \\ y &= m\,x + b \end{aligned} \tag{1}$$

Absorbance values (y) are known for the experimental samples and therefore the equation can be solved for the mass of unknown:

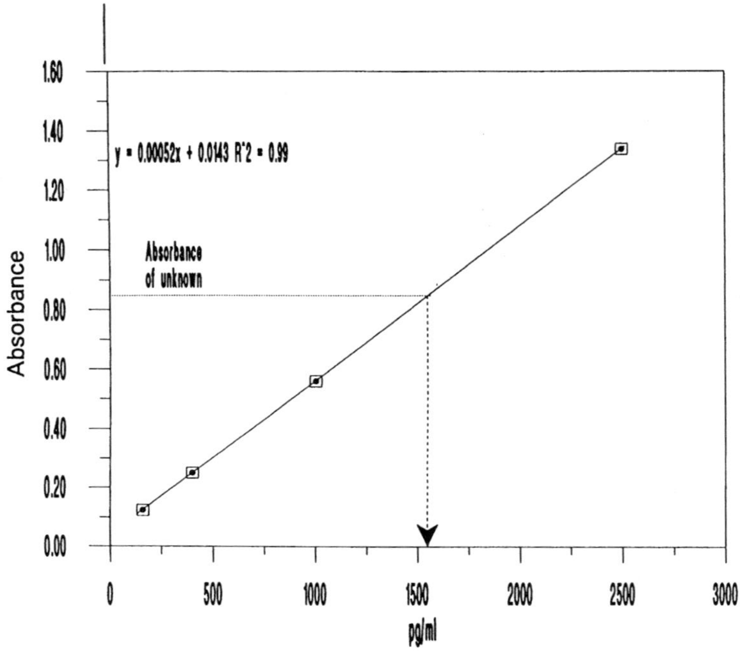

Figure 2 A representative standard curve. An unknown sample concentration of cytokine can be determined by positioning the absorbance value on the standard curve and drawing a vertical line down to intersect with the x-axis or by calculation using the linear regression equation. The measured absorbance is proportional to the amount of cytokine present in the sample.

$$\text{pg/ml} - \frac{\text{Absorbance - y-intercept}}{\text{slope}} \tag{2}$$

For example, the linear regression equation of the standard curve in Figure 2 can be solved as follows:

$$\frac{0.850 - 0.0413}{0.00052} = 1560 \text{ pg/ml} \tag{3}$$

A standard curve with a steep linear slope and a correlation coefficient (R^2) greater than or equal to 0.98 ensures accuracy. The standard curve should never be extrapolated beyond its high or low endpoints, since the assumption of linearity is not valid for EIA standard curves. The limits set by assay sensitivity and solid-phase reaction kinetics cause the slope of the standard curve to flatten at the lower and upper end, respectively. Samples with absorbance values above the standard curve should be diluted. The calculated concentration values of these diluted samples must then be multiplied by the dilution factor.

Every clinical study must determine the expected range of normal values in order to be able to assign statistical relevance to an elevated cytokine or cytokine receptor level observed in a disease state. Circulating levels of cytokines in healthy individuals range from undetectable to low picogram per milliliter values. Cytokine receptors, on the other hand, are normally present in the healthy individual. For example, circulating levels of the soluble IL-2 receptor are detectable in the range of 100 to 500 units/ml (0.33 to 2.0 ng/ml; 0.3 units = 1 pg).[13] Also, the two soluble TNF receptors are detectable in the range of 1 to 3 ng/ml. With a reproducible and specific EIA a cytokine or cytokine receptor level concentration 3 standard deviations (99% confidence level) from the mean normal value can be defined as a statistically significant cut-off value. Cytokine or cytokine receptor levels above this cut-off value are, therefore, abnormally elevated and often indicative of an active disease state. As a last step in data analysis a correlation between cytokine levels and existing methods of rheumatoid arthritis diagnosis (e.g., clinical index rating and synovial fluid leukocyte counts) should be performed.

F. QUALITY CONTROL AND PERFORMANCE CHARACTERISTICS

Performance characteristics such as sensitivity, specificity, precision, and accuracy should be well defined for the EIA kit:

Sensitivity: The value which is two standard deviations above the background absorbance. This criterion permits confidence that low values are statistically significant (95% confidence level) and above background.

Specificity: Assigned after values for a panel of other cytokines or related proteins are less than or equal to the zero control in the assay.

Precision: Index of the assays' ability to yield the same mass value for the same sample. Intra-assay reproducibility is based on replicates run on the sample within the same assay, whereas interassay reproducibility is based on assays run on different days. Reproducibility is reported as the coefficient of variation:

$$\mathrm{CV}(\%) = \frac{\text{Standard Deviation}}{\text{Mean}} \times 100$$

Acceptable performance for an EIA can be characterized by a coefficient of variation of $\leq 10\%$.

Accuracy: Percent recoveries in plasma, serum, or culture supernatants must be performed to qualify an EIA kit for measurement of cytokines or cytokine receptors in biological fluids. Known concentration of cytokine or cytokine receptor must be added to the biological fluid of interest and then compared to values obtained from the standard curve. Percent recoveries can then be calculated as:

$$\frac{\text{concentration derived from the standard curve}}{\text{known concentration of the cytokine or cytokine receptor}} \times 100$$

If synovial fluid is used, the cytokine of interest must be tested in a similar spike and recovery experiment (see Section III.D).

G. LIMITATIONS AND PITFALLS

Since structurally intact or native cytokine is required for cell receptor and antibody recognition, theoretically biologic activity detected by bioassay should correlate with the immunoreactive mass detected by EIA. Indeed this is often the case; however, the measurement of cytokine levels in biological fluids is complicated by the presence of other factors, like soluble binding proteins. Association of cytokines with soluble cytokine receptors or the serum proteins can interfere with cytokine detection in bioassay procedures. Bound cytokines or the inactive monomers of obligatory oligomers (i.e., TNF, IL-5) are not bioactive and will not be detected by bioassay. Yet, if the epitope is still accessible to the antibodies of the immunoassay, then immunoreactivity is preserved and bound cytokine or inactive monomers can be measured. Therefore, differences may be observed upon comparison of immunoassay and bioassay results, since factors exist in biological fluids which can differentially affect biologic activity and immunoreactivity. The technical limitations of the employed assay must be understood in order to interpret the results.

It is also important to consider that cytokine and cytokine receptor levels can be influenced by other factors. For example, infection within the joint, a common complication of rheumatoid arthritis, will generate a different cytokine and cytokine receptor profile from a joint diagnosed solely with rheumatoid arthritis. Moreover, anti-inflammatory treatments may also alter the cytokine and cytokine receptor profile within a sample. Therefore, a thorough knowledge of the patient and sample history should be obtained to assist in the interpretation of the data.

IV. SUMMARY

Cytokines undoubtedly play a role in the pathogenesis of rheumatoid arthritis and contribute to the recruitment and activation of leukocytes, the hyperplasia of the synovium, and progressive destruction of the articular bone and cartilage. Despite the beneficial intentions of cytokine action, such injury to the host often results from the misdirected or excessive production of cytokines. The release of soluble cytokine receptors from activated leukocytes is an immunoregulatory response designed to attenuate the harmful bioactivities of the cytokines.

As the levels of cytokines and cytokine receptors in rheumatoid arthritis continue to be studied, a more complete picture of the cytokine network involved in the pathogenesis of the disease will be formed. Also, the elevation of the cytokine or soluble cytokine receptors may be indicative of the severity and/or prognosis of certain disease states. Research involving the measurement of cytokines and cytokine receptors is still at an early stage. Research to date indicates that IL-6 and soluble IL-2 receptor levels do correlate with other parameters of disease activity. Further studies are warranted, however, and an understanding of the capabilities and limitations of the various assay systems is required in order to implement the one that best fits the needs of the study.

REFERENCES

1. **Smith, J. B., Bocchieri, M. H., Sherbin-Allen, L., Borofsky, M., and Abruzzo, J. L.,** Occurrence of interleukin-1 in human synovial fluid: detection by RIA, bioassay and presence of bioassay-inhibiting factors, *Rheumatol. Int.,* 9, 53, 1989.
2. **Miltenburg, A. M. M., van Laar, J. M., de Kuiper, R., Daha, M. R., and Breedveld, F. C.,** Interleukin-6 activity in paired samples of synovial fluid. Correlation of synovial fluid interleukin-6 levels with clinical and laboratory parameters of inflammation, *Br. J. Rheumatol.,* 30, 186, 1989.
3. **Houssiau, F. A., Devogelaer, J.-P., van Damme, J., Nagant de Deuxchaisnes, C., and van Snick, J.,** Interleukin-6 in synovial fluid and serum of patients with rheumatoid arthritis and other inflammatory arthritides, *Arthritis Rheum.,* 31, 784, 1988.
4. **Miyasaka, N., Sato, K., Hashimoto, J., Kohsaka, H., Yamamoto, K., Goto, M., Inoue, K., Matsuda, T., Hirano, T., Kishimoto, T., and Nishioka, K.,** Constitutive production of interleukin 6/B cell stimulatory factor-2 from inflammatory system, *Clin. Immunol. Immunopathol.,* 52, 238, 1989.
5. **Brennan, F. M., Zacharise, C. O., Chantry, D., Larsen, C. G., Turner, M., Maini, R. N., Matsushima, K., and Feldmann, M.,** Detection of interleukin 8 biological activity in synovial fluids from patients with rheumatoid arthritis and production of interleukin 8 mRNA by isolated synovial cells, *Eur. J. Immunol.,* 20, 2141, 1990.
6. **LaCour, E. G., Grayson, M. H., Ware, C. F., and Pope, R. M.,** Enhanced cytotoxicity in the rheumatoid joint, *Clin. Immunol. Immunopathol.,* 54, 431, 1990.
7. **Lotz, M., Kekow, J., and Carson, D. A.,** Transforming growth factor-β and cellular immune responses in synovial fluids, *J. Immunol.,* 144, 4189, 1990.
8. **Rubin, L. A., Snow, K. M., Kurman, C. C., Nelson, D. L., and Keystone, E. C.,** Serial levels of soluble interleukin 2 receptor in the peripheral blood of patients with rheumatoid arthritis: correlations with disease activity, *J. Rheumatol.,* 17, 597, 1990.
9. **Miossec, P., Elhamiani, M., Chichehian, B., D'Angeac, A. D., Sany, J., and Hirn, M.,** Interleukin 2 (IL2) inhibitor in rheumatoid synovial fluid: correlation with prognosis and soluble IL 2 receptor levels, *J. Clin. Immunol.,* 10, 115, 1991.
10. **Coligan, J. E., Kruisbeek, A. M., Margulies, D. H., Shevach, E. M., and Strober, W., Eds.,** *Current Protocols in Immunology,* Greene Publishing Associates and Wiley-Interscience, New York, 1991.
11. **Balkwill, F. R., Ed.,** *Cytokines, A Practical Approach,* Oxford University Press, New York, 1991.
12. **Aggarwal, B. B. and Gutterman, J. U., Eds.,** *Human Cytokines, Handbook for Basic and Clinical Research,* Blackwell Scientific Publications, Boston, MA, 1992.
13. **Gillis, S., Ferm, M. M., Ou, W., and Smith, K. A.,** T-cell growth factor: parameters of production and a quantitative microassay for activity. *J. Immunol.,* 120, 2027, 1978.
14. **Kitamura, T., Tange, T., Terasawa, T., Chiba, S., Kuwaki, T., Miyagawa, K., Piao, Y.-F., Miyazono, K., Urabe, A., and Takaku, F.,** Establishment and characterization of a unique human cell line that proliferates dependently on GM-CSF, IL-3, or erythropoietin, *J. Cell. Physiol.,* 140, 323, 1989.

15. **Spits, H., Yssel, H., Paliard, X., Kastelein, R., Figdor, C. G., and de Vries, J. E.,** IL-4 inhibits IL-2 mediated induction of human lymphokine activated killer cells, but not the generation of antigen specific cytotoxic T lymphocytes in mixed leukocyte cultures, *J. Immunol.,* 141, 29, 1988.
16. **Aarden, L. A., De Groot, E. R., Schaap, O. L., and Lansdorp, P. M.,** Production of hybridoma growth factor by human monocytes, *Br. J. Immunol.,* 17, 1411, 1987.
17. **Yang, Y.-C., Ricciardi, S., Ciarletta, A., Calvetti, J., Kelleher, K., and Clark, S. C.,** Expression cloning of a cDNA encoding a novel human hematopoietic growth factor: human homologue of murine T cell growth factor P40, *Blood,* 74, 1880, 1989.
18. **Thompson-Snipes, L., Dhar, V., Bond, M. W., Mosmann, T. R., Moore, K. W., and Rennick, D.,** Interleukin-10: a novel stimulatory factor for mast cells and their progenitors, *J. Exp. Med.,* 173, 1625, 1991.
19. **Gately, M. K., Desai, B. B., Wolitzky, A. G., Quinn, P. M., Dywer, C. M., Podlaski, F. J., Familletti, P. C., Sinigaglia, F., Chizonnite, R., Gubler, U., and Stern, A. S.,** Regulation of human lymphocyte proliferation by a heterodimeric cytokine, IL-12 (cytotoxic lymphocyte maturation factor), *J. Immunol.,* 147, 874, 1991.
20. **Metcalf, D., Hilton, D. J., and Nicola, N. A.,** Clonal analysis of the actions of the murine leukemia inhibitory factor, *Nucl. Acids Res.,* 16, 9857, 1988.
21. **Matsushima, K., Larsen, C. G., DeBois, G. C., and Oppenheim, J. J.,** Purification and characterization of a novel monocyte chemotactic and activating factor produced by a human myelomonocytic cell line, *J. Exp. Med.,* 169, 1485, 1989.
22. **Hendrie, P. C., Miyazawa, K., Yang, Y. C., Langefeld, C. D., and Broxmeyer, H. E.,** Mast cell growth factor (*c-kit* ligand) enhances cytokine stimulation of the human factor-dependent cell line, MO7e, *Exp. Hematol.,* 19, 1031, 1991.
23. **Parker, C. W.,** *Radioimmunoassay of Biologically Active Compounds,* Prentice-Hall, Englewood Cliffs NJ, 1976.
24. **Exley, A. R. and Cohen, J.,** Optimal collection of blood samples for the measurement of tumor necrosis factor α, *Cytokine,* 2, 353, 1990.
25. **Engelberts, I., Mollf, A., Schoen, G. J. M., van der Linden, C. J., and Buurman, W. A.,** Evaluation of measurement of human TNF in plasma by ELISA, *Lymphokine Cytokine Res.,* 10, 69, 1991.

Chapter 16

Clinical Value and Limitations of Measuring Cytokines in the Diagnosis and Management of Autoimmune Rheumatic Diseases

Martin Lotz

CONTENTS

I. INTRODUCTION

Laboratory tests are essential in the diagnosis and assessment of disease activity in autoimmune rheumatic disorders. Clinical symptoms in combination with radiographic findings and the particular patterns of autoantibodies constitute the major criteria that are being used in differential diagnosis. Assessment of disease activity and response to therapy also relies on some of these parameters, but more strongly on laboratory tests. Most of these are not specific for a particular disease entity. Commonly used markers are systemic manifestations of the host defense response to inflammatory injury, such as the erythrocyte sedimentation rate (ESR), C-reactive protein (CRP), and albumin as expressions of the hepatic acute-phase response; leukocytosis, thrombocytosis, and anemia as a reflection of bone marrow adaptation; and levels of autoantibodies and complement as the consequence of humoral immune system activation.

Cytokines are the mediators of these biochemical and cellular changes. The value of measuring cytokines and some of their soluble receptors can be seen in two major aspects. First, by establishing correlations between cytokine levels and the presence or magnitude of clinical and laboratory changes the pathogenetic role of cytokines can be substantiated. This approach has already contributed to confirm hypotheses that were

0-8493-5974-1/94/$0.00 + $.50

based on *in vitro* studies of cytokines and their effects on various cellular responses. Second, cytokine measurements have the potential to be useful as markers of disease activity and perhaps aid in differential diagnosis. This applies in particular to systemically active cytokines that are produced by multiple cell types and reach levels in body fluids that are within the sensitivity of available assays. The potential clinical value of cytokine quantification has to be confirmed by studies in which correlations are sought with already established markers of disease activity. This section will summarize the available literature in this area.

II. CYTOKINES PRODUCED BY MULTIPLE CELL TYPES

Diverse cell sources in most organ systems have been identified for this group of cytokines and they include hematopoietic cells, in particular mononuclear phagocytes with the different types of tissue macrophages, endothelial cells, fibroblasts, synoviocytes, and chondrocytes.[1-3] Since these cytokines coordinate systemic manifestations of the inflammatory disease process, they reach levels in body fluids that can be detected by immunoassays as well as by the generally more sensitive bioassays.

A. IL-1

Interleukin (IL)-1 is a cytokine that is involved with several important aspects in the pathogenesis of autoimmune diseases. Together with tumor necrosis factor (TNF), it is the principal factor that causes connective tissue degradation through the induction of proteases and the inhibition of proteoglycan synthesis. IL-1 regulates immune and inflammatory responses and causes systemic changes, including fever, increased hepatic acute protein synthesis, and bone marrow adaptation. The initial studies on IL-1 levels in autoimmune diseases were primarily designed to confirm its role in pathogenesis.

Analysis of plasma extracts by enzyme-linked immunosorbent assay (ELISA) showed that mean levels of IL-1β in rheumatoid arthritis (RA) were approximately twofold higher than in normal controls and this appeared to correlate with clinical and laboratory markers of disease activity.[4] However, in a subsequent study with a tenfold less sensitive radioimmunoassay (RIA), IL-1β could not be detected in RA plasma.[5] The first study on IL-1 in synovial fluids (SF) by Wood et al.[6] demonstrated the presence of IL-1 after isolation by affinity chromatography. IL-1 activity was not detectable in unfractionated fluids, suggesting the presence of inhibitors. The levels were similar in SF from patients with a variety of different arthritides. These findings were confirmed with lymphocyte chemotaxis as a biological assay for IL-1 in SF and this activity was also only detectable after separation from inhibitors.[7] High levels of immunoreactive IL-1β were detected in RA synovial fluids, but these did not correlate with markers of disease activity and there was no difference in SF IL-1β content between RA and osteoarthritis (OA).[5] Other investigators confirmed the presence of IL-1β in RA synovial fluids by ELISA and found higher titers than in OA. In a comparative analysis of synovial fluids in a biological assay and by RIA,[8] small amounts of IL-1 bioactivity and inhibitors were detected. When the same samples were analyzed by RIA, levels were one order of magnitude higher.

From these studies it appears that IL-1β immunoreactivity is present in SF and that IL-1β bioactivity can be demonstrated after separation from inhibitors. These findings are consistent with the detection of IL-1 mRNA in RA synovium.[9] Circulating levels of IL-1β are relatively low and close to the detection limits of the immunoassays and therefore do not represent a reliable marker for use in clinical rheumatology.

IL-1 receptor antagonist (IL-1ra) is a protein that is structurally related to IL-1, competes with IL-1 for receptor binding, and inhibits its biological activities. This protein is an important regulator of immune responses and connective tissue metabolism and is presently under clinical evaluation as a therapeutic agent in RA and other acute and chronic inflammatory diseases.[10] A specific ELISA for IL-1ra that can detect the protein in SF has been developed,[11] but information on the levels of IL-1ra in synovial or other body fluids from patients with autoimmune diseases is not yet available.

B. TNF

TNF-α was detected by ELISA in 7 of 12 RA sera but only in 1 of 11 sera from patients with reactive arthritis.[12] Increased TNF bioactivity was found in a similar percentage of RA sera, with the highest levels in patients with severe disease.[12] Of the same patients' synovial fluids, 6 of 12 RA samples and 3 of 11 samples from patients with reactive arthritis were positive. The highest levels of synovial fluid TNF-α were found in those RA patients with higher ESR and synovial fluid leukocyte count. In the analysis of a larger series of SF, 38% of the samples were positive for TNF.[13] The only correlation with other variables was with disease duration in OA. When measured by ELISA, TNF-α was detected in a higher percentage of RA synovial fluids as compared to non-RA samples. TNF-β was not detectable by bioassay in sera or synovial fluids[14] or only in trace amounts when tested by ELISA.[13] These studies are thus providing similar results on TNF levels in RA, although synovial fluid levels may be underestimated since SF appears to contain inhibitors of TNF activity.[15]

Information on TNF levels in systemic lupus erythematosus (SLE) is more limited. Based on bioassay, most SLE sera contained normal levels of TNF and very high titers were seen in SLE patients with infection.[16] A group of RA sera was tested for comparison and found to have higher titers than the SLE group. Similar findings with elevated TNF in 46% of RA patients and 29% of SLE patients were obtained by RIA.[17]

In these measurements of TNF levels it was not determined to which degree soluble TNF receptors interfered with the detection of TNF.[18] Since soluble TNF receptors are likely to be present in serum or synovial fluids[15] from patients with active autoimmune diseases, this has to be considered in the interpretation of TNF levels.

C. IL-6

Among the diverse biological activities of IL-6, its effects on (auto)antibody formation, the hepatic acute-phase response and hematopoiesis are probably most important to its role in the pathogenesis of autoimmune rheumatic diseases.[1,19] IL-6 is produced in relatively high titers by many cell types *in vitro* and it has been detected in body fluids from patients with diverse disease states. IL-6 levels have been measured in a large number of patients with autoimmune diseases and the available literature suggests that it is of value in assessing disease activity.

There are multiple cellular sources of IL-6 within the joint. Mononuclear phagocytes, endothelial cells,[20] synoviocytes,[21] and chondrocytes[22] can produce IL-6 and the cytokines IL-1 and TNF and bacterial lipopolysaccharides are potent inducers. High levels of IL-6 can be found in synovial fluids from patients with arthritis and there is a good correlation with the intensity of the inflammatory response. IL-6 levels in synovial fluid are higher in samples from patients with inflammatory arthropathies as compared to osteoarthritis. SF IL-6 levels correlate with SF leukocyte count and ESR.[23] A study on a relatively small group of patients specifically analyzed the relationship between SF IL-6 levels and parameters of local disease activity and found a very close correlation between the clinical variables, IL-6 titers and leukocyte content.[24] However, no correlation was found between IL-6 and IgM and IgG concentrations. This lack of correlation was confirmed in a separate study,[25] which found an interesting relationship between SF IL-6 and rheumatoid factors of the IgM, IgG, and IgA isotypes and also with the Lansbury articular index and the ESR. A detailed characterization of the spectrum of autoantibodies to cytoskeletal components showed that synovial fluids from patients with chronic inflammatory arthropathies contained reactivity against vimentin and actin while these autoantibodies were not detectable in sera from the same patients.[26] The titers of these synovial fluid autoantibodies correlated with IL-6 content. Inflammatory microcrystals, including monosodium urate and calcium pyrophosphate dihydrate, but not hydroxyapatite crystals, induce the secretion of IL-6 from mononuclear phagocytes and synoviocytes and high titers of IL-6 can be found in synovial fluids from patients with gout and pseudogout.[27]

Comparative studies of IL-6 levels in RA synovial fluid and serum showed up to 1000-fold higher titers in the joint. SF IL-6 levels correlate with serum IL-6, suggesting that the joint is the source of circulating IL-6.[28] In general, a very good correlation has been found between IL-6 levels in serum and other markers of disease activity. Serum IL-6 correlates with elevated ESR and increased levels of hepatic acute-phase proteins, such as CRP, α1-acid glycoprotein, α1-antitrypsin, haptoglobin, and fibrinogen,[29] or decreased albumin concentrations.[23] The correlation between serum IL-6, ESR, and CRP was also found in a selected group of RA patients with anemia of chronic disease.[30]

SLE sera and cerebrospinal fluids have been shown to contain increased IL-6 levels. Cerebrospinal fluid IL-6 activity was elevated in 10/14 patients with central nervous system (CNS) lupus.[31] All patients showed increased cerebrospinal fluid immunoglobulin levels. Only 1/9 SLE patients without CNS involvement had moderately increased IL-6. IL-6 levels in cerebrospinal fluid decreased markedly during therapy when symptoms improved. Serum titers in CNS lupus patients did not correlate with those in cerebrospinal fluid. A study on a larger series of SLE sera found that most (63/70) contained higher than normal levels of IL-6[32] and titers correlated with disease activity. Similar frequencies of increased IL-6 in active SLE were observed in a study by Stuart et al., who noted that only three of the seven patients with elevated IL-6 had increased levels of CRP.[33] This lack of a correlation between IL-6 and CRP was interpreted to suggest that in SLE there may be a defect in hepatocyte responses to this cytokine. There are no published reports on IL-6 in urine samples from patients with lupus nephritis, but IL-6 levels have been found to be a useful indicator in other kidney diseases. IL-6 may be involved with the pathogenesis of mesangial proliferative glomerulonephritis, since it stimulates mesangial cell proliferation. In 50% of patients with this disorder, urine IL-6 levels were elevated and mesangial cells were shown to be at least in part responsible as a cellular source of IL-6.[34] Urine from normal donors and patients with minimal change nephrotic syndrome did not contain increased IL-6. IL-6 immunoreactivity was also detected in SLE kidney biopsies.[35]

Patients with polymyalgia rheumatica and giant cell arteritis have a strong hepatic acute-phase response and, in a series of 15 untreated patients, all had high serum IL-6 levels.[36] There was, however, no correlation with response to therapy or acute-phase protein levels. Interestingly, six of the patients continued to have increased IL-6 levels

6 months after steroid therapy when hepatic acute-phase proteins had decreased. This observation is important, since it suggests that other cytokines, including IL-11, Leukemia inhibitory factor (LIF), and oncostatin M, that can induce a similar set of acute-phase proteins as IL-6, may be involved. There is only minimal information on the levels of these more recently characterized cytokines in body fluids. We performed a preliminary analysis on LIF activity in synovial fluids and found LIF in higher titers in RA as compared to OA.[37]

Juvenile rheumatoid arthritis (JRA) patients with systemic onset disease had significantly elevated serum IL-6 levels and these decreased during remission.[38] Serum IL-6 levels also correlated with the extent and severity of arthritis and with thrombocytosis.

In all of these studies on IL-6 in different body fluids from patients with rheumatic diseases IL-6 was measured by biological assays. Most commonly used was the B9 hybridoma cell proliferation assay, which is highly sensitive and relatively specific for IL-6. The only known interference of other cytokines is the synergy between IL-2 and IL-6.[39] However, this may not have significant impact for measurements of IL-6 levels in patient samples, since they usually do not contain detectable IL-2 (see below). Some studies also used the hepatocyte stimulating factor assay where the induction of an acute-phase protein is measured in hepatoma cells. This assay, however, is not specific, since IL-1, TNF, IL-11, LIF, and oncostatin M can also induce hepatic acute-phase proteins. The IL-6 protein in synovial fluid has also been demonstrated by western blotting.[40] Only recently an ELISA has been described which has similar sensitivity as the B9 assay and quantification of SF IL-6 gave similar results with both assays.[41]

Collectively these studies support the value of IL-6 in defining disease activity in patients with different autoimmune diseases. With the development of sensitive ELISA or RIA for the detection of IL-6 in body fluids, this cytokine may become a marker that can be introduced into routine laboratory analysis.

D. IL-8

IL-8 is the principal neutrophil chemotactic cytokine and thus of potential importance in the pathogenesis of synovial fluid leukocytosis. Intra-articular sources of IL-8 are synovial cells,[42] fibroblasts, mononuclear phagocytes,[43] and chondrocytes.[44]

In the first study on the presence of IL-8 in synovial fluid, neutrophil chemotactic activity was detected with a biological assay.[45] These measurements did not correlate with the number of neutrophils in synovial fluid, nor with the amount of IL-8 protein and the molecular nature of the chemotactic activity has not been defined. However, more recently it was demonstrated with a specific and sensitive ELISA that RA synovial fluids contain IL-8.[46] In this assay interference of synovial fluid rheumatoid factor with IL-8 measurements was excluded. IL-8 titers were directly related to the number of cells in the joint and to serum levels of CRP. In contrast, IL-8 was not detectable in SF from patients with gout, SLE, and patients with salmonella-induced arthritis. At present it is not known whether IL-8 reaches levels in plasma that can be detected with the available assays.

E. COLONY STIMULATING FACTORS (CSF)

There are four genetically distinct human colony stimulating factors, granulocyte CSF (G-CSF), macrophage CSF (M-CSF), GM-CSF, and multi-CSF (IL-3). RA synovial fluids contain increased titers of GM-CSF as compared to OA samples. IL-3 protein and mRNA were not detected in RA synovial fluid and tissue, but this may be due to the fact that IL-3, in contrast to the other CSF, is only produced by lymphoid cells.[47] The potential pathogenetic significance of elevated synovial fluid GM-CSF may be that it is a factor in addition to IFN-γ that can increase HLA-DR expression.[48] As only very low levels of IFN-γ are present in synovial fluids, GM-CSF may be responsible for the increased HLA DR expression in RA synovial tissue.

F. IFN-α

IFN-α was the first cytokine that has been studied extensively in sera from patients with autoimmune diseases. In 1979 Hooks[49] reported that sera from patients with SLE, Sjögren's syndrome, and RA contained IFN activity as measured in a biological cytopathic effect inhibition assay.[49] IFN titers were found to correlate well with disease activity, levels of autoantibodies and complement, as well as with response to therapy. The IFN activity in patient sera was acid-labile and therefore thought to represent ''immune'' or gamma IFN. However, subsequent studies which performed neutralization with specific antibodies characterized the IFN activity in SLE sera as IFN-α, which therefore represented an unusual, acid-labile species of IFN-α.[50] More recently, it was demonstrated that IFN-α purified from SLE sera is not intrinsically acid-labile,[51] but that a separate activity in serum is responsible for the destruction of IFN-α activity after transient acidification of serum.[52] The biochemical nature of this activity has not yet been defined but its titers correlate with disease activity in SLE. The IFN-like material has also been studied further in RA. The highest levels were found in patients with extra-articular disease manifestations. The IFN was detected by a solid-phase ELISA but when tested in antiviral assays it was found to be inactive. Upon exposure of the RA sera to pH 2 the immunoreactivity in the ELISA was lost.[53] IFN-α in RA synovial fluids was tested in two studies. By RIA less than 4 U/ml were detected in RA and non-RA samples.[54] In a subsequent study with an ELISA using an antibody that recognizes different subtypes of IFN-α, increased titers were found in approximately 25% of RA SF but the majority of the samples were below the detection limit of the assay.[8]

A recent study on IFN-α levels in cerebrospinal fluid from patients with CNS lupus showed increased titers, particularly in patients with lupus psychosis as compared to other manifestations of CNS lupus. IFN-α immunoreactivity and mRNA were detected in neurons. This study suggests that IFN-α produced within the CNS may contribute to the development of lupus psychosis and perhaps become a useful test in the differential diagnosis of psychosis in patients with SLE.[55]

III. CYTOKINES PREDOMINANTLY OF LYMPHOCYTE ORIGIN

A. IL-2, IFN-γ

Activated lymphocytes are the primary source of IL-2 and IFN-γ. IL-2 is relatively restricted with respect to the spectrum of its target cells, which are predominantly within the immune system. In contrast, IFN-γ can induce expression of HLA class II antigens on most cell types. It also acts broadly as an antiviral agent and induces certain hepatic acute-phase proteins. The general experience with measurements of these lymphokines has been that their levels in body fluids from patients are clearly lower than those of the cytokines discussed in the previous section and this is probably one reason for some controversy on the presence or absence of these cytokines in sera or synovial fluids. Some studies found that the IL-2 and IFN-γ levels in different body fluids were below the detection limit of available assays. Their "absence" has led to speculations about the role of IL-2, IFN-γ, and T lymphocytes in autoimmune rheumatic diseases and provided a rationale for studies on therapeutic substitution.

In SLE, peripheral blood T cells express several activation markers and there is evidence for increased serum IL-2 levels. Patients with severe disease had twofold higher serum IL-2 levels than normal controls or lupus patients with mild disease.[56] Representative sera with high IL-2 as measured by ELISA also contained biologically active IL-2 and after chromatographic separation from other serum proteins the IL-2 activity eluted at the expected molecular weight.

There are only few published studies on IL-2 levels in the sera from patients with RA or other rheumatic diseases. RA sera did not contain stimulatory activity when tested for proliferative effects on phytohemagglutinin (PHA) blasts but this IL-2-like activity was found in almost all synovial fluids from different arthritides.[57] The activity was partially characterized with respect to its biochemical properties and found to be consistent with IL-2. Wilkins et al. used an IL-2-dependent cell line and showed that most RA synovial fluids but none of the control samples contained stimulatory activity. The activity was heat-resistant and <50,000 kDa. Both of these studies did not provide definitive support for the identification of the activities as IL-2 and it is now known that several other cytokines can cause stimulation of the cell lines used in these studies. Furthermore, low levels of IL-2-like activity were not neutralized by antibody to IL-2 and all SF were negative for IL-2 when tested by ELISA.[54] SF thus does not appear to contain titers of IL-2 that are within the detection limit of available assays.

Similarly, IFN-γ was not detected, or found to be present only at low titers. When tested in a sensitive RIA, RA synovial fluids were negative for IFN-γ.[54] This appeared to correlate with an absence of IFN-γ mRNA in RA synovial tissue. Similar results were obtained by ELISA where most SF contained no detectable IFN-γ and only low levels were found in some RA SF.[58] In contrast, Saxne et al.[14] detected IFN-γ in synovial fluids and sera from patients with RA by a specific and more sensitive (detection limit: 0.4 ng/ml) ELISA. Five of 12 RA sera and SF contained IFN-γ in titers greater than 1 ng/ml. Synovial fluids and sera from patients with reactive arthritis were negative. In support of this finding, Buchan et al.[59] detected IFN-γ mRNA in 10 of 12 RA synovial mononuclear cell samples. However, only one of these patients contained high levels of this mRNA. Interestingly, upon *in vitro* culture of the synovial cells, levels of IFN-γ mRNA increased, suggesting inhibition of RNA expression *in vivo*.

In summary, IL-2 and IFN-γ, cytokines that are primarily produced by T lymphocytes, are apparently not suitable for diagnostic studies. The finding that their levels are not strongly elevated may be related to their function in a microenvironment rather than systemic fashion like the cytokines discussed in the previous section. The absence of greatly elevated levels of IL-2 and IFN-γ, therefore, does not necessarily argue against their involvement with the disease process.

B. NEOPTERIN

Neopterin is a pyrazino-pyrimidine derivative synthesized from guanosine triphosphate by IFN-γ-activated macrophages. It can easily be measured by commercially available RIA in serum, urine, and synovial fluid. In a wide variety of disease states it has been shown to be a very good indicator of activation of the cellular immune system. In an analysis of a large series of patients it was found that urinary neopterin levels in RA but not OA sera were significantly increased as compared to healthy controls.[60] In RA patients increased neopterin titers were associated with increased disease activity, disease duration, and ESR and correlated with low hemoglobin levels. When RA patients were classified according to clinical disease activity, neopterin levels best discriminated between the different groups. Neopterin levels decreased in response to effective antirheumatic therapy. In synovial fluid the highest levels were seen in RA and gout. OA SF also contained detectable neopterin, but in lower titers.[61]

IV. SOLUBLE CYTOKINE RECEPTORS

A. sIL-2R, TNFR

The soluble form of the IL-2 receptor was discovered by Rubin[62] in culture supernatants of activated lymphocytes. This molecule is a 45-kDa truncated version of the 55-kDa membrane-associated Tac or IL-2Rα subunit. The function of this soluble receptor in the regulation of T cell responses is not clear. It inhibits the biological activity of IL-2 only at high concentrations and this is probably related to its relatively low affinity for IL-2.[62]

Serum levels of sIL-2R were elevated in several autoimmune diseases, including RA, SLE, and systemic sclerosis.[62] Serum as well as synovial fluid levels in OA were lower as compared to RA. High titers were also found in patients with infections, sarcoidosis, or malignancies and it is thus apparent that measurements of sIL-2R in serum are not useful in differential diagnosis.

Earlier studies on relatively small patient populations suggested a correlation between disease activity and sIL-2R in RA. However, a series of more recent studies on larger groups of patients failed to confirm this. A study on 150 patients with refractory RA showed that patients had significantly elevated serum sIL-2R levels at initiation of the trial and that levels fell during treatment.[63] However, there was no correlation between sIL-2R and disease duration, ESR, joint count, or tenderness, nor did sIL-2R levels discriminate between responders or nonresponders to therapy. In a study on the effects of a sustained-release nonsteroidal anti-inflammatory drug (NSAID) and simultaneous measurements of sIL-2R, sCD4, and sCD8, there was also no correlation between the levels of these three soluble forms of T cell surface receptors, nor between sIL-2R and serological or clinical markers of disease activity.[64]

In SLE there were increased levels of sIL-2R in both patients with active as well as inactive disease.[56] Elevated sIL-2R in SLE were found in a cross-sectional study and this correlated with the titers of anti-dsDNA.[65] However, in a longitudinal study of seven patients there were substantial changes in anti-dsDNA that were not paralleled by similar changes in sIL-2R and in some patients sIL-2R continued to be elevated despite low autoantibody levels. Tokano et al.[66] found that there was no correlation between elevated serum sIL-2R, disease manifestations, anti-dsDNA, or complement. In some patients there seemed to be a correlation with disease activity.[66] In a prospective study, sIL-2R was measured in SLE patients prior to the development of a relapse. In 18 of 21 patients sIL-2R levels were increased during exacerbation and correlated with anti-dsDNA and complement but not with the disease activity score. sIL-2R levels were already elevated prior to exacerbation and decreased after therapy.

Levels of sIL-2R were increased in sera from JRA patients as compared to healthy controls and the highest titers were found in the subset with systemic onset disease. In a study on 16 children who were treated with oral methotrexate there was a good correlation between sIL-2R and therapeutic response.[67]

In Wegener's granulomatosis sIL-2R levels were increased in patients with active disease as compared to those in remission.[68] In patients with disease exacerbation, sIL-2R levels increased earlier than CRP and cytoplasmic anti-neutrophil cytoplasmic antibodies (c-ANCA). In addition, patients with active disease but low CRP and ANCA had increased sIL-2R. This study, which analyzed 102 patients, thus suggests that sIL-2R may be a good marker of disease activity and an early sign of imminent relapse in Wegener's.

A good correlation was observed in polymyositis with response to corticosteroid therapy. In addition, sIL-2R levels increased prior to other laboratory markers in patients who developed a relapse of the disease. In Sjögren's syndrome and in systemic sclerosis the highest levels of sIL-2R were an indicator of disease activity, as well as of prognosis and overall disease severity.[69]

Patients with ankylosing spondylitis (AS) sIL-2R in serum were only slightly higher than in normal controls and there was no difference between patients with inflammatory or noninflammatory AS.[70]

In summary, several studies on large series of patients suggest that levels of sIL-2R do not appear to reflect disease activity in RA. In other rheumatic diseases there are indications that measurements of sIL-2R may have some clinical value, but this will have to be confirmed.

B. sTNFR

Soluble forms of both types of TNFR exist. They bind TNF and inhibit its biological activity. At present there is only limited information on their levels in body fluids from patients with autoimmune rheumatic diseases. Significant levels (>20 ng/ml) were found in RA synovial fluids and these concentrations were higher than in samples from OA and AS patients.[71]

V. SUMMARY

These studies on the presence of cytokines in sera, synovial and cerebrospinal fluids, and urine from patients with autoimmune rheumatic diseases have certainly advanced the understanding of the role of the different cytokines in pathogenesis. Elevated levels of some of the cytokines have supported their contribution to specific local or systemic disease manifestations. The unexpected absence of cytokines, or their presence at very low concentrations, has led to the discovery of cytokine inhibitors and the identification of additional cytokines that can induce a particular biological response.

Several cytokines are clearly not useful as clinical markers. IL-1, TNF, IL-2, and IFN-γ are present at relatively low levels and, with available methods, only a small number of specimens from patients with active disease are positive. Interestingly, neopterin levels, which thus far are known to be increased only by IFN-γ, are a very good and readily testable marker of disease activity, suggesting that very small amounts of IFN-γ are sufficient to cause monocyte activation or that other, as yet unidentified factors can stimulate neopterin production. In contrast, soluble IL-2 receptors are present at levels that are within the sensitivity of ELISA but in RA their levels do not correlate well with disease activity or response to therapy. A large series of studies has documented the value of IL-6 as a good indicator of disease activity and this cytokine has promise to become a widely used marker. The role of cytokine measurements in differential diagnosis is still very limited. In the differential diagnosis of CNS manifestations in

SLE, IL-6 and perhaps IFN-α may be useful. Further studies are needed to explore whether levels of cytokines such as TNF can help to distinguish lupus flares from infection.

REFERENCES

1. **Hirano, T. and Kishimoto, T.,** Interleukin-6: possible implications in human diseases, *Ric. Clin. Lab.*, 19, 1, 1989.
2. **Baggiolini, M., Walz, A., and Kunkel, S. L.,** Neutrophil-activating peptide-1/interleukin-8, a novel cytokine that activates neutrophils, *J. Clin. Invest.*, 84, 1045, 1989.
3. **Le, Y. and Vilcek, J.,** Tumor necrosis factor and interleukin-1: cytokines with multiple overlapping biological activities, *Lab. Invest.*, 56, 234, 1992.
4. **Eastgate, J. A., Symons, J. A., Wood, N. C., Grinlinton, F. M., Di Giovine, F. S., and Duff, G. W.,** Correlation of plasma interleukin-1 levels with disease activity in rheumatoid arthritis, *Lancet*, 2, 706, 1988.
5. **Di Giovine, F. S., Poole, S., Situnayake, R. D., Wadhwa, M., and Duff, G. W.,** Absence of correlations between indices of systemic inflammation and synovial fluid interleukin-1 (alpha and beta) in rheumatic diseases, *Rheum. Int.*, 9, 259, 1990.
6. **Wood, D. D., Ihrie, E. J., Dinarello, C. A., and Cohen, P. L.,** Isolation of an interleukin-1-like factor from human joint effusions, *Arthritis Rheum.*, 26, 975, 1983.
7. **Miossec, P., Dinarello, C. A., and Ziff, M.,** Interleukin-1 lymphocyte chemotactic activity in rheumatoid arthritis synovial fluid, *Arthritis Rheum.*, 29, 461, 1986.
8. **Hopkins, S. J., Humphreys, M., and Jayson, M. I. V.,** Cytokines in synovial fluid. I. The presence of biologically active and immunoreactive IL-1, *Clin. Exp. Immunol.*, 72, 422, 1988.
9. **Firestein, G. S., Alvaro Gracia, J. M., and Maki, R.,** Quantitative analysis of cytokine gene expression in rheumatoid arthritis, *J. Immunol.*, 144, 3347, 1990.
10. **Arend, W. P. and Dayer, J. M.,** Cytokines and cytokine inhibitors or antagonists in rheumatoid arthritis, *Arthritis Rheum.*, 33, 305, 1990.
11. **Malyak, M., Joslin, F. G., Verderber, E. L., Eisenberg, S. P., and Arend, W. P.,** IL-1ra ELISA: reduction and alkylation of synovial fluid eliminates interference by IgM rheumatoid factors, *J. Immunol. Meth.*, 140, 281, 1991.
12. **Tetta, C., Camussi, G., Modena, V., Di Vittorio, C., and Baglioni, C.,** Tumor necrosis factor in serum and synovial fluid of patients with active and severe rheumatoid arthritis, *Ann. Rheum. Dis.*, 49, 665, 1990.
13. **Di Giovine, F. S., Nuki, G., and Duff, G. W.,** Tumor necrosis factor in synovial exudates, *Ann. Rheum. Dis.*, 47, 768, 1988.
14. **Saxne, T., Palladino, M. A., Jr., Heinegard, D., Talal, N., and Wollheim, F. A.,** Detection of tumor necrosis factor alpha but not tumor necrosis factor beta in rheumatoid arthritis synovial fluid and serum, *Arthritis Rheum.*, 31, 1041, 1988.
15. **Neale, M. L., Williams, B. D., and Matthews, N.,** Tumor necrosis factor activity in joint fluids from rheumatoid arthritis patients, *Br. J. Rheumatol.*, 28, 104, 1989.
16. **Maury, C. P. J. and Teppo, A. M.,** Tumor necrosis factor in the serum of patients with systemic lupus erythematosus, *Arthritis Rheum.*, 32, 146, 1989.
17. **Maury, C. P. J. and Teppo, A. M.,** Cachectin/tumor necrosis factor-a in the circulation of patients with rheumatic disease, *Int. J. Tissue Reac.*, 11, 189, 1989.

18. **Engelberts, I., Stephens, S., Francot, G. J. M., van der Linden, C. J., and Buurman, W. A.,** Evidence for different effects of soluble TNF-receptors on various TNF measurements in human biological fluids, *Lancet,* 2, 515, 1991.
19. **Hirano, T.,** Interleukin-6 and its relation to inflammation and disease, *Clin. Immunol. Immunopathol.,* 62, S60, 1992.
20. **Jirik, F. R., Podor, T. J., Hirano, T., Kishimoto, T., Loskutoff, D. J., Carson, D. A., and Lotz, M.,** Bacterial lipopolysaccharide and inflammatory mediators augment IL-6 secretion by human endothelial cells, *J. Immunol.,* 142, 144, 1989.
21. **Guerne, P. A., Zuraw, B. L., Vaughan, J. H., Carson, D. A., and Lotz, M.,** Synovium as a source of interleukin 6 in vitro. Contribution to local and systemic manifestations of arthritis, *J. Clin. Invest.,* 83, 585, 1989.
22. **Guerne, P. A., Carson, D. A., and Lotz, M.,** IL-6 production by human articular chondrocytes. Modulation of its synthesis by cytokines, growth factors, and hormones in vitro, *J. Immunol.,* 144, 499, 1990.
23. **Waage, A., Kaufmann, C., Espevik, T., and Husby, G.,** Interleukin-6 in synovial fluid from patients with arthritis, *Clin. Immunol. Immunopathol.,* 50, 394, 1989.
24. **Miltenburg, A. M., van Laar, J. M., de Kuiper, R., Daha, M. R., and Breedveld, F. C.,** Interleukin-6 activity in paired samples of synovial fluid. Correlation of synovial fluid interleukin-6 levels with clinical and laboratory parameters of inflammation, *Br. J. Rheumatol.,* 30, 186, 1991.
25. **Sawada, T., Hirohata, S., Inoue, T., and Ito, K.,** Correlation between rheumatoid factor and IL-6 activity in synovial fluids from patients with rheumatoid arthritis, *Clin. Exp. Rheumatol.,* 9, 363, 1991.
26. **Mayet, W. J., Hermann, E., Bachmann, M., Manns, M., and Meyer zum Buschenfelde, K. H.,** Correlation of anti-cytoskeleton antibody activities in synovial fluid with interleukin-6 in patients with osteoarthritis and inflammatory joint disease, *Klin. Wochenschr.,* 68, 685, 1990.
27. **Guerne, P. A., Terkeltaub, R., Zuraw, B., and Lotz, M.,** Inflammatory microcrystals stimulate interleukin-6 production and secretion by human monocytes and synoviocytes, *Arthritis Rheum.,* 32, 1443, 1989.
28. **Swaak, A. J., van Rooyen, A., Nieuwenhuis, E., and Aarden, L. A.,** Interleukin-6 (IL-6) in synovial fluid and serum of patients with rheumatic diseases, *Scand. J. Rheumatol.,* 17, 469, 1988.
29. **Houssiau, F. A., Devogelaer, J. P., Van Damme, J., de Deuxchaisnes, C. N., and Van Snick, J.,** Interleukin-6 in synovial fluid and serum of patients with rheumatoid arthritis and other inflammatory arthritides, *Arthritis Rheum.,* 31, 784, 1988.
30. **Vreugdenhil, G., Lowenberg, B., van Eijk, H. G., and Swaak, A. J.,** Anaemia of chronic disease in rheumatoid arthritis. Raised serum interleukin-6 (IL-6) levels and effects of IL-6 and anti-IL-6 on in vitro erythropoiesis, *Rheumatol. Int.,* 10, 127, 1990.
31. **Hirohata, S. and Miyamoto, T.,** Elevated levels of interleukin-6 in cerebrospinal fluid from patients with systemic lupus erythematosus and central nervous system involvement, *Arthritis Rheum.,* 33, 644, 1990.
32. **Linker-Israeli, M., Deans, R. J., Wallace, D. J., Prehn, J., Ozeri-Chen, T., and Klinenberg, J. R.,** Elevated levels of endogenous IL-6 in systemic lupus erythematosus. A putative role in pathogenesis, *J. Immunol.,* 147, 117, 1991.
33. **Stuart, R. A., Littlewood, A., Maddison, P. J., and Hall, N. D.,** Elevated serum interleukin-6 (IL-6) levels associated with active disease in systemic connective tissue disorders, *Arthritis Rheum.,* 34, s109, 1991.

34. **Horii, Y., Muraguchi, A., Iwano, M., Matsuda, T., Hirayama, T., Yamada, H., Fujii, Y., Dohi, K., Ishikawa, H., and Ohmoto, Y.,** Involvement of IL-6 in mesangial proliferative glomerulonephritis, *J. Immunol.,* 143, 3949, 1989.
35. **Linker-Israeli, M., Prehn, W. J., Ozeri-Chen, T., and Klinenberg, J. R.,** Elevated levels of endogenous IL-6 in systemic lupus erythematosus: a putative role in pathogenesis, *Arthritis Rheum.,* 34, s141, 1991.
36. **Dasgupta, B. and Panayi, G. S.,** Interleukin-6 in serum of patients with polymyalgia rheumatica and giant cell arteritis, *Br. J. Rheumatol.,* 29, 456, 1990.
37. **Lotz, M., Moats, T., and Villiger, P. M.,** Leukemia inhibitory factor is expressed in cartilage and synovium and can contribute to the pathogenesis of arthritis, *J. Clin. Invest.,* 91, 1575, 1993.
38. **De Benedetti, F., Massa, M., Robbioni, P., Ravelli, A., Burgio, G. R., and Martini, A.,** Correlation of serum interleukin-6 levels with joint involvement and thrombocytosis in systemic juvenile rheumatoid arthritis, *Arthritis Rheum.,* 34, 1158, 1991.
39. **Chirmule, N., Oyaizu, N., Kalyanaraman, V. S., and Pahwa, S.,** Misinterpretation of results of cytokine bioassays, *J. Immunol. Meth.,* 137, 141, 1991.
40. **Bhardwaj, N., Santhanam, U., Lau, L. L., Tatter, S. B., Ghrayeb, J., Rivelis, M., Steinman, R. M., Sehgal, P. B., and May, L. T.,** IL-6/IFN-beta 2 in synovial effusions of patients with rheumatoid arthritis and other arthritides. Identification of several isoforms and studies of cellular sources, *J. Immunol.,* 143, 2153, 1989.
41. **Helle, M., Boeije, L., de Groot, E., de Vos, A., and Aarden, L.,** Sensitive ELISA for interleukin-6. Detection of IL-6 in biological fluids: synovial fluids and sera, *J. Immunol. Meth.,* 138, 47, 1991.
42. **Seitz, M., Dewald, B., Gerber, N., and Baggiolini, M.,** Enhanced production of neutrophil-activating peptide-1/interleukin-8 in rheumatoid arthritis, *J. Clin. Invest.,* 87, 463, 1991.
43. **Koch, A. E., Kunkel, S. L., Burrows, J. C., Evanoff, H. L., Haines, G. K., Pope, R. M., and Strieter, R. M.,** Synovial tissue macrophage as a source of the chemotactic cytokine IL-8, *J. Immunol.,* 147, 2187, 1991.
44. **Lotz, M., Terkeltaub, R., and Villiger, P. M.,** Cartilage and joint inflammation. Regulation of IL-8 expression by human articular chondrocytes, *J. Immunol.,* 148, 466, 1992.
45. **Brennan, F. M., Zachariae, C. O., Chantry, D., Larsen, C. G., Turner, M., Maini, R. N., Matsushima, K., and Feldmann, M.,** Detection of interleukin 8 biological activity in synovial fluids from patients with rheumatoid arthritis and production of interleukin 8 mRNA by isolated synovial cells, *Eur. J. Immunol.,* 20, 2141, 1990.
46. **Peichl, P., Ceska, M., Effenberger, F., Haberhauer, G., Broell, H., and Lindley, I. J.,** Presence of NAP-1/IL-8 in synovial fluids indicates a possible pathogenic role in rheumatoid arthritis, *Scand. J. Immunol.,* 34, 333, 1991.
47. **Xu, W. D., Firestein, G. S., Taetle, R., Kaushansky, K., and Zvaifler, N. J.,** Cytokines in chronic inflammatory arthritis. II. Granulocyte-macrophage colony-stimulating factor in rheumatoid synovial effusions, *J. Clin. Invest.,* 83, 876, 1989.
48. **Alvaro-Gracia, J. M., Zvaifler, N. J., and Firestein, G. S.,** Cytokines in chronic inflammatory arthritis. IV. Granulocyte/macrophage colony-stimulating factor-mediated induction of class II MHC antigen on human monocytes: a possible role in rheumatoid arthritis, *J. Exp. Med.,* 170, 865, 1989.

49. **Hooks, J. J.,** Immune interferon in the circulation of patients with autoimmune disease, *N. Engl. J. Med.,* 301, 5, 1992.
50. **Preble, O. T.,** Systemic lupus erythematosus: presence in human serum of an unusual leukocyte interferon, *Science,* 216, 429, 1982.
51. **Yee, A. M., Buyon, J. P., and Yip, Y. K.,** Interferon alpha associated with systemic lupus erythematosus is not intrinsically acid labile, *J. Exp. Med.,* 169, 987, 1989.
52. **Ronnblom, L. E., Alm, G. V., and Oberg, K. E.,** Autoimmunity after alpha-interferon therapy for malignant carcinoid tumors, *Ann. Intern. Med.,* 115, 178, 1991.
53. **Hasler, F.,** Immunoreactive circulating alpha-interferon in rheumatoid arthritis [letter], *Br. J. Rheumatol.,* 29, 315, 1990.
54. **Firestein, G. S., Xu, W. D., Townsend, K., Broide, D., Alvaro-Gracia, J., Glasebrook, A., and Zvaifler, N. J.,** Cytokines in chronic inflammatory arthritis. I. Failure to detect T cell lymphokines (interleukin 2 and interleukin 3) and presence of macrophage colony-stimulating factor (CSF-1) and a novel mast cell growth factor in rheumatoid synovitis, *J. Exp. Med.,* 168, 1573, 1988.
55. **Shiozawa, S., Kuroki, Y., Kim, M., Hirohata, S., and Ogino, T.,** Interferon-alpha in lupus psychosis, *Arthritis Rheum.,* 35, 417, 1992.
56. **Huang, Y. P., Perrin, L. H., Miescher, P. A., and Zubler, R. H.,** Correlation of T and B cell activities in vitro and serum IL-2 levels in systemic lupus erythematosus, *J. Immunol.,* 141, 827, 1988.
57. **Nouri, A. M. and Panayi, G. S.,** Cytokines and the chronic inflammation of rheumatic disease. III. Deficient interleukin-2 production in rheumatoid arthritis is not due to suppressor mechanisms, *J. Rheumatol.,* 14, 902, 1987.
57a. **Wilkins, J. A., Warrington, R. J., Sigurdson, S. L., Rutherford, W. J.,** The demonstration of an interleukin-2 like activity in the synovial fluids of rheumatoid arthritis patients. *J. Rheumatol.,* 10, 109, 1983.
58. **Hopkins, S. J. and Meager, A.,** Cytokines in synovial fluid. II. The presence of tumor necrosis factor and interferon, *Clin. Exp. Immunol.,* 73, 88, 1988.
59. **Buchan, G., Barrett, K., Fujita, T., Taniguchi, T., Maini, R., and Feldmann, M.,** Detection of activated T cell products in the rheumatoid joint using cDNA probes to interleukin-2 (IL-2) IL-2 receptor and IFN-gamma, *Clin. Exp. Immunol.,* 71, 295, 1988.
60. **Reibnegger, G., Egg, D., Fuchs, D., Gunther, R., Hausen, A., Werner, E. R., and Wachter, H.,** Urinary neopterin reflects clinical activity in patients with rheumatoid arthritis, *Arthritis Rheum.,* 29, 1063, 1986.
61. **Krause, A., Protz, H., and Goebel, K. M.,** Correlation between synovial neopterin and inflammatory activity in rheumatoid arthritis, *Ann. Rheum. Dis.,* 48, 636, 1989.
62. **Rubin, L. A.,** The soluble IL-2 receptor in rheumatic disease, *Arthritis Rheum.,* 33, 1145, 1990.
63. **Dooley, M. A., Pisetsky, D. S., Dawson, D. V., and Polisson, R. P.,** Soluble serum IL-2 receptor levels in refractory RA: trends during MTX therapy, *Arthritis Rheum.,* 34, s36, 1991.
64. **Dooley, M. A., Dawson, D. V., Cush, J. J., Lipsky, P., and Pistesky, D. S.,** Soluble serum IL-2 receptor, CD4 and CD8 levels in early RA: lack of correlation with disease activity, *Arthritis Rheum.,* 34, s90, 1991.

65. **Ward, M. M., Doley, A. M., Christenson, V. D., and Pisetsky, D. S.,** The relationship between soluble interleukin-2 receptor levels and antidouble stranded DNA antibody levels in patients with systemic lupus erythematosus, *J. Rheumatol.*, 18, 235, 1991.
66. **Tokano, Y., Murashima, A., Takasaki, Y., Hashimoto, H., Okumura, K., and Hirose, S.,** Relation between soluble interleukin 2 receptor and clinical findings in patients with systemic lupus erythematosus, *Ann. Rheum. Dis.*, 48, 803, 1989.
67. **Rose, C. D., Singsen, B. H., Gibney, K., Doughty, R. A., and Fawcett, P. T.,** Soluble interleukin-2 receptor levels in methotrexate-treated JRA, *Arthritis Rheum.*, 34, s152, 1991.
68. **Hoosen, C., Rautman, A., and Gross, W. L.,** Elevated serum levels of soluble interleukin-2 receptor (sIL-2R) in Wegener's granulomatosis: evidence for T cell activation, *Arthritis Rheum.*, 34, s71, 1991.
69. **Manousskis, M. N., Papadopoulos, G. K., Drosos, A. A., and Moutsopoulos, H. M.,** Soluble interleukin-2 receptor molecules in the serum of patients with autoimmune diseases, *Clin. Immunol. Immunopathol.*, 50, 321, 1989.
70. **Wendling, D., Radadot, E., and Viel, J. F.,** Soluble interleukin-2 receptor in patients with ankylosing spondylitis, *Arthritis Rheum.*, 34, 1622, 1991.
71. **Ruox-Lombard, P. and Dayer, J. M.,** Soluble tumor necrosis factor receptors in human inflammatory synovial fluids, *Arthritis Rheum.*, 34, s47, 1991.

VII. Immunogenetic Background of Patients with Rheumatic Diseases

Chapter 17

The Organization of the Major Histocompatibility Complex

John D. Reveille

CONTENTS

I. INTRODUCTION

The development and application of molecular genetic technology has seen a veritable explosion in our understanding of the organization of the major histocompatibility complex (MHC). At the beginning of the 1980s, all that was known of this set of immunologically relevant genes was that there was a group on linked genes on the short arm of chromosome six that included three genes encoding proteins important in transplantation immunology (HLA-A, -B, and -C) associated with the so-called ''immune response'' genes (HLA-DR). Most of the speculation of other genes that might be located here came from investigations into inbred strains of mice. We now know the MHC to contain a large cassette of immunologically relevant genes involved with the processing, intracellular transport, and presentation of a variety of antigens, both those synthesized from within the cell and those taken up from the environment, to the T cell receptor.

0-8493-5974-1/94/$0.00 + $.50

Located within this same gene complex are a variety of newly recognized genes whose immunological function has yet to be determined. In this chapter, we will review the organization of the MHC as it is currently understood. How the gene polymorphisms within the MHC are detected and their relevance to disease will be the subject of subsequent chapters.

II. SOME BASIC DEFINITIONS

Before discussing MHC genes and disease susceptibility, it is necessary to define some basic terms that are commonly used. A *locus* is the site on a chromosome occupied by a gene. An *allele* is the designation given the alternative forms of a gene at any given locus. For example, there are currently 41 HLA-DRB1 alleles, or alternative forms of HLA-DRB1, that are known to exist at the HLA-DRB1 locus. A *heterodimer* in the context of HLA refers to a protein composed of two paired polypeptide chains, usually referring to HLA class II gene products. An HLA *specificity* is the protein as expressed on the cell surface, comprised of the sum of its respective gene products. The HLA-B27 specificity refers to the HLA-B27 polypeptide complexed with β_2-microglobulin, whereas the HLA-DR3 specificity refers to the heterodimer composed of a DRα and DRβ chains, each being products of the HLA-DRA and -DRB1 genes, respectively.

Linkage refers to two genes being located on the same chromosome, causing the respective alleles of the two linked genes to be inherited together. A *haplotype* is a set of linked loci on the same chromosome. These linked genes would tend to be passed *en bloc* from generation to generation. *Linkage disequilibrium* is the tendency for certain HLA alleles of linked loci to occur more frequently on the same haplotype than would be expected by chance alone. For example, in Caucasians, HLA-A1, -B8, -DR3, and -DQw2.1 tend to occur together on the same haplotype much more commonly than would be expected by the product of their respective gene frequencies. Finally, *recombination* refers to the formation of new combinations of linked genes, or haplotypes, by the crossing over of genetic material between an individual's homologous chromosomes.

III. THE STRUCTURE AND FUNCTION OF MHC CLASS I AND CLASS II GENE PRODUCTS

MHC class I genes encode a polypeptide of 42,000 kDa which is expressed on the surface of all nucleated cells whose function is the presentation of endogenous peptides derived from intracellular antigens to the α:β T cell receptors (TCR) on CD8+ (presumably cytotoxic) T lymphocytes.[1] CD8-positive T lymphocytes then kill the target cells that present these antigens that are recognized as "nonself" (usually tumor or viral antigens). The class I polypeptide is a membrane-bound glycoprotein which is noncovalently complexed with β_2-microglobulin, which it requires for its conformational stability. Class I molecules take up peptides derived from proteins synthesized within the antigen-presenting cell (APC) itself early in the course of biosynthesis, which then undergo degradation or processing in the cytosol,[2] combine with the class I peptide and β_2-microglobulin in the endoplasmic reticulum, and are expressed subsequently on the cell surface for presentation of the peptide to the TCR (Figure 1).

The class II MHC molecule is a heterodimer consisting of an alpha or "heavy" chain of 34,000 kDa and a beta or "light" chain of 29,000 kDa in mass. The purpose

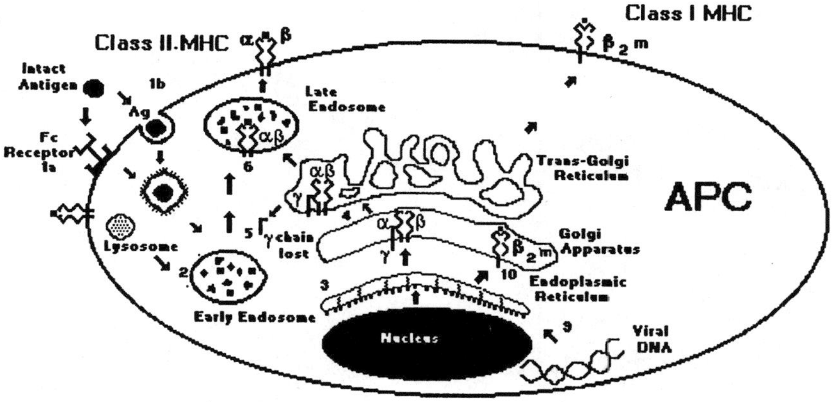

Figure 1 The steps in processing of exogenous and endogenous antigens within an antigen-presenting cell (APC) such as a macrophage: **(1)** in the processing of exogenous antigen, the protein is internalized by either receptor-mediated endocytosis, such as through the Fc receptor **(1a),** or by pinocytosis **(1b).** Protein is internalized in a so-called "coated pit", which **(2)** fuses with a lysosome to form the early endosome, an acidic compartment where proteolysis occurs. Meanwhile, the HLA-class II α and β chains are formed in the endoplasmic reticulum (ER) **(3),** and are transported complexed with the "γ" or invariant chain to the Golgi apparatus and through the trans-Golgi reticulum (TGR) **(4).** On transport between the TGR and the late endosome, the γ chain is cleaved off the class II heterodimer, which is now free to combine with the processed antigenic peptides in the late endosome **(6),** and the complex of class II heterodimer: processed antigen is then transported to the cell surface, where it can engage in presentation of processed exogenous antigen to the T cell receptor on CD4+ (helper) T cells **(7).** For MHC or HLA class I antigen processing, endogenous proteins produced inside the cell, perhaps from viral DNA, are degraded in the cytosol and transported to the ER **(9),** where the peptide binds degraded endogenous peptides. The bimolecular complex is then transferred to the cell surface after travelling through the Golgi apparatus **(10),** where antigen presentation can occur to the α:β TCR on CD8+ (cytotoxic) T cells.

of class II MHC heterodimers is to present exogenous antigen to the α:β TCR of CD4-positive or "helper" T lymphocytes. MHC class II heterodimers are expressed on a more limited variety of cells than class I, usually those of bone marrow origin, such as macrophages, B lymphocytes, dendritic cells, Langerhans cells of the skin, and Kupffer cells in the liver. Inside the "late endosomes" of the APC, the MHC class II heterodimers come into contact with exogenous antigen, which previously internalized into the APC by pinocytosis or receptor-mediated endocytosis and degraded in endosomes by a variety of proteases, and the complex of MHC class II heterodimer and processed (auto) antigenic peptide is then transported to the cell surface for presentation to the α:β TCR (Figure 1, Figure 2).

The three-dimensional structure of certain MHC class I molecules has been determined by X-ray crystallization studies, including HLA-A2, -Aw68, and -B27.[3] The schema derived from these studies has been extrapolated for all class I and class II

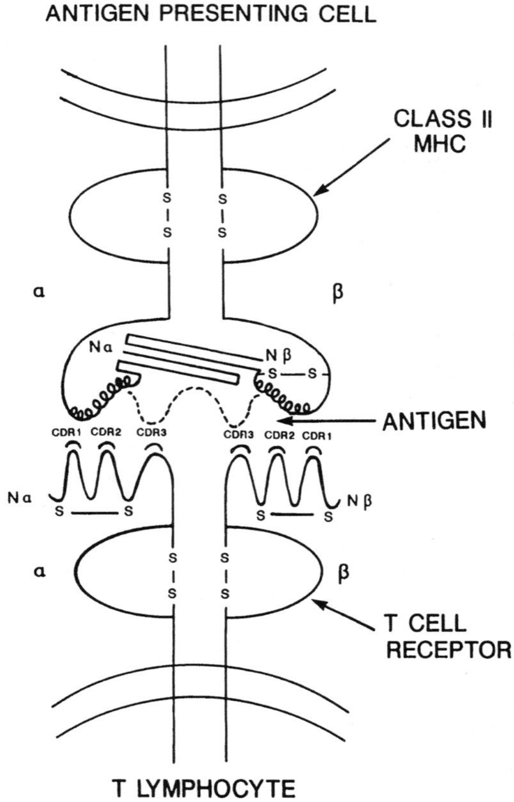

Figure 2 The trimolecular complex of MHC class II heterodimer (on top, expressed on the surface of an antigen-presenting cell), processed antigen (in the middle, indicated by a dotted line) and α:β T cell receptor (TCR) (on the bottom, protruding from the surface of a T lymphocyte). The double bars over the loops of the TCR that contact antigen and the class II heterodimer indicate the three hypervariable, or *c*omplementarity *d*etermining *r*egions (CDR1, CDR2 and CDR3) of the outermost domains of the TCR.

MHC protein: processed antigen:TCR structural models.[4] Basically, processed antigen is presented to the α:β TCR in a cleft or groove, formed by two α-helices that sit on a platform comprised of a β-pleated sheet[3] (Figure 3). This cleft is formed by the first and second domains in a class I MHC molecule and by the first or outermost domains of the class II heterodimer. It is no surprise that most of the amino acid residues that are responsible for the allelic polymorphism of class I and II MHC alleles are located either in these α-helices comprising the walls or in the portion of the β-pleated sheet forming the floors of the antigen-binding cleft.

The peptides within the antigen-binding cleft in class I MHC molecules is nine amino acids in length.[5] A variety of different peptides can fit in this antigen-binding cleft, which share among themselves specific antigen-binding motifs (certain amino acid residues occurring at specific locations along the peptide) that vary between different class I molecules. These specific amino acid residues are critical in interacting with pockets in the cleft that are critical in anchoring the peptide therein (Figure 3). In the case of HLA-B27, for example, over 10,000 different peptide combinations have been found that contain the specific amino acids at the critical positions to fit in the cleft.[5] Many of these peptides have been found to be a variety of intracellular "self" peptides whose presentation does not lead to an immune response. In contrast to peptides bound to MHC class I molecules, however, those bound to class II heterodimers show sig-

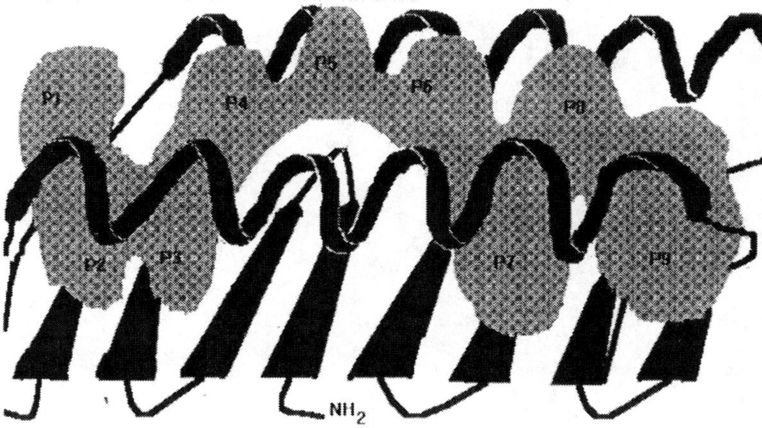

Figure 3 An illustration of the nonameric peptide (amino acid residues indicated by P1–P9), inside the antigen-binding cleft of the HLA-B27 molecule, with the orientation of the amino acid side chains directed toward whether they point into the cleft (P2, P3, P7, and P9) or outward toward the T cell receptor (P4, P5, P6, P8).

nificant heterogeneity in length. They tend to be longer, usually 13 to 15 amino acids in length or longer, probably due to the fact that the ends of the antigen-binding cleft are open (as opposed to the closed ends seen in HLA class I molecules).[6] This has given rise to speculation that the heterogeneity observed may be due to protection of the bound peptides from further degradation in the acid milieu of the late endosome, and that the class II MHC molecules may play an active role in not only antigen presentation to the TCR but also in the very process of antigen processing.

The effect of antigen presentation has implications for both the APC and the T cell. For example, if the APC is a macrophage, the result of antigen presentation is the release of a variety of cytokines, including interleukin-1 (IL-1) and tumor necrosis factor (TNF)-α, the former promoting T cell activation and both having inflammatory properties. The T cell undergoes DNA replication and secretes such cytokines as IL-2, which has important regulatory functions (reviewed elsewhere), IL-4, and γ-interferon, leading ultimately to antibody production by plasma cells and to the expansion of relevant T cell clones.

IV. THE CLASS I REGION OF THE MHC

A. ORGANIZATION

The HLA or MHC class I genes are located within a two million base pair (bp) region comprising the telomeric half of the human MHC (Figure 4). At least 18 distinct class I gene sequences have been identified.[7] Three of these encode the classical transplantation antigens HLA-A, -B, and -C and three more, the recently described and less polymorphic HLA-E, -F, and -G genes. In addition to these are four full-length pseudogenes and eight abbreviated pseudogenes, including three containing a single intron-exon fragment.[8] The introduction of yeast artificial cloning (YAC) has brought about the elucidation of the gene order and organization of most of the class I region of the

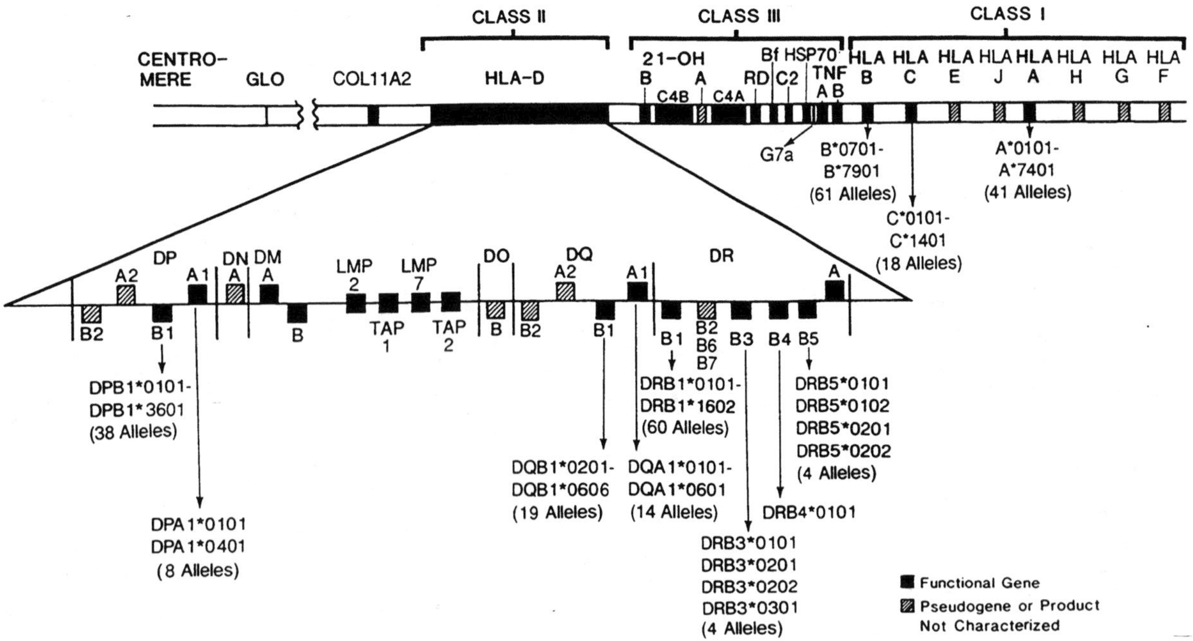

Figure 4 The organization of the major histocompatibility complex on the short arm of chromosome 6. Genes encoding a known protein product are indicated by black boxes; genes whose product has not been well characterized or pseudogenes are indicated by stippled boxes. The class II region of the MHC is further expanded and illustrated below. The number of alleles and their current nomenclature are indicated below each functional locus.

MHC.[9-11] For example, a truncated pseudogene has been found close to HLA-B. A full-length pseudogene has been mapped between HLA-C and HLA-E, provisionally designated HLA-X. More recently, a large number of genes have been mapped around the HLA-A locus, including the functional HLA-F and HLA-G genes, the full-length pseudogenes now designated HLA-H and HLA-J, and a number of pseudogenes. Of particular interest, however, is the finding of a highly polymorphic region between HLA-A and HLA-G of which greater than 50 kb appears to have been deleted on certain HLA haplotypes.[11] The putative genetic instability of this region has led some to propose this to comprise a recombinant hot spot.[11,12]

B. HLA-A

The most telomeric of the ''classical'' class I loci, HLA-A is flanked by numerous newly recognized class I genes whose function (if any) is only now being elicited (Figure 4). There are over 41 alleles of HLA-A currently recognized (Table 1),[12] falling into five different families which share within themselves significant sequence homology: the A2/28 (A*6801, *6802, and *6901) group, including the over 12 subtypes of HLA-A2 that have been described and probably the most ubiquitous in geographic distribution; the A1/3/11 group, with A1 and A3 primarily occurring in Caucasians and A11 in Orientals; and the less frequently occurring A19 (comprising A*2901–A*3301 and A*7401 and occurring mostly in non-Europeans), A9 (A*2301, *2401, *2402), and A10 (A*2501, *2601, *3401, *3402, *6601, and *6602) groups.[12] The HLA-A locus has been remarkably conserved evolutionarily, with HLA-A alleles remarkably similar in sequence to class I-like families of histocompatibility antigens in the great apes.[13]

C. HLA-B

Located closest to the class III region of the MHC, the HLA-B locus is even more polymorphic than HLA-A, with over 61 alleles currently recognized (Table 1). Little homology has been found of HLA-B with class I genes in other species, and significant differences in HLA-B polymorphisms exist between different ethnic groups, suggesting the HLA-B locus to be evolving more rapidly than HLA-A, perhaps in response to stresses imposed by the environment.[14,15]

D. HLA-C

The last of the so-called ''classical'' class I loci to be described, HLA-C is located approximately 100 kb telomeric to HLA-B. There are 18 alleles currently described. Given its lower expression at the cell surface[16] and less efficient association with β_2-microglobulin,[17] some have speculated whether HLA-C has functional significance. However, one recent study found HLA-C to effectively present a viral peptide.[18]

E. OTHER FUNCTIONAL CLASS I GENES

1. HLA-E — This class I locus is located about halfway between HLA and HLA-C, approximately 200 kb telomeric to the HLA-X locus. HLA-E expression has been detected by Northern blot analysis and RNase protection in a variety of cell types.[19,20] It has limited polymorphism, although four alleles are currently known to exist[12] at the DNA level. The function of HLA-E is unknown.
2. HLA-F — This is the most telomeric locus known to exist within the MHC. Limited data available suggest HLA-F to be nonpolymorphic, and its RNA transcripts, like those of HLA-E, are found in both lymphoid and nonlymphoid tissues.[20,21]

Table 1 **Currently Recognized HLA-Class I Alleles and Specificities**

HLA-A		HLA-B		HLA-B		HLA-C	
Allele	**Specificity**	**Allele**	**Specificity**	**Allele**	**Specificity**	**Allele**	**Specificity**
A*0101	A1	B*0701	B7	B*4701	B47	Cw*0101	Cw1
A*0201	A2	B*0702	B7	B*4801	B48	Cw*0102	Cw1
A*0202	A2	B*0703	B703	B*4901	B49(21)	Cw*0201	Cw2
A*0203	A203	B*0801	B8	B*5001	B50(21)	Cw*02021	Cw2
A*0204	A2	B*1301	B13	B*5101	B51(5)	Cw*02022	Cw2
A*0205	A2	B*1302	B13	B*5102	B5102	Cw*0301	Cw3
A*0206	A2	B*1401	B14	B*5103	B5103	Cw*0302	Cw3
A*0207	A2	B*1402	B65(14)	B*5201	B52(5)	Cw*0401	Cw4
A*0208	A2	B*1501	B62(15)	B*5301	B53	Cw*0501	Cw5
A*0209	A2	B*1502	B75(15)	B*5401	B54(22)	Cw*0601	Cw6
A*0210	A210	B*1503	B72(70)	B*5501	B55(22)	Cw*0701	Cw7
A*0211	A2	B*1504	B62(15)	B*5502	B55(22)	Cw*0702	Cw7
A*0212	A2	B*1801	B18	B*5601	B56(22)	Cw*0801	Cw8
A*0301	A3	B*2701	B27	B*5602	B56(22)	Cw*0802	Cw8
A*0302	A3	B*2702	B27	B*5701	B57(17)	Cw*1201	—
A*1101	A11	B*2703	B27	B*5702	B57(17)	Cw*1202	—
A*1102	A11	B*2704	B27	B*5801	B58(17)	Cw*1301	—
A*2301	A23(9)	B*2705	B27	B*7801	B7801	Cw*1401	—
A*2401	A24(9)	B*2706	B27	B*7901	—		
A*2402	A24(9)	B*2707	B27				
A*2403	A2403	B*3501	B35				
A*2501	A25(10)	B*3502	B35				
A*2601	A26(10)	B*3503	B35				
A*2901	A29(19)	B*3504	B35				
A*2902	A29(19)	B*3505	B35				
A*3001	A30(19)	B*3506	B35				
A*3002	A30(19)	B*3701	B37				
A*31011	A31(19)	B*3801	B38(16)				
A*31012	A31(19)	B*3901	B3901				
A*3201	A32(19)	B*3902	B3902				
A*3301	A33(19)	B*4001	B60(40)				
A*3401	A34(10)	B*4002	B40				
A*3402	A34(10)	B*4003	B40				
A*3601	A36	B*4004	B40				
A*4301	A43	B*4005	B4005				
A*6601	A66(10)	B*4101	B41				
A*6602	A66(10)	B*4201	B42				
A*6801	A68(28)	B*4401	B44(12)				
A*6802	A68(28)	B*4402	B44(12)				
A*6901	A69(28)	B*4403	B44(12)				
A*7401	A74(19)	B*4501	B45(12)				
		B*4601	B46				

Data from Bodmer et al.[12]; with permission.

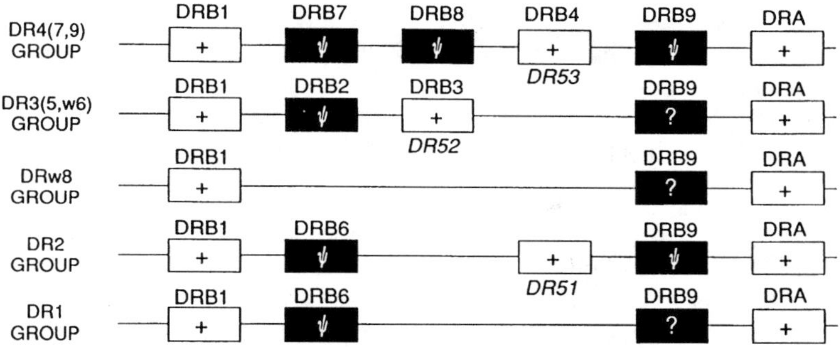

Figure 5 A representation of the varying numbers of HLA-DRB1 genes on different haplotypes. Functional genes are indicated by a "+" inside a white box (such as the HLA-DRB1 gene on all haplotypes). Pseudogenes are designated by a white "ψ" inside a black box (such as the DRB9 gene on HLA-DR4(7,9) or DR2 group haplotypes). Genes whose presence has not been definitely established on the haplotype in question are designated by a "?" inside a black box (such as a DRB9 gene on a DR3(5,w6) group haplotype).

3. HLA-G — The HLA-G locus is located between HLA-A and HLA-F. Unlike other class I genes, the HLA-G has a very restricted tissue pattern of expression,[20,22] with detectable levels of HLA-G RNA found only in placental and extravillous membrane tissue. Although its actual function is unknown, these data suggest HLA-G to have a role in embryonic development or in the fetal-maternal immune response.[20]

V. THE CLASS II REGION OF THE MHC

A. ORGANIZATION

The class II region lies most centromeric within the MHC and spans approximately one million bp of DNA. It contains four families of genes, including HLA-DP, -DQ, -DR, and, most recently described, -DM[23] (Figure 4). In addition, two additional groups of genes have been mapped in this region, including a cluster centromeric to DP that includes a collagen gene (type 11A2)[24] and five genes of unknown function.[25] Between HLA-DNA and DOB another cluster has been identified, originally designated RING 3, 4, 6, 7, 9, 10, 11, and 12.[23,26-31] RING 6 and RING 7 have been renamed HLA-DMA and -DMB, respectively. RING 4 and RING 11 are now called TAP1 and TAP2 (*t*ransporter of *a*ntigen *p*eptides), newly described ABC (ATP binding cassette) transporters.[12,26-29] RING 10 and RING 12 are now called LMP 7 and LMP 2 (*l*arge *m*ultifunction *p*roteases), respectively, and encode proteasome-related sequences involved in antigen processing.[12,30,31]

B. THE HLA-DR SUBREGION

The earliest of the class II subregions to be recognized, this contains a single DRA gene and a number of DRB genes that vary on different haplotypes[12] (Figure 5). The DR1- and DRw10-bearing haplotypes are known to contain two genes, of which one encodes the serologically recognized determinant DR1 (DRB1*01) and the other, DRB6, being a pseudogene. HLA-DR2-DRB subregions contain two functional DRB genes: HLA-

DRB1, with five alleles (DRB1*1501–*1602) and HLA-DRB5, with four alleles (DRB5*0101–*0202), as well as the DRB6 pseudogene. HLA-DR3, -DR5, and -DRw6 haplotypes contain two functional DRB genes; DRB1, encoding the β chain of the DR3, 5, or 6 subtype itself and DRB3, which encode the β chain of the associated DRw52 specificity. There are currently 60 DRB1 alleles recognized (DRB1*0101–1602) and four DRB3 alleles (DRB3*0101–*0202) (Table 2). There lies between them DRB2, which is a pseudogene that is missing exon 2.[32] HLA-DR4, -DR7, and -DR9 haplotypes contain four DRB genes, including HLA-DRB1, encoding HLA-DR4, 7, and 9 DRB1 alleles and DRB4, encoding the β chain of the nonpolymorphic DRw53 determinant. Also found on these haplotypes are pseudogenes, designated DRB7, which contains all six exons of a functioning DRB gene, but is rendered nonfunctional by abnormal splice junctions, premature stop signals, and a translational reading frame shift,[32] and DRB8, which lacks the entire 5′ end of the DRB gene, including exons 1 and 2 as well as a 4.2-kb repeat in exon 6 rendering expression impossible.[32] In addition, an additional DRB pseudogene that has been found on HLA-DR2 and DR4, 7, 9-bearing haplotypes, designated DRB9, which consists of an isolated DRB exon located next to DRA.[33]

Striking differences for HLA-DRB1 allele frequencies have been described in different ethnic groups. The DRB1*1503 subtype of HLA-DR2 and the DRB1*0302 subtype of HLA-DR3, for example, are uniquely found in blacks.[34,35] Similarly, HLA-DRB1*1304, which is extremely rare in Caucasians, is the predominant HLA-DRw6 subtype in certain groups of Western Africans.[36] Newly recognized subtypes of HLA-DRw6 (DRw14), namely DRB1*1403–1410, have been described that occur not uncommonly in Australian aborigines and New Guinea natives but not in European Caucasians.[37,38]

C. THE HLA-DQ SUBREGION

Located between HLA-DRB and -DOB, this subregion contains two functional genes (HLA-DQA1, -DQB1) which encode the α and β chains of the classic HLA-DQ heterodimer, as well as another DQα-related chain sequence (DQA2) and two additional DQβ-related chain sequences (DQB2 and DQB3), which are as yet not known to be expressed. There are currently 14 alleles described at the DQA1 locus.[12] HLA-DQB1 is slightly more polymorphic, with 19 alleles currently described.[12]

D. THE HLA-DP SUBREGION

The last of the "classical" MHC class II loci to be described, the HLA-DP specificities are expressed less efficiently at the cell surface, requiring the use of primed lymphocyte testing for analysis.[39,40] This and the relative lack of disease associations (the only convincing ones being with pauciarticular JRA and HLA-DPB1*0201[41,42] and seronegative polyarticular JRA with DPB1*0301[43]) leads one to speculate about the functional significance of the HLA-DP subregion. Yet there is enormous polymorphism here described, with eight alleles now known to exist at HLA-DPA1 and 38 alleles at DPB1.[12] As with other MHC class II loci, ethnic differences are seen with HLA-DPB1 alleles.

The HLA-DP locus is located between the collagen 11A2 gene locus and HLA-DNA, spanning less than 150 kb. Aside from the functional α and β chain genes described above, there are an additional set of DPα and DPβ chain-related pseudogenes (DPA2 and DPB2, respectively).

Table 2 **Currently Recognized HLA Class II Alleles**

DRB1

*0101(DR1/Dw1)[a]
*0102(DR1/Dw20)
*0103(DR1/DwBON)
*1501(DR2/Dw2)
*1502(DR2/Dw12)
*1503(DR2)
*1601(DR2/Dw21)
*1602(DR2/Dw22)
*0301(DR3/Dw3)
*0302(DR3/DwRSH)
*0303(DR3)
*0401(DR4/Dw4)
*0402(DR4/Dw10)
*0403(DR4/Dw13)
*0404(DR4/Dw14)
*0405(DR4/Dw15)
*0406(DR4/DwKT2)
*0407(DR4/Dw13)
*0408(DR4/Dw14)
*0409(DR4)
*0410(DR4)
*0411(DR4)
*11011(DR11/Dw5)
*11012(DR11/Dw5)
*1102(DR11/DwJVM)
*1103(DR11)
*11041(DR11/DwFS)
*11042(DR11)
*1105(DR11)
*1201(DR12/DwDB6)
*1202(DR12)
*1301(DR13/Dw18)
*1302(DR13/Dw19)
*1303(DR13/DwHAG)
*1304(DR13)
*1305(DR13)
*1306(DR13)
*1401(DR14/Dw9)
*1402(D14R/Dw16)
*1403(DR14)
*1404(DR14)
*1405(DR14)
*08032(DR8/Dw8.3)
*0804(DR8)
*0805(DR8)
*09011(DR9/Dw23)
*09012(DR9/Dw23)
*1011(DR10)

DRB3

*0101(DR52a)
*0201(DR52b)
*0202(DR52b)
*0301(DR52c)

DRB4

*0101(DR53)

DRB5

*0101(DR51)
*0102(DR51)
*0201(DR51)
*0202(DR51)

DQA1

*0101(DQw5)
*0102(DQw5,6)
*0103(DQw6)
*0201(DQw2.2,9)
*3011(DQw7,8)
*03012(DQw9)
*0302(DQw9)
*0401(DQw4)
*0501(DQw2.1,7)
*05011(DQw2.1)
*05012(DQw7)
*05013(DQw7)
*0601(DQw6)

DQB1

*0501(DQw5)
*0201(DQw2.1,2.2)
*0301(DQw7)
*0302(DQw8)
*0303(DQw9)
*0304(DQw7)
*0401(DQw4)
*0402(DQw4)

DPA1

*0101
*0102
*0103
*0201
*02021
*02022
*0301
*0401

DPB1

*0101(DPw1)
*0201(DPw2)
*02011(DPw2)
*02012(DPw2)
*0202(DPw2)
*0301(DPw3)
*04001(DPw4)
*0402(DPw4)
*0501(DPw5)
*0601(DPw6)
*0801
*0901
*1001
*1101
*1301
*1401
*1501
*1601
*1701
*1801
*1901
*2001
*2101

Table 2 **Currently Recognized HLA Class II Alleles (Continued)**

*1406(DR14)	*0502(DQw5)	*2201
*1407(DR14)	*0503(DQw5)	*2301
*1408(DR14)	*05031(DQw5)	*2401
*1409(DR14)	*05032(DQw5)	*2501
*1410(DR14)	*0504(DQw5)	*2601
*0701(DR7/Dw17)	*0601(DQw6)	*2701
*0702(DR7/DwDB1)	*0602(DQw6)	*2801
*0801(DR8/Dw8.1)	*0603(DQw6)	*2901
*0802(DR8/Dw8.2)	*0604(DQw6)	*3001
*08022(DR8/Dw8.2)	*0605(DQw6)	*3101
*08031(DR8/Dw8.3)	*0606(DQw6)	*3201
		*3301
		*3401
		*3501
		*3601

[a]Parentheses contain HLA-DR/Dw (or DR alone), -DQ, or -DP specificities corresponding to the respective DRB, DQB, or DPB1 alleles.
Data from Bodmer et al.[12]

E. OTHER FUNCTIONAL CLASS II REGION GENES

1. HLA-DM — Formerly known as RING 6 and RING 7, these two genes encode proteins of 261 and 263 amino acids respectively, which are of domain configurations similar to those of a class II heterodimer. The $\alpha2$ domain of DMA is more related to class II α chains and β_2-microglobulin, and DMB, although overall significantly different in sequence, contains short motifs characteristic of class II β chain sequences.[23] The presence of multiple cysteine residues in the DMA and DMB outermost domains suggests restricted peptide-binding capacity. The DMA and DMB genes are remarkably different from other class II sequences overall, yet are highly conserved between human and mouse,[23] suggesting that this heterodimer might perform an important function that predates divergence of class I and class II.
2. TAP1 and TAP2 — Formerly called RING 4 and RING 11, respectively, it has been hypothesized that the products of these genes form a heterodimer.[26-29] The TAP heterodimer is felt to be responsible for transporting fragments of endogenous antigen, produced by degradation of the endogenous antigen in the cytoplasm, into the lumen of the endoplasmic reticulum,[26-29] where they will ultimately come into contact with a class I polypeptide and be presented at the cell surface to the TCR of CD8-positive lymphocytes.
3. LMP2, LMP7 — These were formerly called RING 12 and RING 10, respectively, and encode two proteasome-related proteins.[12,30,31] Sequence analysis of cDNAs from these loci has revealed proteins of 272 and 219 amino acids in length, respectively, to be encoded, with sequences similar to a component of human proteasome (a large intracellular protease with broad specificity).

VI. THE CLASS III REGION OF THE MHC

A. ORGANIZATION

In the 680-kb stretch of DNA located between the class I and class II gene clusters, at least 36 genes are now known to be located (Figure 1).[44] These include a number of genes of unrelated function. The first and best known of these gene clusters include the early components of the classical (C2 and C4) and alternative (properdin factor B) complement pathways, which are the functional genes most centromeric (and closest to HLA-DR) in the class III region. Located immediately telomeric thereto are the C2 and properdin factor β genes and closely associated with them the "RD" gene, which encodes a 42-kDa intracellular protein characterized by a dipeptide repeat made up of a basic residue (arginine or lysine) next to an acidic one (aspartic or glutamic acid) stretching over 52 amino acids.[45-47] Of particular interest is a gene encoded on the opposite strand of that encoding steroid 21 hydroxylase B, called appropriately OSG (opposite strand gene). This gene appears to encode a protein of unknown function characterized by the presence of at least three repeats of approximately 100 amino acids.[47,48]

B. C2, C4, AND FACTOR B

The C4-21 hydroxylase gene cluster includes C4 and 21 hydroxylase genes that have been duplicated in tandem: 21-hydroxylase B, C4B, the pseudogene 21-hydroxylase A, and C4A. C4A and C4B are two nonallelic isotypes of C4 that exhibit significant allelic polymorphism. As of the VIth Complement Genetics Workshop and Conference in 1989, at least 13 C4A and 16 C4B allotypes, as well as nonexpressed or deleted genes at each C4 locus, were recognized.[49] Even though they are 99% homologous in sequence, C4A and C4B differ slightly in their biologic activity, with C4A binding protein antigens (i.e., immune complexes) more efficiently and C4B better adhering to polysaccharides on cell surfaces.[50] The organization of the C4 and 21 hydroxylase genes varies on different HLA haplotypes (Figure 6).[51]

The C2 and properdin factor B gene cluster lies telomeric to C4. They are postulated to have arisen from a gene duplication; both function as serine proteases and share approximately 37% sequence homology. The C2 gene spans 18 kb and produces an mRNA that is 2.9 kb in length.[52] Although not as polymorphic as C4, nevertheless nine alleles have been described, with one, C2C, found in 97% of all populations studied.[51] The factor B gene lies only 421 bp centromeric to C2. It is 6 kb in length, encodes a mRNA of 2.6 kb, which translates a 764 amino acid peptide.[52] Only three alleles have been described thus far.

C. HSP-70

The family of heat shock proteins (HSP) are expressed in response to heat shock and a variety of other stimuli, including oxidative free radicals and toxic metal ions.[53-57] HSP-70, the most predominant, is remarkably conserved through evolution, sharing 60 to 78% sequence homology among different eukaryote species. The HSP-70 cluster consists of three highly homologous genes between the C2 and the tumor necrosis factor (TNF) loci that presumably arose from gene duplications.[53-57] HSP70-1 and 70-2 are intronless genes that encode an identical protein product of 641 amino acids.[57] The eight

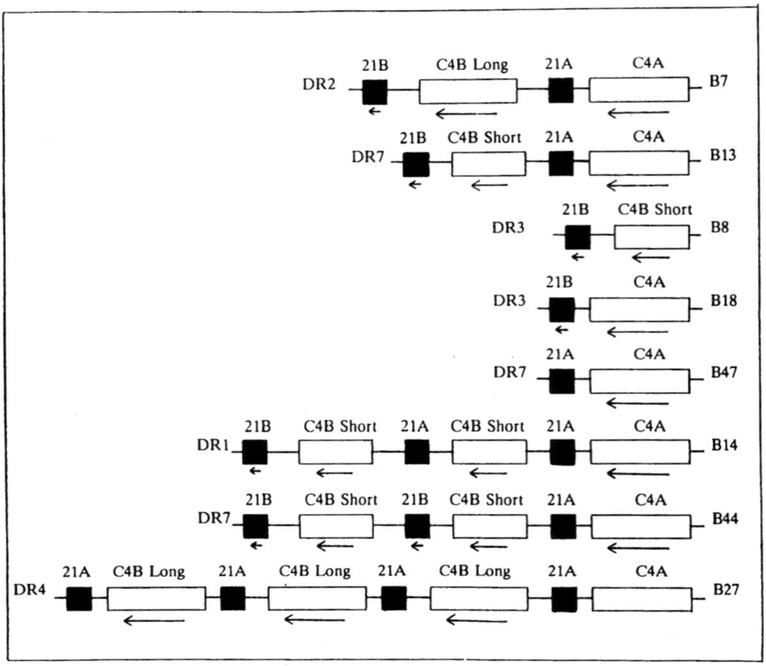

Figure 6 The organization of the C4, 21-hydroxylase (21-OH) gene cluster on different HLA-B, DR haplotypes, illustrating C4, 21-OH gene duplications and deletions, varying from the HLA-B8, DR3 haplotype, where there is a C4A, 21-OHA gene deletion, to certain HLA-B27, DR4 haplotypes, where three copies of the C4B gene are found (a gene triplication)

nucleotide differences between the two genes do not result in amino acid differences. There is considerable nucleotide sequence difference between these in the 3′-untranslated region, although the functional significance of this is unclear.

The third gene in this cluster, HSP70-Hom (homologous) is also intronless and encodes a 641 amino acid polypeptide that is 90% similar to HSP70-1 and 70-2, with the greatest sequence divergence at the C-terminal, which results in a protein that is more basic than that of HSP70-1 and 70-2. The most significant difference between HSP70-Hom and the other HSP genes is that it is not heat inducible (nor is transcription affected by 2-deoxy-D-glucose treatment or starvation), which drastically affects the level of message from other HSP genes.[57]

Immediately telomeric to HSP70-Hom lies a gene previously called G7a, which encodes valyl-tRNA-synthetase, whose relationship to the immune system is unclear.[58-60]

D. TUMOR NECROSIS FACTOR A AND B

The tumor necrosis factors A and B are located at a considerable distance telomeric from the other MHC class III gene clusters, approximately 230 kb from HLA-B.[61-63] TNFA and B are produced by macrophages and T lymphocytes, and play a variety of roles in the inflammatory response, as well as inhibiting lipoprotein lipase and stimulating the transcription of class I genes.

E. OTHER CLASS III GENES

Aside from those class III genes already described, a number of other genes have been recently identified whose products, if any, have not been well characterized. For example, seven genes have been found between HLA-DRA and 21-hydroxylase B,[64] as well as one between C4A and RD,[45] four between C2 and HSP70.2,[45,47] and nine between G7a (valyl-tRNA synthetase) and TNFA.[46] Of this latter group, two, BAT2 (G2) and BAT3 (G3), encode large proline-rich proteins with molecular masses of 228 and 110 kDa, respectively.[65] Finally, one additional gene (BAT1) has been located between TNFB and HLA-B.[47,66]

VII. CONCLUSION

Ongoing studies of the structure and function of the genes contained within the MHC are being published in recent literature so rapidly that it is a challenge to even keep current with the new knowledge. There is little doubt that the function and immunologic relevance of the new MHC genes described above will become clear in the very near future. How they function in disease susceptibility is another matter entirely. This is important, because such understanding ultimately has potential therapeutic implications, which will be discussed in another chapter. Thus, for the clinician, learning what genes actually comprise the MHC and how they function has relevance that will ultimately translate to the patient's bedside, affecting not only how we understand our patients' diseases but also offering new approaches to therapy.

REFERENCES

1. **Bjorkman, P. J. and Parham, P.,** Structure, function, and diversity of class I major histocompatibility complex molecules, *Annu. Rev. Biochem.,* 59, 253, 1990.
2. **Monaco, J. J.,** A molecular model of MHC class-I-restricted antigen processing, *Immunol. Today,* 13, 173, 1992.
3. **Madden, D. R., Gorga, J. C., Strominger, J. L., and Wiley, D. C.,** The structure of HLA-B27 reveals nonamer self-peptides bound in an extended conformation, *Nature,* 353, 321, 1991.
4. **Booth, P. B., Jenkins, W. J., and Marsh, W. L.,** Anti-I^T: a new antibody of the I blood-group system occurring in certain Melanesian sera, *Br. J. Haematol.,* 12, 341, 1966.
5. **Jardetzky, T. S., Lane, W. S., Robinson, R. A., Madden, D. R., and Wiley, D. C.,** Identification of self peptides bound to purified HLA-B27, *Nature,* 353, 326, 1991.
6. **Chicz, R. M., Urban, R. G., Lane, W. S., Gorga, J. C., Stern, L. J., Vignali, D. A. A., and Strominger, J. L.,** Predominant naturally processed peptides bound to HLA-DR1 are derived from MHC-related molecules and are heterogeneous in size, *Nature,* 358, 764, 1992.
7. **Koller, B. H., Geraghty, D. E., DeMars, R., Duvick, L., Rich, S. S., and Orr, H. T.,** Chromosomal organization of the human major histocompatibility complex class I gene family, *J. Exp. Med.,* 169, 469, 1989.
8. **Geraghty, D. E.,** *HLA,* Vol. 2, Sasazuki, A., Ed., Oxford University Press, Oxford, 1992.

9. **Geraghty, D. E., Pei, J., Lipsky, B., Hansen, J. A., Taillon-Miller, P., Bronson, S. K., and Chaplin, D. D.,** Cloning and physical mapping of the HLA-class I region spanning HLA-E-to-HLA-F interval by using yeast artificial chromosomes, *Proc. Natl. Acad. Sci. U.S.A.,* 89, 2669, 1992.
10. **Bronson, S. K., Pei, J., Taillon-Miller, P., Chorney, M. J., Geraghty, D. E., and Chaplin, D. D.,** Isolation and characterization of yeast artificial chromosome clones linking the HLA-B and HLA-C loci, *Proc. Natl. Acad. Sci. U.S.A.,* 88, 1676, 1991.
11. **Chimini, G., Borretto, J., Marquet, D., Lanau, F., Lauquin, G., and Pontarotti, P.,** Molecular analysis of the human MHC class I region using yeast artificial chromosome clones, *Immunogenetics,* 32, 419, 1990.
12. **Bodmer, J. G., Marsh, S. G. E., Albert, E. D. et al.,** Nomenclature for factors of the HLA system, 1991, *Tissue Antigens,* 39, 161, 1992.
13. **Kuhner, M. K., Lawlor, D. A., Ennis, P. D., and Parham, P.,** Gene conversion in the evolution of the human and chimpanzee MHC class I loci, *Tissue Antigens,* 38, 152, 1991.
14. **Belich, M. P., Madrigal, J. A., Hildebrand, W. H., Zemmour, J., Williams, R. C., Luz, R., Petzl-Erler, M. L., and Parham, P.,** Unusual HLA-B alleles in two tribes of Brazilian Indians, *Nature,* 357, 326, 1992.
15. **Watkins, D. I., McAdam, S. N., Liu, X., Strang, C. R., Milford, E. L., Levine, C. G., Garber, T. L., Dogon, A. L., Lord, C. I., Ghim, S. H., Troup, G. M., Hughes, A. L., and Letvin, N. L.,** New recombinant HLA-B alleles in a tribe of South American Amerindians indicate rapid evolution of MHC class I loci, *Nature,* 357, 329, 1992.
16. **Snary, D., Barnstable, C. J., Bodmer, W. F., and Crumpton, M. J.,** Molecular structure of human histocompatibility antigens, *Eur. J. Immunol.,* 7, 580, 1977.
17. **Gusson, D., Rein, R. S., Mejer, I., de Hoog, W., Seemann, G. H. A., Hochstenbach, M., and Ploegh, H. L.,** Isolation, expression and the primary structure of HLA-Cw1 and HLA-Cw2 genes: evolutionary aspects, *Immunogenetics,* 25, 313, 1987.
18. **Dill, O., Kievits, F., Koch, S., Ivanyi, P., and Hammerling, G. J.,** Immunological function of HLA-C antigens in HLA-Cw3 transgenic mice, *Proc. Natl. Acad. Sci. U.S.A.,* 85, 5664, 1988.
19. **Koller, B. H., Geraghty, D., DeMars, R., and Orr, H. T.,** HLA-E: a novel HLA-class I gene expressed in resting T lymphocytes, *J. Immunol.,* 141, 897, 1988.
20. **Mizuno, S., Trapani, J. A., Koller, B. H., Dupont, B., and Yang, S. Y.,** Isolation and nucleotide sequence of a cDNA clone encoding a novel HLA class I gene, *J. Immunol.,* 140, 4024, 1988.
21. **Schmidt, C. M. and Orr, H. T.,** A physical linkage map of HLA-A, -G, -7.5p, and F, *Hum. Immunol.,* 31, 180, 1991.
22. **Wei, X. and Orr, H. T.,** Differential expression of HLA-E, HLA-F, and HLA-G transcripts in human tissue, *Hum. Immunol.,* 29, 131, 1990.
23. **Kelly, A. P., Monaco, J. J., Cho, S., and Trowsdale, J.,** A new human HLA class II-related locus, DM, *Nature,* 353, 571, 1991.
24. **Hanson, I. M., Gorman, P., Lui, V. C. H., Cheah, K. S. E., Solomon, E., and Trowsdale, J.,** The human alpha 2 (XI) collagen gene (col 11A2) maps to the centromeric border of the major histocompatibility complex on chromosome 6, *Genomics,* 5, 925, 1989.

25. **Janatipour, M., Naumov, Y., Ando, A., Sugimura, K., Okamoto, N., Tsuji, K., Abe, K., and Inoko, H.,** Search for MHC-associated genes in humans: five new genes centromeric to HLA-DP with yet unknown functions, *Immunogenetics,* 35, 272, 1992.
26. **Spies, T., Bresnahan, M., Bahram, S., Arnold, D., Blanck, G., Mellins, E., Pious, D., and DeMars, R.,** A gene in the human major histocompatibility complex class II region controlling the class I antigen presentation pathway, *Nature,* 348, 744, 1990.
27. **Trowsdale, J., Hanson, I., Mockridge, I., Beck, S., Townsend, A., and Kelly, A.,** Sequences encoded in the class II region of the MHC related to the 'ABC' super family of transporters, *Nature,* 348, 741, 1990.
28. **Deverson, E. V., Gow, I. R., Coadwell, W. J., Monaco, J. J., Butcher, G. W., and Howard, J. D.,** MHC class II region encoding proteins related to the multidrug resistance family of transmembrane transporters, *Nature,* 348, 738, 1990.
29. **Powis, S. H., Mockridge, I., Kelly, A., Kerr, L.-A., Glynne, R., Gileadi, U., Beck, S., and Trowsdale, J.,** Polymorphism in a second ABC transporter gene located within the class II region of the human major histocompatibility complex, *Proc. Natl. Acad. Sci. U.S.A.,* 89, 1463, 1992.
30. **Glynne, R., Powis, S. H., Beck, S., Kelly, A., Kerr, L.-A., and Trowsdale, J.,** A proteasome-related gene between the two ABC transporter loci in the class II region of the human MHC, *Nature,* 353, 357, 1991.
31. **Kelly, A., Powis, S. H., Glynne, R., Radley, E., and Beck, S.,** Second proteosome-related gene in the human MHC class II region, *Nature,* 353, 667, 1991.
32. **Vincek, V., Klein, D., Figueroa, F., Hauptfeld, V., Kasahara, M., O'Huigin, C., Mach, B., and Klein, J.,** The evolutionary origin of the HLA-DR3 haplotype, *Immunogenetics,* 35, 263, 1992.
33. **Rollini, P., Mach, B., and Gorski, J.,** Linkage map of three HLA-DR beta-chain genes: evidence for a recent duplication event, *Proc. Natl. Acad. Sci. U.S.A.,* 82, 7197, 1985.
34. **Moraes, M. E., Fernandez-Vina, M., and Stastny, P.,** DNA typing for class II HLA antigens with allele-specific or group-specific amplification. IV. Typing for alleles of the HLA-DR2 group, *Hum. Immunol.,* 31, 139, 1991.
35. **Demopulos, J. T., Hodge, T. W., Wooten, W., and Acton, R. T.,** A novel DRB1 allele in DR2-positive American blacks, *Hum. Immunol.,* 30, 41, 1991.
36. **Hill, A. V. S., Allsopp, C. E. M., Kwiatkowski, D., Taylor, T. E., Yates, S. N. R., Anstey, N. M., Wirima, J. J., Brewster, D. R., McMichael, A. J., Molyneux, M. E., and Greenwood, M. M.,** Extensive genetic diversity in the HLA class II region of Africans, with a focally predominant allele, HLA-DRB1*1304, *Proc. Natl. Acad. Sci. U.S.A.,* 89, 2277, 1992.
37. **Petersdorf, E. W., Smith, A. G., Haase, A. M., and Hansen, J. A.,** Polymorphism of HLA-DRw52-associated DRB1 genes as defined by sequence-specific oligonucleotide probe hybridization and sequencing, *Tissue Antigens,* 28, 169, 1991.
38. **Dong, R. P., Kimura, A., and Sasazuki, T.,** Sequence analysis of three novel DRw14-DRB1 alleles, *Immunogenetics,* 36, 130, 1992.
39. **Shaw, S., Johnson, A. H., and Shearer, G. M.,** Evidence for a new segregant series of B-cell antigens that are encoded in the HLA-D region and that stimulate secondary allogenic proliferative and cytotoxic responses, *J. Exp. Med.,* 152, 565, 1980.

40. **Wan, K. R. and Schendel, D.,** Genetic analysis of HLA-D region products defined by PLT, in *Histocompatibility Testing 1984,* Albert, E. D., Barr, M. P., and Mayr, W. R., Eds., Springer-Verlag, Berlin, 1984, 289.
41. **Begovich, A. B., Bugawan, T. L., Nepom, B. S., Klitz, W., Nepom, G. T., and Erlich, H. A.,** A specific HLA-DPB allele is associated with pauciarticular juvenile rheumatoid arthritis but not adult rheumatoid arthritis, *Proc. Natl. Acad. Sci. U.S.A.,* 88, 9489, 1989.
42. **Barron, K. S., Joseph, A., MacLeod, M., Owerbach, D., and Reveille, J. D.,** DNA analysis of HLA-DR, DQ and DP genes in pauciarticular juvenile rheumatoid arthritis, *J. Rheumatol.,* 18, 1723, 1991.
43. **Fernandez-Vina, M. A., Fink, C. W., and Stastny, P.,** HLA antigens in juvenile arthritis. Pauciarticular and polyarticular juvenile arthritis are immunogenetically distinct, *Arthritis Rheum.,* 33, 1787, 1990.
44. **Zemmour, J. and Parham, P.,** HLA class I nucleotide sequences, 1991, *Hum. Immunol.,* 31, 195, 1991.
45. **Sargent, C. A., Dunham, I., and Campbell, R. D.,** Identification of multiple HTF-island associated genes in the human major histocompatibility complex class III region, *EMBO J.,* 8, 2305, 1989.
46. **Levi-Strauss, M., Carroll, M. C., Steinmetz, M., and Meo, T.,** A previously undetected MHC gene with an unusual periodic structure, *Science,* 240, 242, 1988.
47. **Spence, M. A., Spurr, N. K., and Field, L. L.,** Report of the committee on the genetic constitution of chromosome 6, *Cytogenet. Cell Genet.,* 51, 149, 1989.
48. **Morel, Y., Bristow, J., Gitelman, S. E., and Miller, W. L.,** Transcript encoded on the opposite strand of the human steroid 21-hydroxylase/complement component C4 gene locus, *Proc. Natl. Acad. Sci. U.S.A.,* 86, 6582, 1989.
49. **Mauff, G., Brenden, M., Braun-Stilwell, M., Doxiadis, G., Giles, C. M., Hauptman, G., Rittner, C., Schneider, P. M., Stradmann-Bellinghausen, B., and Uring-Lambert, B.,** C4 reference typing report, *Complement Inflamm.,* 7, 193, 1990.
50. **Isenman, D. E. and Young, J. R.,** Comparison of functional properties of the human C4 isotypes. The molecular basis for the difference in immune hemolysis activity of the Chido and Rodgers isotypes of human complement component, *J. Immunol.,* 132, 3019, 1984.
51. **Moreley, B. A. and Campbell, R. D.,** Internal homologies of the B alpha fragment from human complement component factor B, a class III MHC antigen, *EMBO J.,* 3, 153, 1984.
52. **Jahn, I., Uring-Lambert, B., Arnold, D., Clememceau, S., and Hauptmann, G.,** C2 reference typing report, *Complement Inflamm.,* 7, 175, 1990.
53. **Lindquist, S.,** The heat shock response, *Annu. Rev. Biochem.,* 55, 1151, 1986.
54. **Lindquist, S. and Craig, E. A.,** The heat shock proteins, *Annu. Rev. Genet.,* 22, 631, 1988.
55. **Sargent, C. A., Dunham, I., Trowsdale, J., and Campbell, R. D.,** Human major histocompatibility complex contains genes for the major heat shock protein HSP70, *Proc. Natl. Acad. Sci. U.S.A.,* 86, 1968, 1989.
56. **Hunt, C. and Morimoto, R. I.,** Conserved features of eukaryotic hsp70 genes revealed by comparison with the nucleotide sequence of human hsp70, *Proc. Natl. Acad. Sci. U.S.A.,* 82, 6455, 1985.
57. **Milner, C. M. and Campbell, R. D.,** Structure and expression of the three MHC-linked HSP70 genes, *Immunogenetics,* 32, 242, 1990.

58. **Hsieh, S. L. and Campbell, R. D.,** Evidence that the gene G7a in the human major histocompatibility complex encodes valyl-tRNA synthetase, *Biochem. J.*, 278, 809, 1991.
59. **Spies, T., Bresnahan, M., and Strominger, J. L.,** Human major histocompatibility complex contains a minimum of 19 genes between the complement cluster and HLA-B, *Proc. Natl. Acad. Sci. U.S.A.*, 86, 8955, 1989.
60. **Dunham, I., Sargent, C. A., Kendall, E., and Campbell, R. D.,** Characterization of the class III region in different MHC haplotypes by pulsed-field gel electrophoresis, *Immunogenetics,* 32, 175, 1990.
61. **Spies, T., Morton, C. C., Nedaspasov, S. A., Fiers, W., Pious, D., and Strominger, J. L.,** Genes for tumor necrosis factors alpha and beta are linked to the human major histocompatibility complex, *Proc. Natl. Acad. Sci. U.S.A.*, 83, 8699, 1986.
62. **Dunham, I., Sargent, C. A., Trowsdale, J., and Campbell, R. D.,** Molecular mapping of the human histocompatibility complex by pulsed-field gel electrophoresis, *Proc. Natl. Acad. Sci. U.S.A.*, 84, 7237, 1987.
63. **Carroll, M. C., Katzman, P., Alicot, E. M., Koller, B. H., Geraghty, D. E., Orr, H. T., Strominger, J. L., and Spies, T.,** Linkage map of the human major histocompatibility complex including the tumor necrosis factor genes, *Proc. Natl. Acad. Sci. U.S.A.*, 84, 8535, 1987.
64. **Marsh, S. G. and Bodmer, J. G.,** HLA class II nucleotide sequences, 1991, *Hum. Immunol.*, 31, 207, 1991.
65. **Banerji, J., Sands, J., Strominger, J. L., and Spies, T.,** A gene pair from the human major histocompatibility complex encodes large proline rich proteins with multiple repeat motifs and a single ubiquitin-like domain, *Proc. Natl. Acad. Sci. U.S.A.*, 87, 2374, 1990.
66. **Spies, T., Blanck, G., Bresnahan, M., Sands, J., and Strominger, J. L.,** A new cluster of genes within the human major histocompatibility complex, *Science,* 243, 214, 1989.

Chapter 18

Serologic Typing for MHC Antigens

Velta A. Lazda

CONTENTS

I. INTRODUCTION

The serologic typing for the products of the major histocompatibility complex (MHC) genes, directly analogous to using antibodies to type red blood cells, began in the 1950s. In 1954 Dausset observed that leucoagglutinins were present in polytransfused patients but not in nontransfused patients, thus providing the first evidence for leucocyte blood groups.[1] Using seven sera from multiply transfused patients, Dausset defined the first antigen of the human leucocyte antigen (HLA) system, termed MAC,[2] now known as HLA-A2. Following the discovery in 1958[3,4] that anti-leukocyte antibodies also could be induced by pregnancies and were rather frequent in the sera of multiparous women, a rich source of reagents for typing became available. Over the years, the list of HLA antigens has grown to more than 100 serologically defined specificities (Table 1).[5] Through International Histocompatibility Workshops (eleven held since 1964) and the International Cell and Sera Exchange program,[6] the HLA specificities have been standardized and new variants identified.

0-8493-5974-1/94/$0.00 + $.50

Table 1 **Complete Listing of Recognized HLA Specificities**

A	%	B	%	C	DR	%	DQ	%	DP
A1	98	B5		Cwl	DR1	90	DQ1	97	DPw1
					DR103				
A2	100	B7	95	Cw2	DR2	96	DQ2	90	DPw2
A203		B703							
A210									
A3	100	B8	98	Cw3	DR3	88	DQ3	98	DPw3
A9		B12		Cw4	DR4	94	DQ4	59	DPw4
A10		B13	96	Cw5	DR5	92	DQ5(1)	10	DPw5
A11	99	B14	98	Cw6	DR6	78	DQ6(1)	45	DPw6
A19		B15		Cw7	DR7	96	DQ7(3)	68	
A23(9)	98	B16		Cw8	DR8	70	DQ8(3)	10	
A24(9)	99	B17		Cw9(w3)	DR9	90	DQ9(3)	11	
A25(10)	85	B18		Cw10(w3)	DR10				
A26(10)		B21			DR11(5)	85			
A28	97	B22			DR12(5)				
A29(19)	98	B27	97		DR13(w6)	31			
A30(19)	97	B35	92		DR14(w6)	32			
					DR1403				
					DR1404				
A31(19)	94	B37			DR15(2)	54			
A32(19)	96	B38(16)	89		DR16(2)				
A33(19)	89	B39(16)	87		DR17(3)	11			
		B3901							
		B3902							
A34(10)	78	B40			DR18(3)	28			
		B4005							
A36	83	B41	93						
A43		B42	92		DR52	96			
A66(10)		B44(12)	99		DR53	96			
A68(28)	54	B45(12)	91						
A69(28)	50	B46							
A74(19)	41	B47	91						
		B48	89						
		B49(21)	97						
		B50(21)	84						
		B51(5)	94						
		B5102							
		B5103							
		B52(5)	74						
		B53	87						
		B54(22)	74						
		B55(22)							
		B56(22)							
		B57(17)	89						
		B58(17)	81						

Table 1 **Complete Listing of Recognized HLA Specificities (Continued)**

A	%	B	%	C	DR	%	DQ	%	DP
		B59	87						
		B60(40)	95						
		B61(40)							
		B62(15)	83						
		B63(15)	88						
		B64(14)							
		B65(14)							
		B67	57						
		B70	77						
		B71(70)							
		B72(70)							
		B73	68						
		B75(15)	37						
		B76(15)							
		B77(15)							
		B7801							
		Bw4							
		Bw6							

% = Percentage of laboratories participating in the 1991 International Cell Exchange that detected a given specificity.[6]

Specificities in parenthesis are broad antigens from which the split antigens were derived.

Data from Reference 5.

Figure 1 schematically depicts our current concept of the HLA complex, showing the genetic regions containing the HLA loci. The six genetic loci whose gene products are identified by HLA typing are HLA-A, HLA-B, and HLA-C, which determine class I antigens, and HLA-DR, HLA-DQ, and HLA-DP, which determine class II antigens. Of major tissue typing importance, class I antigens occur on both T and B lymphocytes and virtually every nucleated cell of the body. Class II antigens, however, have a restricted tissue distribution, being present on B lymphocytes, monocytes, some macrophages, epidermal Langerhans' cells, and dentritic cells. The DQ antigens are not expressed on all monocytes, only a subset of these cells.[7] Class II antigens are not expressed on platelets or T lymphocytes, unless the T cells are activated.

HLA typing is used primarily for the determination of HLA compatibility prior to transplantation, for paternity testing, for anthropological studies, and for establishing HLA-disease associations.

II. PRINCIPLES OF SEROLOGICAL TYPING FOR HLA

The principle in serological typing for HLA is to visualize or detect that an antigen-antibody reaction has taken place. The antibody is contained in the selected immune sera of individuals immunized primarily through pregnancy and blood transfusions; the antigen source has been cells with a high density of HLA antigens on their cell surface, such as lymphocytes.

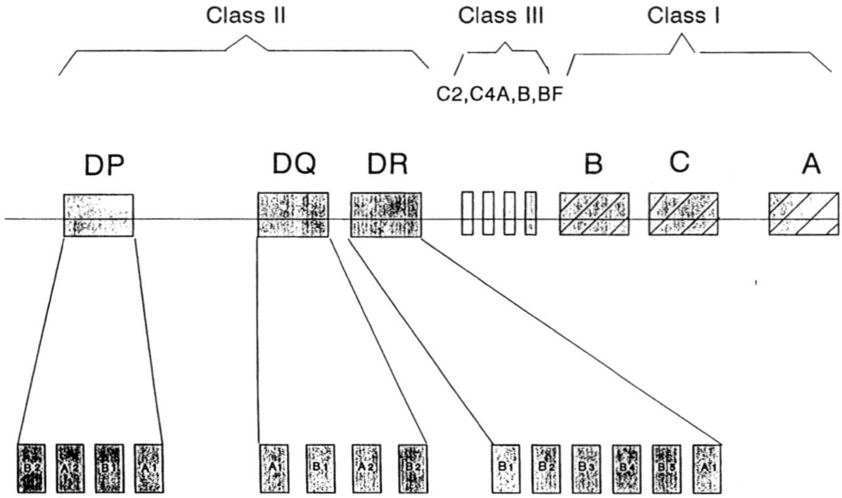

Figure 1 The HLA complex consists of a class I region with genes encoding HLA-A, HLA-B, and HLA-C; a class II region with genes encoding HLA-DR, HLA-DQ, and HLA-DP, with each subregion containing a tandem set of genes for one or more alpha and beta chains of the class II molecules. The class III region contains genes encoding a variety of factors, such as complement factors.

A. LYMPHOCYTOTOXICITY

Introduced in 1964 by Terasaki and McClelland,[8] the microlymphocytotoxicity test, or complement-dependent cytotoxicity (CDC), provided a technique that overcame many of the disadvantages of leukoagglutination used previously. Not only was the test more reproducible, but many tests could be performed with minimal amounts of cells and sera.

The microlymphocytotoxicity test is a complement-dependent, serological test that detects cell death due to the binding of antibodies to target cells, which in turn activates the complement to lyse the cells (Figure 2). If there is sufficient binding of antibody to its specific HLA molecule, e.g., anti-B27 binding to HLA-B27, the complement cascade is activated, leading to membrane damage. Damaged membranes become leaky and lose their ability to retain or exclude molecules. The percent of injured cells can be visually determined by the addition of stains that leak into the cells, so-called vital dyes, e.g., trypan blue, eosin-Y, and ethidium bromide. Cells from an individual to be HLA typed are tested against panels of defined HLA antibodies. The specific HLA types expressed on the cells is deduced from noting which HLA antisera caused cell injury or death.

There are many technical variants of the lymphocytotoxic test. The one that has been most widely adapted is the two-step procedure (NIH test),[9] in which lymphocytes and antibody are preincubated before complement is added for greater sensitivity. Instead of vital dyes (e.g., eosin-Y), it is also possible to use labels that are taken up by living cells and released by dead ones, e.g., fluorescein diacetate[10] or radioactive chromium.[11]

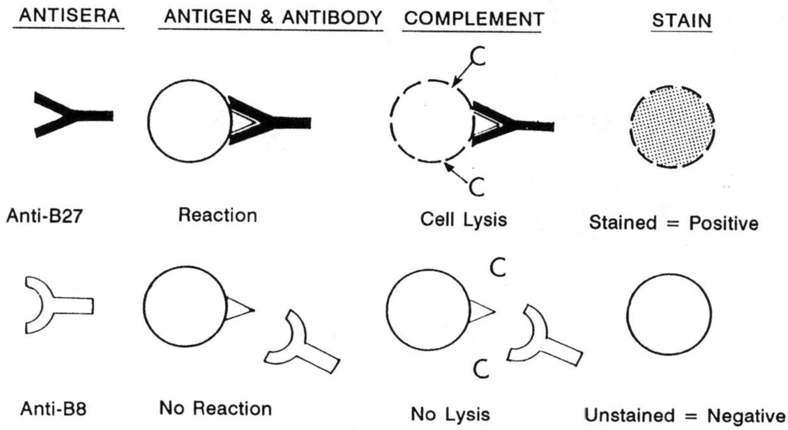

Figure 2 Principle of the lymphocytotoxicity test illustrated schematically.

B. COMPLEMENT-FIXATION TEST WITH PLATELETS

Although rarely done any more, the complement-fixation test with platelets can also be used to serologically type for HLA-A, -B, -C.[12] The principle of this test is measurement of complement consumption in the assay using sheep erythrocytes sensitized with anti-sheep erythrocyte antibody as the indicator cells. If the latter cells remain intact, this indicates that the complement added initially has been consumed by antibody combining with antigen on the platelets, i.e., a positive reaction. The main advantage of this test is that the platelets, unlike lymphocytes, need not be alive when typed. The disadvantages are that not all antisera are suitable to use in the complement-fixation test and the test is not as sensitive as the lymphocytotoxic test.

C. IMMUNOFLUORESCENCE

The expression, or presence, of HLA molecules on the cell surface, in principle, can also be visualized using fluorescent staining methods and flow cytometric analysis. This can be accomplished either by ''direct'' staining, where flourochromes, such as fluorescein or phycoerythrin, are conjugated to the antibody which binds to the cell surface determinant; and ''indirect'' staining, where the antibody which binds to the surface determinant is not fluorescenated and its binding is demonstrated by the binding of a second-step fluorescenated antibody reagent specific for the determinants of the non-fluorescent first-step antibody. For complete HLA phenotyping, immunofluorescence methods would be extremely cumbersome, given the large panel of specific antibody reagents that have to be tested, but are feasible where the presence or absence of only one particular HLA molecule, e.g., HLA-B27, on a cell is to be determined. The advantage of assays that are not complement-dependent, is that nonspecific killing that may occur with cells overly sensitive to complement can be avoided.

III. ANTISERA FOR HLA TYPING

A. PROCUREMENT AND PREPARATION

Serologic typing for HLA is dependent on the availability of typing reagents, the most common source being pregnancy sera. Although a substantial percentage of parous

Table 2 **Major Public Epitopes Present on HLA-A and HLA-B Gene Products**

CREG[a]	Associated Private Epitopes
A1C	A1, A3, A11, A10, A19, A9, A28
A2C	A2, A28, A9, B17, A10, A33
B5C	B5, B53, B35, B18, B15, B17, B70, B49
B7C	B7, B27, B22, B42, B48, B40, B41, B13, B47
B8C	B8, B14, B16, B22, B52
B12C	B12, B21, B40, B41, B13
Bw4	B5, B53, B44, B49, B37, B63, B17, B38, B59, B13, B47, B27
Bw6	B35, B18, B70, B45, B50, B62, B46, B39, B8, B14, B40, B41, B73, B7, B48, B42, B22, B67

[a]CREG, cross-reactive group.
Data from Reference 17.

females, 10 to 19% of primigravidae and 20 to 30% of those with two or more children,[13-15] make an HLA antibody, only about 1 to 2% of them will make an antibody sufficiently specific to be used as a typing reagent for the private HLA specificities. Consequently, large numbers of sera must be screened in order to find quality reagents. At the most only about 10% of the samples screened can be expected to be useful reagents. Konoeda et al.[16] tested placenta extracts from 50,000 pregnancies in the Oriental and Caucasian populations and found only 5% with lymphocytotoxic antibodies. Most of the specificities found were directed against the public epitopes[17] (Table 2). Antibodies directed against the B-locus private specificities occurred in 41% of the positive sera and were more frequent than those against the A-locus (24%) or C-locus (3%).

In recent years the possibility of making monoclonal antibodies for use as tissue typing reagents has been pursued, since monoclonal antibodies could provide virtually an endless source of large quantities of specific cytotoxic antibody. Attempts to produce monoclonal antibodies to HLA antigens from hybridomas of tumor cells and immunized mouse lymphocytes have only been partially successful, since mice often fail to produce antibodies to the epitopes identified by human alloantisera.

B. CHARACTERIZATION OF ANTIBODIES

The specificity(s) of antibodies in antisera is determined by screening the sera against an HLA-typed cell panel. The composition of the HLA-typed target cell panel is an important consideration for characterizing antibodies. Ideally, one would hope to have each HLA antigen represented on the panel at least twice.

When screening sera for HLA class II (DR, DQ) antibodies, the sera must first be absorbed with pooled (at least 100 donors), packed platelets to remove HLA class I antibodies, if any, as these will also react with B lymphocyte targets. Platelet-absorbed sera must be retested for the presence of any residual HLA-A, -B, or -C antibodies. Antibodies toward HLA-C and some -B groups (e.g., B8 and B12) are very difficult to remove because of their variable expression on platelets.[18,19]

C. CROSS REACTIVITY

There is extensive serologic cross reactivity among different alleles at each HLA locus, especially HLA-A (Figure 3) and HLA-B (Figure 4). This requires detailed characterization of anti-HLA antibodies for their use as typing reagents and complicates the detection of some HLA antigens. Cross reactivity may be due to sharing of public epitopes,[20] as illustrated schematically in Figure 5. Other cross reactivity may be due to structural similarity between the antigenic determinants themselves. Many of the so-called monospecific alloantisera in reality are only "operationally" monospecific. That is, when conditions for testing are such that cross reactivity is minimized, the alloantiserum detects one distinct HLA epitope.

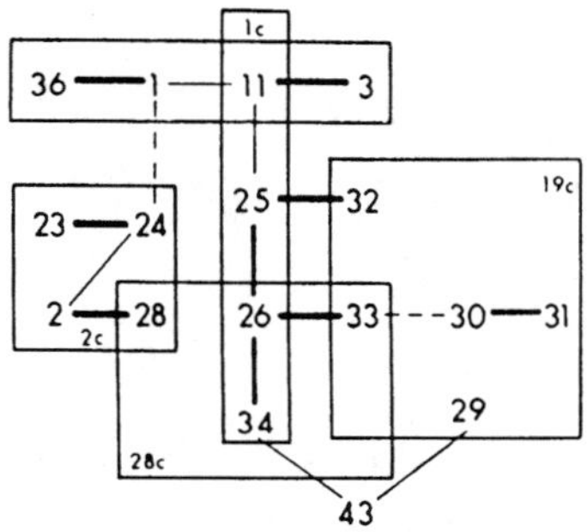

Figure 3 Scheme illustrating major serological cross-reactivity patterns among HLA-A locus molecules. Squares and rectangles are putative public epitopes shared by more than one HLA molecule. Publics are designated 1C, 2C, 28C, and 19C. Additional serological cross-reactivity is indicated by thick (strong) and thin (moderate) lines. "W" prefixes of provisional specificities are omitted for simplicity. (From Rodey, G. E. and Fuller, T. C., *Crit. Rev. Immunol.,* 7, 229, 1987. With permission.)

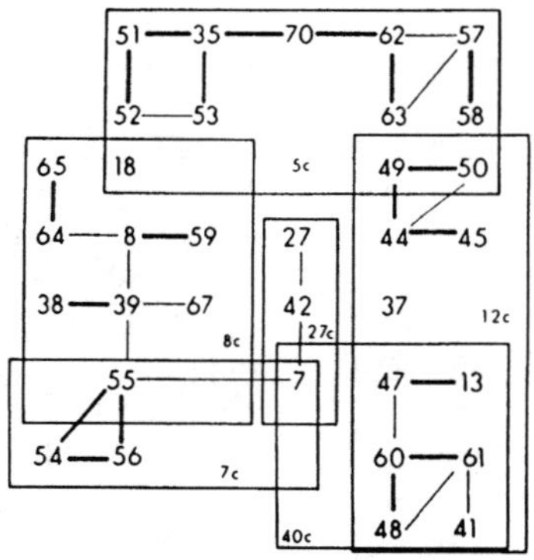

Figure 4 Scheme illustrating major serological cross-reactivity patterns among HLA-B locus molecules. Squares and rectangles are putative public epitopes shared by more than one HLA molecule. Publics are designated 5C, 7C, 8C, 27C, 40C, and 12C. Additional serological cross-reactivity is indicated by thick (strong) and thin (moderate) lines. "W" prefixes of provisional specificities are omitted for simplicity. (From Rodey, G. E. and Fuller, T. C., *Crit. Rev. Immunol.,* 7, 229, 1987. With permission.)

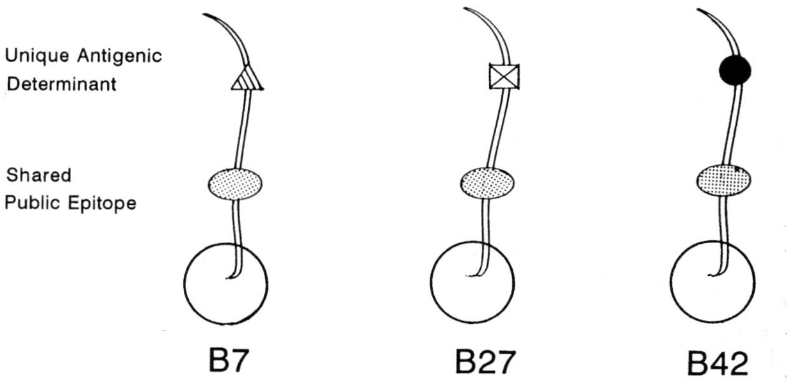

Figure 5 Schematic illustration of cross-reactivity due to a shared public epitope (public B27c) on B7, B27, and B42 cross reacting HLA molecules.

IV. TECHNICAL ASPECTS OF HLA TYPING

A. SPECIMEN COLLECTION, HANDLING, AND STORAGE

Peripheral blood is generally the source of lymphocytes for serologic HLA typing. In the case of cadaver organ donors, however, the availability of lymph nodes (inguinal or mesenteric) and spleen, as well as the ease of separation and higher yield of lymphocytes, particularly B lymphocytes, make these tissues the preferred specimens.

Peripheral blood for HLA typing is drawn by venipuncture into a suitable anticoagulant, e.g., heparin or ACD (acid-citrated dextrose). Ethylene diamine tetraacetate (EDTA)-preserved blood, however, cannot be used with the cytotoxicity test. One 10-ml tube of blood is sufficient for HLA-A, -B, or -C typing and two tubes enough for complete (HLA-A, -B, -C, -DR, -DQ) typing. However, it is wise to collect about five tubes (50 ml) of peripheral blood, in the event that a patient may have a low lymphocyte count. Once drawn, the blood should be thoroughly, but gently, mixed with the anticoagulant and each tube properly labeled with the name of the individual and the date blood was drawn and stored at room temperature (22°C). The more recently the blood is drawn prior to typing, the more likely a pure and viable lymphocyte preparation is obtained. When blood is shipped, a courier service should be used to insure delivery within 24 to 48 h and the specimens should be packaged in an insulated container to prevent freezing during air shipment.

B. DEFIBRINATION OF BLOOD

Defibrination of blood is ideal as platelets are removed initially and do not have to be sedimented later. Removal of platelets is important. If the cell suspension contains too many platelets, false-negative reactions may be seen with weak HLA antisera. This is caused by platelets, which express HLA-A, -B, and -C antigens, absorbing the antibodies, which are then unavailable for reacting with lymphocytes. Blood drawn in ACD anticoagulant is ideal for defibrination. If the blood is not freshly drawn, it should first be warmed for 5 to 10 min at 37°C. For defibrination, five 3-mm glass beads, 2.5 units of thrombin and 0.3 ml of 10% $CaCl_2$ are added to each tube of blood. The blood is mixed by end-to-end rotation at 30 rpm for 10 min and fibrin clots that form are removed with wooden applicator sticks.

C. LYMPHOCYTE ISOLATION BY FLOTATION

A high level of lymphocyte purity is required for HLA typing. Ficoll-Hypaque centrifugation of blood separates mononuclear cells from unwanted granulocytes and red blood cells.[21] Heparinized or defibrinated blood is diluted with at least an equal volume of buffer, e.g., phosphate-buffered saline (PBS), and 5-ml aliquots are layered over 2.5 ml of Ficoll-Hypaque (density = 1.077 g/ml) and centrifuged at $400 \times g$ for 30 min or $1000 \times g$ for 15 min. The mononuclear cells at the interface are carefully collected using a Pasteur pipette, washed with PBS twice, and centrifuged. The yield of lymphocytes from an average healthy individual is approximately 5 to 10×10^6 cells per 10 ml of defibrinated blood.

D. T AND B LYMPHOCYTE SEPARATION

For HLA-A, -B, -C typing T lymphocytes are preferred. The absence of B lymphocytes assures that interference due to anti-class II antibodies in the typing sera, if any, will be avoided. For HLA-DR, -DQ typing B lymphocytes are required, since T lymphocytes lack class II antigens. Nylon wool can be used to separate B and T lymphocytes from one another.[22] B lymphocytes, because of their cell surface properties, are adherent and will stick to nylon wool, while T lymphocytes are washed off. This separation method will yield 70 to 80% enrichment in B lymphocytes. Columns are prepared using common plastic drinking straws cut to 12–14 cm in length and heat-sealed at a 45° angle at one end. Each column is packed with 0.1 g of nylon wool, soaked in Hank's Balanced Salt Solution (HBSS), packing the nylon wool into the straw little by little and evenly, to a height of approximately 6 cm. Using a 25-g hypodermic, a small hole is punched in the bottom sealed tip of the straw to allow media to slowly drip through as the column is first washed with 5 ml of medium (McCoy's + 5% fetal calf serum). Lymphocytes, up to 20 million suspended in 0.5 ml of medium, are added to the top of the column, allowing the cells to move all the way into the nylon wool and 0.2 ml of medium is added to prevent the column from drying out. The column is placed in a horizontal position and incubated for 30 min at 37°C. T cells are obtained by collecting the nonadherent cells as they are removed from the column by allowing 5 ml of warm medium to pass slowly through the column. The column then is rinsed with 10 ml of warm medium. The B cell-rich adherent cells are recovered from the column by adding 5 ml of cold medium little by little to the column and repeatedly squeezing the straw vigorously at the level of the wool while the media passes through. The T and B lymphocytes are washed twice with medium, counted, and adjusted to proper concentration. If not used right away, the lymphocyte preparations are best stored at 4°C in medium containing penicillin/streptomycin to prevent microbial growth.

T and B lymphocyte separation can also be achieved using immunomagnetic beads (Dynal) and the separation can be done using whole blood.[23] The beads are precoated with a monoclonal antibody, e.g., monomorphic anti-class II for isolating class II-positive cells (B lymphocytes) or anti-CD8 for isolating a subset of T lymphocytes. This method is especially suitable for isolating B lymphocytes of good quality and purity for HLA-DR, -DQ typing. One 10-ml tube of ACD blood is centrifuged, the plasma is removed, and the volume made up to 5 ml using PBS (PBS with 0.1% bovine serum albumin and 0.1% sodium azide). The blood is chilled to 4°C. Using a micropipettor, 0.1 ml of beads are added, and the blood is mixed by rotating the tube gently at 4°C for 3 min. PBS (5 ml) is then added, the blood is mixed, and a magnet is applied to the side of the tube to hold cells attached to the beads in place while the remainder of the blood and unattached cells are removed by washing four times. The isolated cells remain attached to the beads as rosettes and are used as such for HLA-DR, -DQ typing.

Other B cell separation methods include the use of appropriately prepared monoclonal antibody and complement (Lympho-Kwik method). Here the monoclonal antibody preparation has complement pre-added in a viscous medium. By incubating with specific monoclonal antibody, the cell type not required (e.g., T cells) is lysed by the complement and removed by washing. This method produces relatively pure B cell suspension.

E. TARGET CELL VIABILITY AND PURITY

For HLA typing by lymphocytotoxicity, it is critical that the target cells have good viability and purity. Contamination with too many granulocytes can lead to false-positive reactions, since these cells are killed by rabbit serum alone, and platelet contamination can lead to false-negative reactions due to antibody depletion. Starting with lymphocytes of poor viability (<80%) will make it difficult to judge reactions against a high background of dead cells. Therefore, it is prudent to remove nonviable cells from target cell preparation prior to starting the test.

F. MICROLYMPHOCYTOTOXICITY TEST

1. Typing for HLA-A, -B, and -C Antigens

Lymphocytes, preferably isolated T lymphocytes, are adjusted in medium, e.g., McCoy's + 5% fetal calf serum, to a concentration of 2.0 to 2.5 million lymphocytes per milliliter. Using too many cells (twice or more the optimum concentration) could result in antigen excess and cause false-negative reactions. The viability of the lymphocytes should exceed 90%.

Terasaki microtiter trays prepared in advance with antisera specific for all known HLA-A, -B, and -C specificities are used. These typing trays are either obtained commercially or prepared locally and stored at −70°C until use. The typing trays must have at least two operationally monospecific sera, or three partially nonoverlapping multispecific sera for each HLA-A, HLA-B, and HLA-C antigen.[24] The trays contain 1 μl of the antiserum placed in the bottom of the well and each serum is overlaid with 5 μl of mineral oil to prevent the serum from drying out. In addition to the alloantisera, each tray has negative and positive control sera. The negative control serum is normal human serum obtained from nontransfused, blood group AB males. The positive serum generally is an anti-human lymphocyte serum that reacts with 100% of the lymphocytes. In addition, the typing trays contain monoclonal antibodies specific for various cells, e.g., T lymphocytes, B lymphocytes, monocytes, and granulocytes to check for the purity of the cell preparation.

The cell suspension for HLA typing is thoroughly mixed and, using a microliter syringe with a repeating dispenser or an automated cell dispenser, 1 μl of cells is added to each well, being careful not to touch the serum in any one well, so as not to carry it over to the next well. The sera and cells are mixed by vortexing the tray and incubated at room temperature (22°C) for 30 min. Pretested rabbit complement is then added at 5 μl per well and incubation continued for 60 min at room temperature. The cells are then stained using a vital dye. If eosin is used, 2 μl of 5% eosin-Y is added, followed by 5 μl of pH-adjusted (pH 7.2 to 7.4) formaldehyde to stop the reaction and fix the cells. A 50 × 75 mm microscope slide then is lowered onto the wells in order to flatten the top of the droplet, and after the cells have settled, the reactions are read using an inverted phase contrast microscope. Living cells are small and refractile, whereas dead cells appear larger and are stained dark.

If trypan blue is used, the excess complement must first be removed from each well by "flicking" the trays, otherwise the excess protein (albumin) will bind trypan blue and inhibit staining. Each well is filled with 0.25% trypan blue in 2% EDTA and, after allowing the cells to settle for 10 min, the trypan blue is flicked off, mineral oil is added, and the reactions are read using a bright-field microscope. The nonviable cells are stained blue, while the live cells are colorless. Fluorescent dyes of contrasting colors, e.g., acridine orange (stains live cells greenish-yellow) and ethidium bromide (stains dead cells red) are also suitable, simple to use, and stained live and dead cells easy to distinguish. One μl of the two fluorescent dyes in solution (0.3 mg/ml of acridine orange and 1 mg/ml of ethidium bromide stock solution diluted 1:10 in 5% EDTA, pH 7.0) is added to each well, followed by 1 μl of bovine hemoglobin (0.1 g/ml in 5% EDTA, pH 7.0, ultracentrifuged at 20,000 × *g* for 45 min) to quench the reaction. The reactions are read using an inverted fluorescent microscope.

2. Typing for HLA-DR, -DQ

B lymphocytes must be used as the target cells for HLA-DR, -DQ typing, unless a technique, such as two-color fluorescence,[25] is used that distinguishes T and B lymphocytes.

Typing for HLA-DR, -DQ[26] is carried out in the same manner as for HLA-A, -B, -C, except for the following:

1. Antisera must be platelet-absorbed and specific for HLA-DR and DQ.
2. There must be at least three operationally monospecific sera, or five partially nonoverlapping multispecific sera for each DR and DQ specificity.[24]
3. An anti-B lymphocyte serum is used as the positive control.
4. Incubation times are lengthened and generally are 60 min with serum and 120 min with complement, except when immunomagnetic bead-separated B lymphocytes are used (30 min with serum and 60 min with complement) or the two-color fluorescence test is used (60 min with serum and 60 min with complement).
5. Complement is selected and tested for specific use with B lymphocytes which are more sensitive target cells.

3. Scoring

The reactions in each well of the microlymphocytotoxicity test as they are viewed under the microscope are scored based on the percentage of killed cells on a scale of 1 to 8, as follows:

Score	Percent Dead	Interpretation
1	0–10	Negative
2	11–20	Doubtful negative
4	21–50	Weak positive
6	51–80	Positive
8	81–100	Strongly positive
0		Not readable, e.g., no serum, no cells, etc.

The negative control establishes the level of spontaneous cell death, so-called ''background''. A very high background, negative well scored >4, will generally invalidate the test, since reading and interpretation become difficult.

The positive control should be definitely positive (score of 6 or 8), otherwise the test results are questionable. For HLA-DR, -DQ typing, the level of lysis in the positive B lymphocyte control is particularly critical, since this is a measure of the B cell enrichment of the test cells.

V. INTERPRETATION OF RESULTS AND REPORTING

Assignment of an HLA phenotype based on the test results requires considerable experience, knowledge of HLA cross reactivity, HLA frequency differences in various

Table 3 **HLA Phenotypes of Renal Transplant Candidates and Kidney Donors**

	Frequency (%)			
	Blacks		Caucasians	
HLA	Patients ($N = 303$)	Donors ($N = 74$)	Patients ($N = 358$)	Donors ($N = 399$)
A1	7.3	6.8	30.7	32.1
A11	2.0	1.4	11.2	11.0
A23	21.5	17.6	5.6	4.0
A30	26.1	28.4	5.6	4.5
A33	16.2	16.2	2.5	2.0
A34	10.2	9.5	0.6	0.2
A36	4.3	6.8	0	0
A74	2.3	2.7	0	0
B8	6.9	8.1	21.5	23.6
B22	1.3	0	7.3	4.8
B62	0.7	4.1	11.7	13.5
B42	11.2	17.6	0	0
B45	9.6	8.1	2.8	1.3
B53	22.4	17.6	0.3	0.8
B58	11.2	10.8	1.1	2.5
B63	6.6	10.8	1.1	0.8
B70	15.2	16.3	1.1	0.5
DR4	10.5	11.1	38.0	29.9
DR8	12.9	22.2	6.3	6.8

Note: Frequencies of these phenotypes are significantly different in blacks and Caucasians.
Data from Reference 29.

races and common HLA haplotypes, as well as familiarity with the reactivity of the antisera being used.

When analyzing the typing reactions, one assigns antigens bearing in mind that there can be no more than two private HLA epitopes per locus: -A, -B, -C, -DR, -DQ, etc. However, for some individuals only one antigen may be serologically detectable, either due to homozygosity (the same antigen is inherited from both parents) or inability to define the second antigen because of unavailability of antisera defining the unknown specificity. Homozygous cells often can present problems, since they react more strongly and have a wider range of cross reactions than heterozygous cells.[27] It is possible, therefore, for example, for cells that are homozygous B7, B7, to react with all of the B7 antisera as well as all of the B27 antisera. Therefore, one runs the risk of mistakenly assigning this individual B7, B27. This problem can be avoided when a large battery of well-characterized antisera, both with heterozygous and homozygous panel cells, is used and there is familiarity with how the antisera react and knowledge of the more common haplotypes which have a higher frequency of being homozygous.[28]

Different races differ markedly in the frequency of HLA antigens (Table 3).[29] Sera that are concordant in their reactions with cells from Caucasians may give discordant reactions in non-Caucasians. Sometimes the anomalous reactions are against antigens absent from, or rare in, Caucasians. HLA typing of non-Caucasians often requires using antisera that have been standardized in the specific population, so-called ''black trays'' or ''oriental trays''.

VI. LIMITATIONS AND PITFALLS

Patients who receive frequent blood transfusions and from whom blood is drawn for tissue typing too soon after a transfusion, may present a confusing picture. If the cell donor has been transfused within the previous 7 d, results are acceptable only if antigens are unequivocally defined, with no more than two antigens per locus.[24] Otherwise, another specimen needs to be obtained.

As already mentioned, impure cell preparations may create problems. Excess granulocytes and platelets can compete with test lymphocytes for binding of antibodies, resulting in false-negative reaction. The physiological and pathological condition of the cell donor may also give rise to variation in test results. Apparent loss of HLA class I antigens from lymphocytes with subsequent recovery has been reported for patients during chloramphenicol treatment.[30] Glucocorticoids decrease the expression of class II antigens.[31] Cyclosporine prevents the induction of both class I and class II antigens.[32] Decreased expression of HLA antigens on target cells will make it extremely difficult, if not impossible, to type these cells.

VII. QUALITY CONTROL

To ensure reliable test results, quality control is a necessary component in a laboratory performing HLA typing. There must be quality control for the test components, e.g., reagents, controls, equipment, facilities, as well as personnel.

Negative serum — Normal serum to be acceptable as a negative control for serologic HLA typing must be pretested and determined to be noncytotoxic when screened against a lymphocyte panel using the lymphocytotoxicity assay.

Positive serum — The purpose of the positive control is to demonstrate that conditions were adequate for a positive reaction to occur. This control should be an antibody that will kill all of the cells in the prescribed test situation, in the presence, but not in the absence, of complement. The positive control should be titrated and used at a dilution that is in the approximate range of reactivity of test sera. A positive control that is too concentrated may give a positive reaction when the complement is too weak or the incubation too short for any HLA antisera to react, thus giving one a false impression of suitable test conditions.

Complement — Because complement is extremely labile, the laboratory must establish and adhere to strict rules for handling complement to minimize the possibility of decreasing the activity of this reagent. The complement, when received frozen from commercial sources in larger volumes than required for a single use, is thawed at 37°C, kept at 4°C while it is dispensed into smaller volumes for storage at −70°C. Complement is thawed just before use and used only once, i.e., never refrozen. Each batch of complement must be evaluated for efficacy, the evaluation being done under the same conditions as those used for actual tests. Each batch of complement must be tested to determine that it mediates cytotoxicity in the presence of specific antibody, but is not cytotoxic in the absence of this antibody. The test should employ multiple dilutions of complement to ensure that it is maximally active at least one dilution beyond that intended for use. The test should be carried out with at least two antibodies which should react with at least two different test cells and at least one cell which should not react. A strong and weak antibody should be selected for the test, or serial dilutions of a single serum may be used. Complement should be tested separately for use with each type of target cell, since a different dilution or preparation may be required for optimal performance.[24]

Antisera — Specificity of individual sera received from other laboratories or commercial sources must be confirmed to ensure that they reveal the same specificities in the receiving laboratory. Each lot of new commercial trays must be evaluated by testing either with at least five different cells of known phenotype representing major specificities or in parallel with previously evaluated trays.[24]

Other reagents — It is a requirement that all new reagents, including buffers, stains, etc., be tested in parallel with old reagent, before they are placed in routine use.

REFERENCES

1. **Dausset, J.,** Leuco-agglutinins. IX. Leuco-agglutinins and blood transfusion, *Vox Sang.,* 4, 190, 1954.
2. **Dausset, J.,** Iso-leuco-anticorps, *Acta Haematol.,* 20, 156, 1958.
3. **Payne, R. and Rolfs, M. R.,** Fetomaternal leukocyte incompatibility, *J. Clin. Invest.,* 37, 1756, 1958.
4. **van Rood, J. J., van Leeuwen, A., and Eernisse, J. G.,** Leucocyte antibodies in sera of pregnant women, *Vox Sang.,* 4, 427, 1959.
5. **Bodmer, J. G., Marsh, S. G. E., Albert, E. D., Bodmer, W. F., Dupont, B., Erlich, H. A., Mach, B., Mayr, W. R., Parham, P., Sasazuki, T., Schreuder, G. M. T., Strominger, J. L., Svejgaard, A., and Terasaki, P. I.,** Nomenclature for factors of the HLA system, 1991, *Tissue Antigens,* 39, 161, 1992.
6. **Lau, M., Terasaki, P., Park, M. S., and Barbetti, A.,** International cell exchange 1991, in *Clinical Transplants 1991,* Terasaki, P., Ed., UCLA Tissue Typing Laboratory, Los Angeles, CA.
7. **Nunez, G., Giles, R. C., Ball, E. J., Hurley, C. K., Capra, J. D., and Stastny, P.,** Expression of HLA-DR, MB, MT and SB antigens on human mononuclear cells: identification of two predominantly distinct monocyte populations, *J. Immunol.,* 133, 1300, 1984.
8. **Terasaki, P. I. and McClelland, J. D.,** Microdroplet assay of human serum cytotoxins, *Nature (London),* 204, 998, 1964.
9. Staff, Transplantation and Immunology Branch, NIH lymphocytotoxicity technique, NIAID Manual of Tissue Typing Techniques, NIH Publication No. 80–545. Ray, J. G., Jr., Ed., 1979–1980.
10. **Bodmer, W., Tripp, M., and Bodmer, J.,** Application of a fluorochromatic assay to human leukocyte typing, in *Histocompatibility Testing 1967,* Curtoni, E. S., Mattiuz, P. L., Tosi, R. M., Eds., Munksgaard, Copenhagen, 1967, 341.
11. **Rogentine, C. N. and Plocinik, B. A.,** Application of the ^{51}Cr cytotoxicity technique to the analysis of human lymphocyte isoantigens, *Transplantation,* 5, 1323, 1967.
12. **Colombani, J., D'Amaro, J., Gabb, J., Smith, G., and Svejgaard, A.,** International agreement on a micro-technique of platelet complement fixation, *Transplant. Proc.,* 3, 121, 1971.

13. **Ahrons, S.,** Leukocyte antibodies: occurrence in primigravidae, *Tissue Antigens,* 1, 178, 1971.
14. **Doughty, R. W. and Gesthorpe, K.,** Some parameters of lymphocyte antibody activity through pregnancy and further eluates of placental material, *Tissue Antigens,* 8, 43, 1976.
15. **Vives, J., Gelabert, A., and Castillo, R.,** HLA antibodies and period of gestation: decline in frequency of positive sera during last trimester, *Tissue Antigens,* 7, 209, 1976.
16. **Konoeda, Y., Terasaki, P. I., Wakiosaka, A., Park, M. S., and Mickey, M. R.,** Public determinants of HLA indicated by pregnancy antibodies, *Transplantation,* 41, 253, 1986.
17. **Rodey, G., Terasaki, P., Park, M. S., Fuler, T., Kostyu, D., Phelan, D., Fuller, A., Schroeder, M., Zhao, T., Chandanayingyong, D., Duquesnoy, R., Marrari, M., Cambon-Thomsen, A., Calot, M., Gebel, H., and Hunter, J.,** Antigen Society #33 Report (Public Epitopes), in *Immunobiology of HLA,* Vol. I, Dupont, B., Ed., Springer-Verlag, New York, 1989, 288.
18. **Thorsby, E., Helgesen, A., and Gjemdal, T.,** Repeated platelet transfusions from HL-A compatible unrelated sibling donors, *Tissue Antigens,* 2, 397, 1972.
19. **Astes, R. H., Szatkowski, N., Liebert, M., and Duquesnoy, R. J.,** Expression of HLA-B12, B8, w4, w6 on platelets, *Transplant. Proc.,* 9, 1695, 1977.
20. **Rodey, G. E. and Fuller, T. C.,** Public epitopes and the antigenic structure of the HLA molecules, *Crit. Rev. Immunol.,* 7, 229, 1987.
21. **Boyum, A.,** Separation of lymphocytes, lymphocyte subgroups and monocytes: a review, *Lymphology,* 10, 71, 1977.
22. **Danilovs, J. A., Terasaki, P. I., Park, M. S., and Ayoub, G. B.,** B lymphocyte isolation by thrombin-nylon wool, in *Histocompatibility Testing 1980,* Terasaki, P. I., Ed., UCLA Tissue Typing Laboratory, Los Angeles, 1980, 287.
23. **Vartdal, F., Gaudernack, G., Funderud, S., Bratlie, A., Lea, T., Ungelstad, J., and Thorsby, E.,** HLA class I and II typing using cells positively selected from blood by immunomagnetic isolation — a fast and reliable technique, *Tissue Antigens,* 28, 301, 1986.
24. American Society for Histocompatibility and Immunogenetics, *Standards for Histocompatibility Testing,* Revised March, 1990, ASHI Quarterly, 14, 1, 1990.
25. **van Rood, J. J., van Leeuwen, A., and Ploem, J. S.,** Simultaneous detection of two cell populations by two-colour fluorescence and application to the recognition of B-cell determinants, *Nature (London),* 262, 795, 1976.
26. **Bodmer, J. G., Pickbourne, P., and Richard, S.,** Ia serology, in *Histocompatibility Testing 1977,* Bodmer, J. G., Batchelor, J. B., Bodmer, W. F., Festenstein, H., and Morris, P. J., Eds., Munksgaard, Copenhagen, 1977, 38.
27. **Gantan, Z. P. and Perkins, H. A.,** Differential reactions of HLA typing sera with cells homozygous for crossreacting antigens, *Transfusion,* 30, 631, 1990.
28. **Lee, T. D.,** Distribution of HLA antigens. Distribution of HLA antigens in North American caucasians, North American blacks and orientals, in *The HLA System, A New Approach,* Lee, J., Ed., Springer-Verlag, New York, 1990, 141.
29. **Lazda, V. A.,** The impact of HLA frequency differences in races on the access to optimally HLA-matched cadaver renal transplants, *Transplantation,* 53, 352, 1992.
30. **Ben-David, A., Orgad, S., Danon, Y., and Michaeli, D.,** HL-A antigen changes in patients treated with chloramphenicol, *Tissue Antigens,* 3, 378, 1973.

31. **Madsen, M., Kissmeyer-Nielsen, F., Rasmussen, P., and Anderson, P.,** Decreased expression of HLA-DR antigens on peripheral blood B lymphocytes during glucocorticoid treatment, *Tissue Antigens,* 17, 195, 1981.
32. **Leapman, S. B., Strong, D. M., Filo, R. S., Smith, E. J., and Brandt, G. L.,** Cyclosporin A prevents the appearance of cell surface ''activation'' antigens, *Transplantation,* 34, 94, 1982.

Chapter 19

DNA Typing for MHC Alleles

John D. Reveille

CONTENTS

I. INTRODUCTION

The "standard" method for determining HLA antigens, that of serologic typing, has already been covered in the previous chapter. Over the past 10 years, however, a number of alternative methods have been developed to determine HLA alleles, primarily those utilizing DNA typing. These techniques have a number of advantages over serologic typing. First of all, DNA typing usually utilizes genomic DNA, which can be extracted from peripheral blood leukocytes. Once genomic DNA is thus extracted, it is quite stable at 4°C (at the temperature of a standard refrigerator).[1] This nicely gets around the time constraints of serologic typing, which requires the use of fresh, living cells and allows for the more easy performance of studies on populations. Another very important advantage is the increased sensitivity of DNA analyses, particularly oligonucleotide typing, which allows the precise determination of the markedly expanded polymorphism that has been recognized in class I and class II MHC alleles.[2] Third, the quality and number of the cells to be used in serologic typing is often poor in chronically ill individuals, particularly in those with diseases such as systemic lupus erythematosus (SLE), where the patients are often on corticosteroids and immunosuppressive medications[3,4] and in whom anti-lymphocytotoxic antibodies are often found,[5] which can all affect the number and quality of lymphocytes to be typed.

0-8493-5974-1/94/$0.00 + $.50

II. RFLP ANALYSIS OF GENOMIC DNA

A. TECHNIQUE

In this technique, DNA (here genomic DNA) is cut at specific nucleotide sequences by restriction enzymes, which bind specifically to and cleave double-stranded DNA at specific sites within or adjacent to a particular sequence, known as the recognition sequence.[6] Most of the restriction enzymes used in restriction fragment length polymorphism (RFLP) analysis recognize specific sequences that are four, five, or six nucleotides in length and display twofold symmetry. An example of this is *PvuII,* which recognizes the sequence 5′-CAGCTG-3′ (which would read exactly the same on the opposite DNA strand) wherever it occurs in the genome, and cleaves in the middle between the G and the C. The resultant DNA fragments are size-separated by electrophoresis through an agarose gel (usually overnight, depending on the amount of separation desired), the gel then washed in alkali (to denature the double-stranded DNA fragments contained therein), and the DNA transferred onto a nitrocellulose or nylon filter either electrophoretically or passively by the method of Southern[7] (hence the term "Southern blot"). The DNA is "fixed" or stabilized onto the filter, either by baking in a vacuum oven or by ultra-violet (UV) cross-linking.

At this point the endonuclease-digested, size-separated DNA contained on the filter can be hybridized to a DNA probe corresponding to the gene of interest. These DNA probes are usually either genomic segments obtained from genomic DNA libraries or, instead, are of cDNA, which is a DNA copy generated from the RNA of cells that synthesize a known gene product, using the enzyme reverse transcriptase. Usually these genomic or cDNA probes range in length between a few hundred to a few thousand (kilobases or kb). The DNA probes are detected either by labeling with^{32} P-GTP or -ATP by nick translation[8] or by random primer labeling,[9] or, instead, biotinylated and then hybridized to the filter overnight at the appropriate temperature, washed with the appropriate stringency (usually a factor of salt concentration and temperature), and autoradiography carried out at -70°C (to reduce scatter of the radioactive particles and hence reduce blurring of the bands) for up to several days. A representative Southern blot is shown in Figure 1.

B. APPLICATION

Since the early to mid-1980s, RFLP analysis has been developed as an alternative technique to serologic HLA typing.[10,11] At the Xth International Histocompatibility Workshop, which met in New York City in 1987, these RFLPs were standardized to the HLA-DR and -DQ specificities then recognized.[12]

The restriction endonuclease that has probably been utilized the most in HLA class II typing has been *TaqI.*[13,14] With this enzyme and DRβ probe[15] hybridization alone, one can identify RFLPs specific for HLA-DR1, -DR2(DRw15), -DR2(DRw16), -DR4, -DR5(DRw11), -DR5(DRw12), -DR7/9, -DRw8, -DRw52b (now called DRB3*0201/0202), and -DRw53 (now called DRB4*0101)[2,12,14] (Figure 1). Linkage disequilibrium with DQα[16] and DQβ[17] probes furthermore allows, at least in Caucasians, the determination of HLA-DR3(DRw17) and, in blacks, DR3(DRw18),[18] and the DRB1*1301, *1302, *1401, and *1402 subtypes of HLA-DRw6.[19,20] In our own laboratory, we have been most successful in determining HLA-DQ specificities with *BamHI* endonuclease digestion and DQβ probe hybridization,[21] since the DQβ probe hybridizes only weakly to RFLPs less than 4 kb in size on *TaqI* blots.[22]

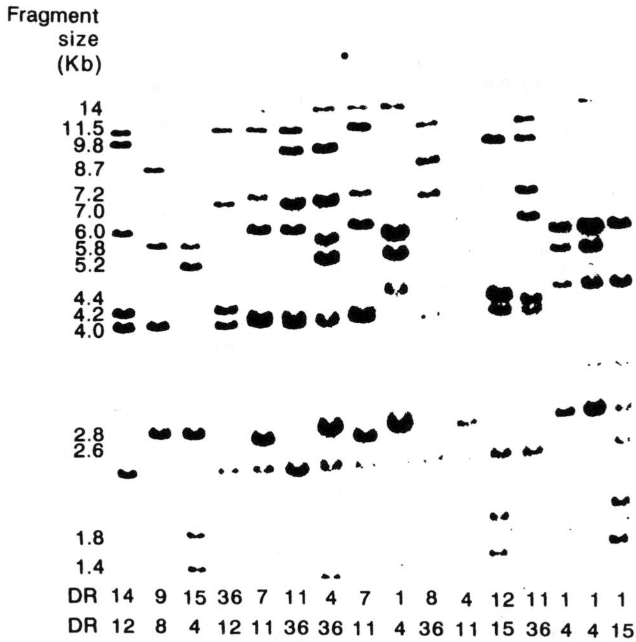

Figure 1 An autoradiograph of a Southern blot of *TaqI* digested genomic DNA hybridized to a full-length DRB1 cDNA probe from 16 different individuals. The size of the DNA fragments in kilobases (kb) represented by the bands in each lane is indicated on the left. The HLA-DR types for each of individual is indicated below each lane. For example, the subject's DNA in the farthest right lane types as HLA-DR1, DR15.

C. ADVANTAGES AND DISADVANTAGES OF RFLP ANALYSIS

The principal advantage of this technique is that it allows the easily readable and reproducible determination of HLA class II alleles (especially HLA-DQA1, -DQB1, and many -DRB1 alleles). And for some situations, such as in the determination of C4A gene deletions, RFLP analysis is as good as, if not superior to, other currently available techniques. RFLP analysis, however, is not as sensitive as some of the newer techniques in the determination of the marked polymorphism now known to lie at DRB1. For example, there are now 12 subtypes of HLA-DR4 known to exist at DRB1. Yet these subtypes would all share similar RFLP bands. Moreover, the linkage disequilibrium with DQα and DQβ RFLPs that is used to define HLA-DRw13 and DRw14 alleles was done initially in Caucasians.[20] More recent data suggest that this linkage disequilibrium may not be present in other racial groups, nor can the expanded polymorphism recently described in non-Caucasians in HLA-DRw13 and -DRw14 alleles be detected by RFLP analysis of genomic DNA.[2] The principal problem with RFLP analysis is the time necessary to carry it out. First of all, only 20 to 30 samples (depending on the comb used) can be tested on a given gel. Also, the restriction digest usually requires an overnight incubation, and the electrophoresis another 24 h. The Southern transfer likewise is usually carried out overnight (although more recent modifications allow for the transfer to be carried out in a few hours). The filters containing the transferred DNA are then usually hybridized to the radiolabeled cDNA probe overnight, and the autoradiography carried out over 3 to 5 d. Moreover, there are a number of important variables which can (and not infrequently do) go wrong, which require repetition of the analysis, such as the completion of the restriction endonuclease digestion (affected by the amount and purity of the genomic DNA and the quality of the restriction enzyme used), and the quality of the cDNA probe used in the hybridization (which tends to be less stable at 4°C than the shorter oligonucleotide probes). For these reasons RFLP analysis has been largely replaced by newer techniques.

III. THE POLYMERASE CHAIN REACTION

Probably one of the most important and innovative developments in molecular biology in the last decade is the development and automation of the polymerase chain reaction (PCR). The PCR represents an *in vitro* method for the enzymatic synthesis of specific DNA sequences, using two oligonucleotide primers that hybridize to opposite strands and flank the region of interest in the target DNA.[23] Basically, this amplification of the DNA segment of interest involves a repetitive series of cycles including template denaturation, primer annealing, and the extension of the annealed primers by DNA polymerase (the most frequently used being the thermostable DNA polymerase isolated from *Thermus aquaticus,* called *Taq* polymerase) that results in the exponential accumulation of a specific fragment whose termini are defined by the 5′ ends of the primers. To manually carry out these cycles (usually about 25 to 30 for a given set of amplifications) would be cumbersome and tedious, and a number of automated thermocyclers (or thermocycler-like machines) are currently being marketed — the biggest marketer being Perkin-Elmer-Cetus, Inc. (Emeryville, CA).

The application of PCR to molecular biology has made possible a variety of applications previously difficult or even impossible, including the generation of large amounts of DNA for genotyping by sequence-specific oligonucleotide probe hybridization or RFLP analysis (see below), with applications to studies of disease association, forensic medicine, analysis of mutations or evolutionary analysis; or for direct DNA sequencing, site-directed mutagenesis,[24] or chromosome crawling.[23,25]

IV. RFLP ANALYSIS OF PCR-AMPLIFIED DNA (PCR-RFLP)

The PCR-RFLP method is a simple and practical technique based on digestion of PCR-amplified DNA with sequence-specific restriction enzymes. The result is that the amplified NA fragment is cut into one or more DNA fragments (depending on the number of times the recognition sequence occurs in the fragment), which can be separated by electrophoresis through an agarose or polyacrylamide gel, stained with ethidium bromide, and photographed. This technique has already been applied to the determination of DRB1, DRB3, DRB5, DQA1, DQB1, and DPB1 alleles.[26-29]

V. SEQUENCE-SPECIFIC OLIGONUCLEOTIDE PROBE HYBRIDIZATION OF PCR-AMPLIFIED DNA

A. TECHNIQUES

Oligonucleotide probes have been used in hybridizations of genomic DNA for several years, with some success.[30] The ease with which they can be generated by currently available automated synthesis, now widely commercially available, as well as their ability to, under appropriately stringent conditions, detect one-base pair differences in the nucleotide sequence makes their use a considerable advantage over cDNA or genomic probes. The problem, however, is that these shorter probes are technically more difficult to use than the longer genomic or cDNA probes on genomic DNA digests, because of the weaker signal generated on the autoradiograph. This problem has been circumvented by the use of PCR, which can generate large quantities of the gene of interest, making the use of sequence-specific oligonucleotides (SSOs) practical and easy.

Basically, the technique involved is straightforward. An aliquot of the amplified DNA (usually about 50 ng) is denatured by either heating to over 80°C or by adding 0.4 *N* NaOH and 25 n*M* EDTA and is blotted onto a nylon membrane filter using either a dot blot or slot blot manifold apparatus, which will vacuum-pull the sample through the filter, fixing the DNA thereon. The DNA sample is affixed onto the filter either by baking for 1 h at 80°C or by UV cross-linking.

The filters can then be hybridized to oligonucleotide probes, most frequently 17 to 20 bp in length. The probes are either labeled with γ^{32}P-ATP (usually of specific activity of 4500 Ci/mmol or greater), using polynucleotide kinase, or with a variety of nonradioactive labeling reagents, such as digoxigenin-UTP. Hybridization and washing conditions are determined by the length of the oligo and the GC content. A recent modification in the SSO typing technique that has made the use of multiple SSOs much easier is the use of tetramethylammonium chloride (3 *M*) in the hybridization solution and washes, which allows for greater uniformity in the hybridization and washing temperatures, regardless of the GC content of the probe and is even less influenced by the length thereof. Autoradiography is carried out over 15 min to several hours (Figure 2), depending on the probe (we usually do two exposures, to ease typing with less avid probes or where the PCR reaction may not have yielded as much DNA in certain individuals).

The PCR-SSO technique was recently utilized at the 11th International HLA Workshop to study disease associations and anthropological relationships between various ethnic groups of HLA-DRB1, -DRB3, -DQA1, -DQB1, -DPA1, and -DPB1 genes, an endeavor which has utilized much useful information in this regard. Similarly, as publications over the past few years have defined the SSOs and conditions for such studies,[31-35] studies of class II HLA genes and ethnic differences and disease associations determined by SSO typing are and will figure prominently in the published literature.

SSO typing of class I HLA alleles is less well developed, due to the multiplicity of class I genes and sequence homology (greater than class II). However, the use of a polymerase enhancer (Stratagene, La Jolla, CA) and careful adjustment of the annealing temperature in the PCR reaction for every primer used is now resulting in success in differentiating subtypes of class I alleles not discernable by serologic methods.[36]

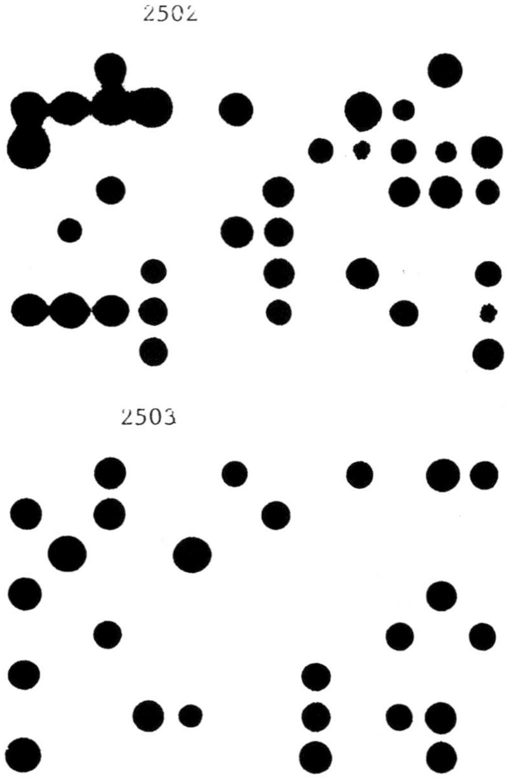

Figure 2 Two dot blots, containing the PCR-amplified second exon of the HLA-DQA1 gene, from 96 different individuals and hybridized to ^{32}P-labelled eighteenmer probes corresponding to variable sequences around position 25 of the HLA-DQA1 outermost domain. The dot blot on top was hybridized to the probe 2502, which hybridizes to sequences shared by HLA-DQA1*0103, 0201, and *0601. The dot blot on the bottom was hybridized to the probe 2503, which hybridizes to HLA-DQA1*03.

B. ADVANTAGES AND DISADVANTAGES

The principal advantage of this technique is the high specificity for the individual polymorphisms now known to exist at the MHC class II alleles and the speed at which large numbers of individuals can be typed. However, because of the allelic diversity at some of the HLA loci, the typing procedure becomes more complicated, requiring the use of numerous filters and numerous oligonucleotide probe labelings/hybridizations, requiring the technician to handle relatively large amounts of ^{32}P and utilizing large amounts of polynucleotide kinase. When small numbers of individuals are to be typed, such as for transplantation matching, this becomes especially impractical.

C. REVERSE DOT BLOT TYPING

To get around the technical difficulty of genotyping a small number of individuals when a large number of SSOs are necessary at a given locus, the "reverse dot blot typing" technique has been developed.[37] Here, the SSO probes are immobilized in a spatial array and the amplified PCR product itself is labeled either with a radionuclide or with biotinylated primers and a streptavidin-horseradish peroxidase conjugate with either chromogenic or luminescent substrates.[37] This approach not only may be much more practical when typing of small numbers of individuals is desired, such as for transplantation cross-matching or forensic medicine, but also avoids such potential difficulties of standard SSO typing as differences of specific activity of the labeled probes, because only the PCR product is labeled. "Kits" containing immobilized probes on filters for typing at a single locus, such as HLA-DQA1, are currently commercially available.

Clearly, when typing large numbers of individuals is desired, such as for disease-association or population studies, this technique is less practical.

VI. PCR FINGERPRINTING

This technique uses the formation of mismatched DNA hybrids (heteroduplexes), which are formed at the end of each PCR cycle between coamplified products of the HLA-DRB1, -DRB3, -DRB4, and -DRB5 second exons (as well as those of the respective DRB pseudogenes found on the DR haplotype).[38,39] During the annealing stage of each cycle of the PCR, a proportion of coding strands of each DRB locus may anneal to noncoding strands of a different DRB locus. Regions of nucleotide sequence complementarity are double stranded, but regions of nucleotide sequence mismatch form single-stranded loops along the length of the molecule. The number, size, and position of the single-stranded loops vary for each DR haplotype and combination of haplotypes in both HLA-DR homozygous and heterozygous individuals. The heteroduplexes can be separated from each other and from corresponding homoduplexes (which would be obtained from an individual homozygous at the HLA-DR locus) by gel retardation analysis in nondenaturing polyacrylamide gels. The result is that haplotype-specific gel banding patterns (PCR fingerprints) are observed. If two individuals thus tested had a matching pattern, this would indicate HLA-DR identity between the two. On the other hand, differences between two individuals at the HLA-DR loci would result in a mismatched pattern. However, most individuals are heterozygous at their respective DR loci. Their PCR fingerprints may be reproduced by mixing DNAs from two corresponding HLA-DR homozygous typing cells (HTCs) prior to the PCR. The result of such a mixture will be additional bands not present in either of the patterns from the HTCs resulting from heteroduplex formation in *trans,* that is from PCR products from two different haplotypes.

A variant of this technique is the DNA cross-match test. Here, genomic DNAs from two different individuals are amplified by PCR in the same tube. The resulting PCR fingerprint is compared with those from the separate PCRs from each individual. Matching fingerprints between all three would indicate HLA-DR identity, whereas the formation of new heteroduplexes or mismatching would indicate nonidentity.

A major application of this would be in transplantation, especially in individuals who might appear HLA-identical for class I and serologically defined class II (such as both having HLA-DR4 but different DR4-DRB1 alleles, i.e., DR4-DRB1*0401 and DR4-DRB1*0404). An advantage of this technique is that it can be performed in one day, probably quicker than PCR-SSO typing. One recent study showed PCR fingerprinting and DNA cross-matching to be more informative than DNA-RFLP analysis alone, and equivalent to RFLP analysis supplemented with PCR-SSO typing.[40]

VII. SINGLE-STRAND CONFORMATIONAL POLYMORPHISM ANALYSIS BY PCR (PCR-SSCP)

In this technique, PCR products are heat-denatured in the presence of formamide and separated by electrophoresis through a polyacrylamide gel to observe single-stranded conformational polymorphism. Different alleles at a given locus are distinguished by

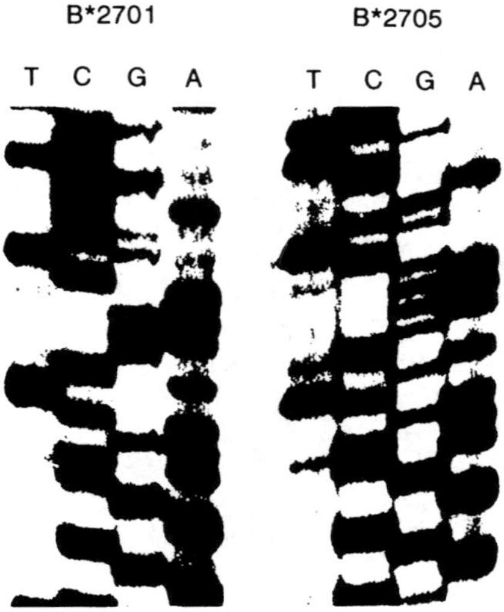

Figure 3 A portion of a nucleotide sequencing gel, depicting sequences in the third hypervariable region of the second exon distinguishing HLA-B*2701 from B*2705. (Genomic DNA from an individual with HLA-B*2701 was kindly supplied by Dr. S. Y. Choo.) The sequence from the gel in the illustration would read (reading from the bottom to the top), "AAGGCCAAGGCACAC ... etc" for both individuals. One of the differences between B*2701 and B*2705 is observed in the middle of the photograph, where the sequence for HLA-B*2701 reads "GAGAGAA" and for B*2705 "GAGAGAG".

their different migration rates through the gel. This technique has recently been utilized to type at the HLA-DQA1 and DQB1 loci.[41]

VIII. DETERMINATION OF HLA POLYMORPHISMS BY NUCLEOTIDE SEQUENCE ANALYSIS

Differences in HLA alleles, to our present knowledge, reflect differences in their nucleotide sequence. Therefore, it is no surprise that the gold standard for determining a possible difference between the homologous alleles between two individuals would be to determine the nucleotide sequences of their respective genes. Up until recently, this was an extremely labor-intensive project, involving construction of genomic libraries, screening of the libraries for the desired gene, and subcloning. However with improvements of techniques dealing with direct sequencing of PCR products, the possibility of using the determination of differences between individuals or between patient and control groups by rapid determination of their nucleotide sequences (sequence-based typing [SBT])[42] is becoming more feasible. For each individual, the process would involve five steps: (1) nucleic acid extraction (presumably automated if this is to be practical); (2) synthesis of locus-specific cDNA; (3) enzymatic amplification by PCR; (4) direct sequencing of the amplified product; and (5) analysis of the sequence patterns (Figure 3). As with step 1, the latter two steps would also presumably be automated and computerized. Such a system would allow SBT on a number of individuals in less than 24 h, and would clearly replace the other DNA techniques outlined above.

IX. CONCLUSION

In this chapter we have briefly covered most of the techniques of DNA typing of MHC alleles currently utilized. The technology is evolving rapidly, with the underlying driving forces being accuracy and specificity of the data, as well as speed, safety, and the minimizing of expense. Standard RFLP analysis was "state-of-the art" for several years during the mid- and late 1980s, but the speed and greater specificity of oligotyping has largely replaced this (although in certain applications, such as in the determination of C4 gene deletions, genomic RFLP analysis is still used). Some of the technology, such as the routine use of nucleotide sequence analysis, may not be practical for smaller laboratories, where access to large, expensive equipment such as computer-automated DNA sequencers might be lacking.

This technology has revolutionized the approach to studies of HLA and disease, and an evolving body of data are suggesting that molecular genetic technology will improve the results of organ transplantation, by allowing for more precise matching between organ donors and recipients.

REFERENCES

1. **Blin, N. and Stafford, D. W.,** A general method for isolation of high molecular weight DNA from eukaryotes, *Nucleic Acids Res.*, 3, 2303, 1978.
2. **Bodmer, J. G., Marsh, S. G. E., Albert, E. D. et al.,** Nomenclature for factors of the HLA system, 1991, *Tissue Antigens,* 39, 161, 1992.
3. **Snyder, D. S. and Unanue, E. R.,** Corticosteroids inhibit murine macrophage Ia expression and interleukin 1 production, *J. Immunol.*, 129, 1803, 1982.
4. **Hokland, M., Larsen, B., Heron, I., and Plesner, T.,** Corticosteroids decrease the expression of beta2-microglobulin and histocompatibility antigens on human peripheral blood lymphocytes in vitro, *Clin. Exp. Immunol.*, 44, 239, 1981.
5. **Terasaki, P. I., Mottironi, V. D., and Barnett, E. V.,** Cytotoxins in disease: autocytotoxins in lupus, *N. Engl. J. Med.*, 283, 724, 1970.
6. **McDaniel, D. O., Barger, B. O., Reveille, J. D., Alarcon, G. S., Koopman, W. J., and Acton, R. T.,** Analysis of restriction fragment length polymorphisms in rheumatic diseases, in *Rheumatic Disease Clinics of North America,* Zvaifler, N. J., Ed., W. B. Saunders, Harcourt Brace Jovanovich, Philadelphia, 1987, 353.
7. **Southern, E. M.,** Detection of specific sequences among DNA fragments separated by gel electrophoresis, *J. Mol. Biol.*, 98, 503, 1975.
8. **Rigby, P. W. J., Dieckmann, V., Rhodus, C., and Berg, P.,** Labeling deoxyribonucleic acid to high specific activity in vitro by nick translation with DNA polymerase I, *J. Mol. Biol.*, 113, 237, 1977.
9. **Feinberg, A. P. and Vogelstein, B.,** A technique for radiolabeling DNA restriction fragments to high specific activity, *Anal. Biochem.*, 132, 6, 1983.
10. **Cohen, D., LeGall, I., Marcadet, A., Font, M. P., Lalouel, J. M., and Dausset, J.,** Clusters of HLA class II beta restriction fragments describe allelic series, *Proc. Natl. Acad. Sci. U.S.A.*, 81, 7870, 1984.
11. **Tilanus, M. G. J., vanEggermond, M. C. J. A., vanderBijl, M., Morolli, B., Schreuder, G. M. Th., DeVries, R. R. P., and Giphart, M. J.,** HLA class II DNA analysis by RFLP reveals novel class II polymorphism, *Hum. Immunol.*, 18, 265, 1987.
12. **Simons, M. J., Wheeler, R., Cohen, D., Lalouel, J. M., and Dupont, B.,** Restriction fragment length polymorphism of HLA genes: summary of the Tenth International Workshop Southern blot analysis, in *Immunobiology of HLA.* Vol. I. *Histocompatibility Testing 1987,* Dupont, B., Ed., Springer-Verlag, New York, 1989, 959.

13. **Kohonen-Corish, M. R. J. and Serjeantson, S. W.,** HLA-DR beta gene DNA polymorphisms revealed by taq I correlate with HLA-DR specificities, *Hum. Immunol.,* 15, 263, 1986.
14. **Bidwell, J. L., Bidwell, E. A., Savage, D. A., Middleton, D., Klouda, P. T., and Bradley, B. A.,** A DNA-RFLP typing system that positively identifies serologically well-defined and ill-defined HLA-DR and DQ alleles, including DRw10, *Transplantation,* 45, 640, 1988.
15. **Long, E. O., Wake, C. T., Gorski, J., and Mach, B.,** Complete sequence of an HLA-DR beta chain deduced from a cDNA clone and identification of multiple non allelic DR beta chain genes, *EMBO J.,* 2, 389, 1983.
16. **Spielman, R. S., Lee, J., Bodmer, W. F., Bodmer, J. G., and Trowsdale, J.,** Six HLA-D region alpha-chain genes on human chromosome 6: polymorphisms and associations of DC alpha-related sequences and DR types, *Proc. Natl. Acad. Sci. U.S.A.,* 81, 3461, 1984.
17. **Larhammar, D., Hyldig-Nielsen, J. J., Servenius, B., Anderson, G., Rask, L., and Peterson, P. A.,** Exon-intron organization and complete nucleotide sequence of a human major histocompatibility antigen DC beta gene, *Proc. Natl. Acad. Sci. U.S.A.,* 80, 7313, 1983.
18. **Hurley, C. K., Gregersen, P. K., Gorski, J., Steiner, N., Robbins, F. M., Hartzman, R., Johnson, A. H., and Silver, J.,** The DR3(w18), DQw4 haplotype differs from DR3(w17), DQw2 haplotypes at multiple class II loci, *Hum. Immunol.,* 25, 37, 1989.
19. **Lee, K. W., Hurley, C. K., Hartzman, R., and Johnson, A. H.,** The complexity of DRw6 and DR5 haplotypes in American blacks demonstrated by serology, cellular typing, and restriction fragment length polymorphism analysis, *Hum. Immunol.,* 29, 202, 1990.
20. **Bosch, M. L., Fei, H., Bontrop, R. E., Gerrets, R., Tilanus, M. G. J., Termijtelen, A., and Giphart, M. J.,** Polymorphisms within the HLA-DRw6 haplotype. III. DQ alpha and DQ beta polymorphism associated with HLA-D*, *Hum. Immunol.,* 19, 91, 1987.
21. **Hyldig-Nielsen, J. J., Boehm, B. O., Wood, K. J., Bushell, A. R., Singal, D. P., and Svejgaard, A.,** RFLP standardization report for DQ Beta/BamHI, in *Immunobiology of HLA.* Vol. I. *Histocompatibility Testing 1987,* Dupont, B., Ed., Springer-Verlag, New York, 1989, 634.
22. **Marcadet, A., Martell, M., Cohen, D., Bignon, J. D., Kobayashi, K., Carpenter, C. B., and Walford, R. L.,** RFLP standardization report for DQ Beta/TaqI, in *Immunobiology of HLA.* Vol. I. *Histocompatibility Testing 1987,* Dupont, B., Springer-Verlag, New York, 1989, 620.
23. **Saiki, R. K.,** Basic methodology, in *PCR Technology. Principles and Applications for DNA Amplification,* Erlich, H. A., Ed., Stockton Press, New York, 1989, 7.
24. **Irwin, N.,** In vitro amplification of DNA by the polymerase chain reaction, in *Molecular Cloning. A Laboratory Manual,* Ford, N., Nolan, C., and Ferguson, M., Eds., Cold Spring Harbor Laboratory Press, Cold Spring Harbor, 1989, 14.2.
25. **Irwin, N.,** Site-directed mutagenesis of cloned DNA, in *Molecular Cloning. A Laboratory Manual,* Ford, N., Nolan, C., and Ferguson, M., Eds., Cold Spring Harbor Laboratory Press, Cold Spring Harbor, 1989, 15.2.

26. **Maeda, M., Uryu, N., Murayama, N., Ishii, H., Ota, M., Tsuji, K., and Inoko, H.,** A simple and rapid method for HLA-DP genotyping by digestion of PCR-amplified DNA with allele-specific restriction endonucleases, *Hum. Immunol.,* 27, 111, 1990.
27. **Ota, M., Seki, T., Nomura, N., Sugimura, K., Mizuki, N., Fukushima, H., Tsuji, K., and Inoko, H.,** Modified PCR-RFLP method for HLA-DPB1 and -DQA1 genotyping, *Tissue Antigens,* 38, 60, 1991.
28. **Nomura, N., Ota, M., Tsuji, K., and Inoko, H.,** HLA-DQB1 genotyping by a modified PCR-RFLP method combined with group-specific primers, *Tissue Antigens,* 38, 53, 1991.
29. **Uryu, N., Maeda, M., Ota, M., Tsuji, K., and Inoko, H.,** A simple and rapid method for HLA-DRB and -DQB typing by digestion of PCR-amplified DNA with allele specific restriction endonucleases, *Tissue Antigens,* 35, 20, 1990.
30. **Nepom, B. S., Palmer, J., Kim, S. J., Hansen, J. A., Holbeck, J. A., and Nepom, G. T.,** Specific genomic markers of the HLA-DQ subregion discriminate between DR4+ insulin-dependent diabetes mellitus and DR4+ seropositive rheumatoid arthritis, *J. Exp. Med.,* 164, 345, 1986.
31. **Gao, X., Fernandez-Vina, M., Shumway, W., and Stastny, P.,** DNA typing for class II HLA antigens with allele-specific or group-specific amplification. I. Typing for subsets of HLA-DR4, *Hum. Immunol.,* 27, 40, 1990.
32. **Fernandez-Vina, M., Shumway, W., and Stastny, P.,** DNA typing for class II HLA antigens with allele-specific or group-specific amplification. II. Typing for alleles of the DRw52-associated group, *Hum. Immunol.,* 28, 51, 1990.
33. **Fernandez-Vina, M., Moraes, M. E., and Stastny, P.,** DNA typing for class II HLA antigens with allele-specific or group-specific amplification. III. Typing for 24 alleles of HLA-DP, *Hum. Immunol.,* 30, 60, 1991.
34. **Moraes, M. E., Fernandez-Vina, M., and Stastny, P.,** DNA typing for class II HLA antigens with allele-specific or group-specific amplification. IV. Typing for alleles of the HLA-DR2 group, *Hum. Immunol.,* 31, 139, 1991.
35. **Gao, X., Moraes, J. R., Miller, S., and Stastny, P.,** DNA typing for class II HLA antigens with allele-specific or group-specific amplification. V. Typing for subsets of HLA-DR1 and DR'Br', *Hum. Immunol.,* 30, 147, 1991.
36. **Fernandez-Vina, M. A., Falco, M., Sun, Y., and Stastny, P.,** DNA typing for HLA class I alleles. I. Subsets of HLA-A2 and of -A28, *Hum. Immunol.,* 33, 163, 1992.
37. **Saiki, R., Walsh, P. S., Levenson, C. H., and Erlich, H. A.,** Genetic analysis of amplified DNA with immobilized sequence-specific oligonucleotide probes, *Proc. Natl. Acad. Sci. U.S.A.,* 86, 6215, 1989.
38. **Bidwell, J. L. and Hui, K. M.,** Human HLA-DR/Dw allotype matching by analysis of HLA-DRB gene PCR product polymorphism (PCR "fingerprints"), *Technique,* 2, 92, 1990.
39. **Wood, N. A. P., Clay, T. M., and Bidwell, J. L.,** HLA-DR/Dw matching by PCR fingerprinting; the origin of PCR fingerprints and further applications, *Eur. J. Immunogenet.,* 18, 147, 1991.
40. **Clay, T. M., Bidwell, J. L., and Howard, M. R.,** PCR-fingerprinting for selection of HLA matched unrelated donors, *Lancet,* 337, 1049, 1991.
41. **Carrington, M., Miller, T., White, M., Gerrard, B., Steward, C., Dean, M., and Mann, D.,** Typing of HLA-DQA1 and DQB1 using DNA single-strand conformation polymorphism, *Hum. Immunol.,* 33, 208, 1992.

42. **Santamaria, P., Boyce-Jacino, M. T., Lindstrom, A. L., Barbosa, J. J., Faras, A., and Rich, S. S.,** HLA class II ''typing'': direct sequencing of DRB, DQB, and DQA genes, *Hum. Immunol.*, 33, 69, 1992.

Chapter 20

MHC Genes and Disease Susceptibility

John D. Reveille

CONTENTS

0-8493-5974-1/94/$0.00 + $.50

I. INTRODUCTION

Reports of HLA antigens or genes and disease association have factored heavily in the literature since the early 1970s. Indeed, many a researcher's career has been based (and sometimes foundered) on such examinations, and HLA and disease has probably emerged as one of the "cottage industries" of the latter quarter of the twentieth century. Until fairly recently, the relevance of the myriad studies that have been published regarding HLA and disease associations has not been entirely clear.

The past few years, however, have witnessed remarkable breakthroughs in our understanding of the organization of the major histocompatibility complex (MHC) and the various and often related functions of the gene families contained therein. Now some of the HLA and disease associations, particularly those that transcend racial and ethnic boundaries, can be reexamined and can offer important clues as to disease pathogenesis. Probably the best examples of this are the association of HLA-B27 with ankylosing spondylitis (AS), or of HLA-DR4 with seropositive rheumatoid arthritis (RA), or of C4A null alleles with systemic lupus erythematosus (SLE). On the other hand, other HLA associations are less easy to explain, or even to understand, such as that of HLA-DR2 and narcolepsy, where no autoimmune etiology is apparent, or of HLA-DR2 and multiple sclerosis, an association which only seems to be present in Caucasians. The latter may instead reflect linkage to as yet unidentified genes which are present on different HLA haplotypes in different ethnic groups.

In this chapter, the associations of specific rheumatologic, neurologic, and dermatologic conditions with genes of the MHC will be discussed. The persistence of associations in different racial and ethnic groups will be emphasized in particular, and possible mechanisms for the disease associations explored. Putative associations of HLA and infection of malignancy will not be discussed. Finally, possible clinical applications to determining a patient's MHC gene repertoire will be discussed.

II. CLASS I

A. THE SERONEGATIVE SPONDYLOARTHROPATHIES

1. AS and Reiter's Syndrome

a. Epidemiology

Nearly 20 years have passed since the first reports linking ankylosing spondylitis (AS) and Reiter's syndrome to HLA-B27 in European and North American Caucasians were published.[1-3] These have emerged over time as one of the best examples of a disease association with a hereditary marker. In Caucasians over 90% of patients with AS have

Table 1 **HLA-Class I Specificities and Disease Susceptibility**

		HLA Association	Frequency (%) Patients	Controls	Ref.
Ankylosing spondylitis	Caucasians	B27	90	6–8	1,2
Reiter's syndrome	Caucasians	B27	80	6–8	3
IBD-associated spondylitis	Caucasians	B27	50–60	6–8	61
Psoriasis vulgaris	Caucasians	B17	34	6	46–49,55
	Caucasians	Cw6	72	24	52
	Japanese	Cw6,7,12[a]	81	48	57
	Japanese	Cw11	32	9	56
Psoriatic arthritis	Caucasians	B16(38,39)	17	6	55,58
	Caucasians	B27	24	6–8	59,60
Psoriatic spondylitis	Caucasians	B27	70	6–8	66
Behcet's syndrome	Japanese	B51	62	26	67
	Chinese	B51	51	11	62
	Italians	B51	82	22	72
Takayasu's arteritis	Japanese	B52	53	24	71

[a]HLA-C locus alleles sharing an *alanine* at position 73 of the outermost (α1) domain.

HLA-B27, and over 80% of those with Reiter's syndrome (Table 1). The association of AS with B27 has been confirmed in Chinese,[4] Indians, and Pakistanis,[5] Arabs,[6] Iranians,[7] Israeli Jews,[8] and, in the western hemisphere, Mexicans.[9] There appears to be a gene dosage effect for HLA-B27 in AS,[10] with homozygosity for HLA-B27 associated with more severe disease. Studies in HLA-B27-negative AS patients have found either an excess of the HLA-B7 cross-reactive group which shares antigenic cross-reactivity, including B7 (and its three subtypes B*0701–*0703), HLA-Bw22 (now split into B*5401, *5501, *5502, *5601, and *5602), HLA-B27 (B*2701–*2707), B40 (split now into B*4001–*4005) and HLA-B42 (B*4201) or HLA antigens associated with psoriasis or psoriatic arthritis,[11,12] in which spondylitis also occurs. The same has been seen in Reiter's syndrome.[3]

Among non-Caucasians, the prevalence of AS and Reiter's syndrome varies in proportion to the respective population frequency of HLA-B27. In certain groups of native Americans, for example, the frequency of HLA-B27 is high, as is the prevalence of AS. HLA-B27 occurs in 50% of Haidas and 25% of Bella Coolas, two groups residing in British Columbia in Canada. Sacroiliitis, the earliest lesion in AS, has been reported in 10% and 2% in these groups respectively.[13,14] On the other hand, HLA-B27 occurs in less than 1% of the population in Japan,[15] and the prevalence of AS is about one quarter of that in Caucasians.[16] In African blacks HLA-B27 is rare (occurring in less than 1% of the population), and AS likewise very uncommon.[17] Only eight black AS patients were identified over a 4-year period from a large clinic in South Africa, where in a comparable Caucasian population it was estimated that over 2000 cases of AS would occur. Contributing to this lower frequency of AS in African blacks is the recent description of a HLA-B27 subtype that was not associated with AS in one large population study.[18] This HLA-B27 allele, designated B*2703, differs from other B27 subtypes by a single amino acid substitution, which dramatically alters the charge in the "A" pocket in the antigen-binding cleft of the HLA-B27 molecule, which is felt to be important in "anchoring" the peptide in the cleft.[18] In American blacks, the frequency of HLA-B27 is less than 2%,[19] and AS and Reiter's syndrome are likewise believed to be far less common than in Caucasians,[20] this slightly higher frequency of HLA-B27 felt to reflect Caucasian gene admixture. Moreover, AS is less highly associated with HLA-B27 in blacks, both in a study from South Africa, where only two of nine (22%) black AS patients had HLA-B27,[17] and in others from the U.S. where 50 to 60% of black AS patients were B27-positive.[21,22]

b. Mechanisms and Potential Problems

HLA-B27 occurs in approximately 6 to 8% of the Caucasoid population, yet the population frequency of AS is about 0.2%.[23,24] Furthermore, AS occurs much more frequently in B27-positive relatives of probands with AS (up to 30%) than in B27-positive relatives of controls.[24] This has led some to propose that either a B27 subtype (at least seven are now known to occur) or another gene found on some but not all B27-bearing haplotypes may exist that further increases the risk for AS or Reiter's syndrome.[25] One potential candidate gene was recently identified by restriction fragment length polymorphism (RFLP) analysis,[26,27] found to be linked to specific HLA-A locus alleles[27,28] and peripheral arthritis in AS,[26] although subsequent studies did not confirm this disease association in other populations.[28,29]

The best evidence, however, that HLA-B27 is directly and primarily responsible for AS and Reiter's syndrome comes from a recently developed transgenic rat model for the disease, where HLA-B27 was introduced into an inbred rat line, and most of the rats found to express HLA-B27 subsequently developed lesions typical of AS, Reiter's syndrome, and psoriasis,[30] Nevertheless, the fact that spondyloarthropathy was not produced when B27 was successfully introduced into transgenic mice (as opposed to the rat model)[4] suggests that HLA-B27 functions on a permissive background of other host factors, presumably genetic. What these are remains to be seen.

With the demonstration that HLA-B27 itself plays a role in susceptibility to spondyloarthropathy having been established, determining the precise nature of this role has been a bit more controversial. Molecular mimicry between HLA-B27 and an infectious agent has been proposed as one mechanism.[31] There are two different ways in which this might happen. In one, infection occurs with a microorganism expressing antigens cross-reactive with the HLA-B27 molecules expressed on the surface of a patient's cells, which results in an autoimmune response directed against "self" tissues. In the other, the deletion in the thymus (earlier in development) of T cells reactive against this cross-reactive epitope results in the lack of an appropriate immune response against this microorganism, resulting in persistence of infection and clinical disease.[32] Evidence for the latter is the finding of *Chlamydia trachomatis, Yersinia enterocolitica,* and *Salmonella typhimurium* antigens in synovial phagocytic cells in patients with reactive arthritis (Reiter's syndrome) triggered by these same infectious agents.[33-36] Even more compelling than this has been the demonstration of shared amino acid sequences between the polymorphic and antigen-specific region of HLA-B27 and several bacteria, including *Klebsiella pneumoniae,*[37] and a plasmid found thus far only in arthritogenic strains of *Shigella flexneri.*[38] Whether these examples of molecular mimicry specifically contribute to disease pathogenesis remains to be determined, however.

The fine internal structure of the HLA-B27 molecule has been determined by crystallization studies[39] (Figure 1), and a considerable amount has been learned about the nature of the peptide contained in the antigen-binding cleft. This peptide fragment is nine amino acids in length,[40] and only four of these appear crucial in contacting residues

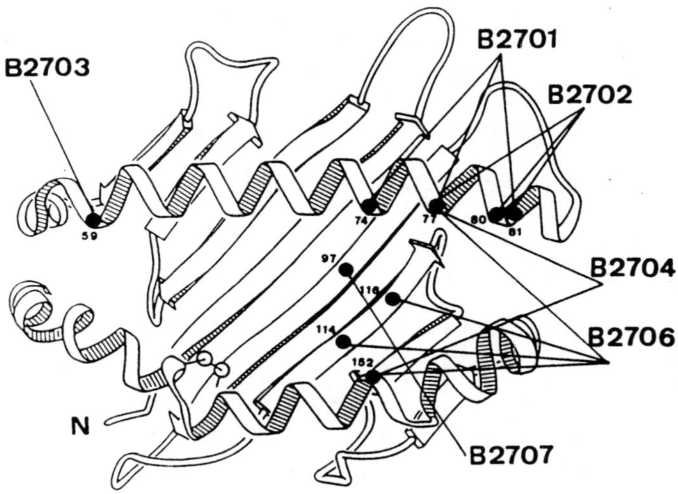

Figure 1 Schematic representation of the three-dimensional structure of the HLA-B*2705 molecule, showing the location of the amino acids distinguishing the other six B27 alleles. (Modified after Reference 42.)

in the B27 molecule.[40,41] The nature of those residues that are crucial in contacting the homologous portion of the T cell receptor remains to be determined. As we now know it, there are over 10,000 different possible peptides that possess the crucial amino acid determinants for B27-binding that exist in nature.[40]

HLA-B27 is unique from other HLA specificities by the presence of two amino acids, a *lysine* residue at position 70 and an *asparginine* at position 97 (the latter replaced by a *serine* in HLA-B*2707).[42,43] Over seven subtypes of HLA-B27 are known to exist (B*2701–B*2707).[44] One of these, B*2705, is by far the most common and found in all groups studied. HLA-B*2702, considerably less common, is found in Caucasians. B*2704 and B*2706 are found exclusively in Orientals and B*2703 is peculiar to African blacks.[18] HLA-B*2701 and B*2707, the most recent B27 subtypes to be described,[43,45] appear to be very rare and have thus far been only described in Caucasians and Asian Indians, respectively.[45a] These B27 subtypes differ among themselves by one to six amino acid substitutions in the outermost two domains (Figure 1). Thus far HLA-B*2701, *2702, *2704, and *2705 have been described in patients with AS. B*2706 and B*2707 appear to be extremely rare, and a true disease association has yet to be described. The possible lack of a disease association of HLA-B*2703 has been described above. Population studies of HLA-B27 subtypes will help to define whether these are truly disease-protective, and if so will better define which epitopes on the B27 molecule are most crucial in susceptibility to spondyloarthropathy.

c. The Clinical Relevance of Typing for HLA-B27

HLA-B27 associations with AS has provided fertile ground for clinical research in the past 20 years. The question arises whether typing for HLA-B27 is a useful clinical tool for the practicing rheumatologist. Probably the two most important questions that any clinician should ask before ordering a laboratory test on any patient is whether the results will either: (1) provide important information that has diagnostic value, or (2) have therapeutic implications. Indeed, there are many who feel that only the latter has any true relevance. As far as therapeutic implications are concerned, the finding that homozygosity for HLA-B27 confers a worse prognosis in AS[10] may have some predictive value, but whether this would have specific therapeutic implications is arguable. Moreover, to prove homozygosity for HLA-B27 may entail performing a family study (given that the individual could have an HLA-B antigen on the other haplotype typing as a blank), and would thus be cumbersome and probably impractical.

The other question, that of diagnostic value for HLA-B27 typing, is relevant. The argument for some time has been that since HLA-B27 is found in 6 to 8% of the Caucasoid population, a false diagnosis of AS or spondyloarthropathy could result in some individuals if too much weight is placed on a positive result. However, one important purpose of a lab test is to confirm a clinical suspicion that is already there. There is little to be gained from routinely HLA-B27 typing all patients with classical AS or Reiter's syndrome, nor would the presence of HLA-B27 have any relevance in a patient with an erosive, symmetric, additive polyarthritis, subcutaneous nodules, positive serum rheumatoid factor but no axial symptoms, or a patient with a malar rash, nephritis, polyarthritis, anti-native DNA and anti-nuclear antibodies, and hypocomplementemia. But for the patient with undiagnosed seronegative peripheral arthritis, who may or may not be found to have other mucocutaneous lesions, the presence of HLA-B27 would provide weight for a diagnosis of spondyloarthropathy, weight that has to be kept in context with other symptoms and signs. Where HLA-B27 typing has probably been most widely misused is in the area of diagnosing low back pain, where people with otherwise straightforward mechanical low back pain have been given a diagnosis of AS on the finding of HLA-B27 positivity. Again, interpretation of the significance of a positive result must be kept in the context of the clinical presentation. Even in the presence of inflammatory low back pain symptoms (morning stiffness, relief with exercise, etc.) the significance of a positive HLA-B27 typing in the absence of frank radiographic abnormalities must be interpreted with caution.

2. Psoriasis, Psoriatic Arthritis, and Psoriatic Spondylitis

Initial reports suggested that psoriasis vulgaris (PV) was linked to HLA-B13 and -B17 (especially the HLA-B57 subtype) as well as HLA-B37, in western European Caucasians[46-48] (Table 1). Subsequent studies confirmed these associations in other groups, including Russians,[49] Asian Indians,[50] and other eastern Asians.[51] However, more recently, an HLA-C locus allele linked to these HLA-B alleles, namely HLA-Cw6, has been implicated in susceptibility to psoriasis vulgaris.[52-55] One recent study from Japan has also implicated HLA-Cw11, and another HLA-Cw6, -Cw7, and -Cw12, the latter three sharing significant sequence homology in the third hypervariable region of the outermost domain.[56,57]

Most patients with psoriatic arthritis have the above-noted HLA alleles associated with psoriasis. On top of this, however, are associations of peripheral psoriatic arthritis and spondylitis with the splits of HLA-B16 (B38, or B*3801, and B39, or B*3901, B*3902).[55,58] Over two thirds of patients with psoriatic spondylitis also have HLA-B27.[59]

Pustular psoriasis has been associated with HLA-B27,[48] as has psoriatic arthritis occurring in the setting of human immunodeficiency virus (HIV) infection, which shares considerable clinical overlap with Reiter's syndrome.[60] Similarly, acute anterior uveitis, which can occur as an isolated phenomenon or in association with AS or Reiter's syndrome, is another HLA-B27-associated disease.[61]

3. Inflammatory Bowel Disease-Associated Spondylitis/Arthritis

Peripheral arthritis, sacroiliitis, and spondylitis occur in association with inflammatory bowel disease (IBD), although only spondylitis has been associated with HLA-B27 (Table 1). No HLA association has been found for IBD-related peripheral arthritis or sacroiliitis.[62,63]

B. OTHER DISEASE ASSOCIATIONS WITH CLASS I ALLELES

1. Behcet's Syndrome

This condition, characterized by painful oral and genital ulcers in association with vasculitis, ocular lesions, meningoencephalitis, and arthritis, occurs most frequently in Asians and Arabs. In studies from Italy, Israel, Japan, and China the most consistent association has been with HLA-B51 (B*5101)[64-67] (Table 1).

2. Takayasu's Arteritis (TA)

Characterized by a pulseless condition occurring most frequently in young females of Asian or South American extraction, this large vessel vasculitis involving the aortic arch and its branches has been most consistently associated with HLA-B52 (B*5201), largely in studies from Japan.[68-71] One study has suggested a more specific association with the haplotype B52, DRB1*1502, DRB5*0102, DQA1*0103, DQB1*0601, DPA1*02, DPB1*0901, and that the haplotype HLA-Bw54, DRB1*0405, DRB4*0101, DQA1*0301, DQB1*0401 may confer resistance to TA.[72] On the other hand, such associations have not been observed in Caucasians, raising the possibility that a heretofore unidentified gene on Japanese HLA-B52 haplotypes may actually be the disease gene, which is not present on Caucasian B52 haplotypes[73] (Table 1).

III. CLASS II AND CLASS III

A. THE RHEUMATIC DISEASES

1. Rheumatoid Arthritis (RA)

The association of rheumatoid arthritis (RA) with HLA-DR4 was first established over 16 years ago in Caucasians.[74] Reports since then have shown the HLA-DR4 association with RA to persist in nearly every racial and ethnic group studied,[75-79] except Israelis and Indians, in whom the association was with HLA-DR1,[80-81] and the Yakima group of native Americans, where the association was with the Dw16 (DRB1*1402) subtype of HLA-DRw6 (DRw14).[82] Recent studies using molecular genetic techniques have suggested the genetic susceptibility to RA to lie with an amino acid sequence in the third hypervariable region of the HLA-DRB1 outermost domain shared by certain HLA-DR4 (DRB1*0401, *0404, *0405, and *0408), -DR1 (DRB1*0101, *0102) subtypes,[83,84] DRw6 (Dw16 or DRB1*1402)[82] and DRw10.[85,86]

This sequence is located between positions 66 and 75 of the DRB1 chain (Figure 2), with certain positions appearing to be particularly important. At positions 70 and 71, HLA-Dw4 (DRB1*0401), Dw14 (DRB1*0404, *0408), and Dw14 (DRB1*0405,

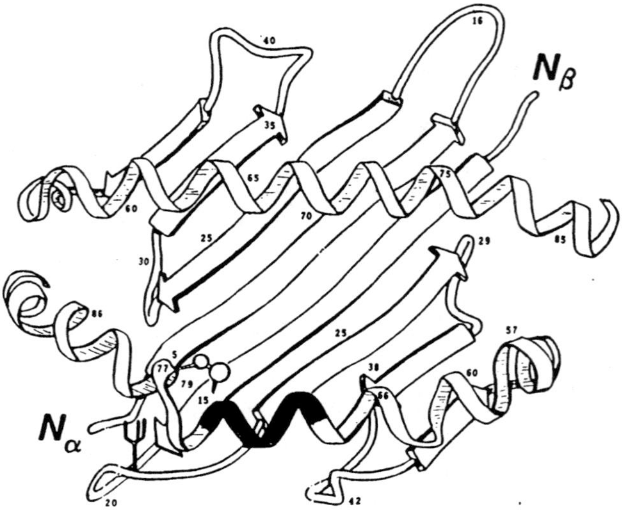

Figure 2 Schematic representation of a proposed model of the MHC or HLA class II molecule. Here the so-called "rheumatoid epitope", spanning residues 70 to 74 on the outermost domain of the HLA-DRB1 chain, is indicated in black.

*0406) have basic amino acids (glutamine and arginine or lysine). HLA-Dw10 (DRB1*0402), which is not associated with RA, has two charged residues here (aspartic acid and glutamic acid) and Dw13 (DRB1*0403, *0407) a glutamic acid residue at position 74, instead of an alanine, which would result in charge differences that could alter the peptide-binding characteristics of the antigen-binding cleft.[87] The potential disease relevance of this sequence in the third hypervariable region becomes even more significant in light of recent data describing significant homology between the sequence at positions 66 to 75 and sequences present in both a bacterial heat shock protein, dnaJ, which is an important epitope for B cell-mediated autoantibody production,[88] and an Epstein-Barr (EBV) virus-encoded protein, gp110.[89] EBV is a potent T cell stimulator. Moreover, T cells or autoantibodies reactive with these exogeneous peptides also cross react with the Dw4 peptide in position 66–75.[90]

It is true that there are probably several genes at work in the pathogenesis of RA. The HLA contribution has been estimated at approximately 30%.[91] Moreover, the population frequency of the so-called ''rheumatoid epitope'' shared by HLA-Dw4 (DRB1*0401), Dw14 (DRB1*0404, *0408), Dw15 (DRB1*0405), DR1 (DRB1*0101, *0102), DRw14 (Dw16-DRB1*1402), and DRw10 in Caucasians is approximately 45%, although only 2% have RA.[92] In fact a growing body of data is suggesting that the presence of the ''rheumatoid epitope'' may in fact influence disease severity. There is little or no association of HLA-DR4 or the ''rheumatoid epitope'' with milder forms of RA.[93,94] On the other hand, homozygosity for HLA-DR4 alleles bearing this ''disease-associated epitope'' has been linked to more rapidly progressive RA, and hence a worse prognosis.[95-97] Thus, typing for HLA-DRB1 alleles may have clinical implications for patients with newly diagnosed RA, where a more aggressive approach to treatment of HLA-DR4-homozygous RA patients may be indicated to forestall and even prevent functional disability.

2. Systemic Lupus Erythematosus (SLE)

a. MHC Class II and Class III Associations in Caucasians

The initial HLA class II associations with SLE emerged in 1978, when HLA-DR2 and -DR3 were first noted to be increased in Caucasian SLE patients.[98,99] Reports since then have varied as to whether HLA-DR2[100] or -DR3[101-105] were more closely associated with SLE. In general the HLA-DR3 associations (usually coinciding with the presence of HLA-B8) came from reports from northwestern Europe or the British Isles,[106] or the U.S., where there was a high proportion of patients of Scotch-Irish (i.e., Celtic) ancestry, such as from northern Alabama.[105] The HLA-DR2 associations were more likely to be seen in central or Eastern Europe,[107] or in U.S. populations containing a high proportion of patients of central or eastern European ancestry, such as in Baltimore, Maryland[100] (Table 2).

The HLA-B8, -DR3 association with SLE takes on a different interpretation when this haplotype was linked to a C4A null allele (C4A*Q0), which in turn was more highly correlated with SLE in reports from Britain,[108] the U.S.,[109,110] and Australia.[111] Subsequent reports have confirmed the HLA-DR3 association with SLE per se to be largely explained by the presence of the C4A gene deletion, linked in Caucasians to the HLA-B8, -DR3 haplotype.[105,112,113] One recent study of an extremely large number of SLE families, in fact, has implicated the presence of the C4A gene deletion and not C4A null alleles *per se* to be the risk factor for SLE.[107]

b. MHC Class II and Class III Associations in American Blacks

Initial reports of serologic typing analyses in small numbers of patients found weak associations with HLA-DR2 and -DR3 in American blacks.[114-116] Subsequent studies examining larger numbers of patients with either serologic typing[117] or RFLP analyses[118] failed to document any HLA-DR association. However, more recent analysis using oligotyping in our own laboratory has suggested that SLE in American blacks is associated with HLA-DRB1*1503, a DR2 subtype unique to blacks.[119-121] However, as in Caucasians, susceptibility to SLE has been associated with C4A null alleles, as well as with the same C4A gene deletion that has been found on HLA-B8, -DR3 haplotypes, although in Blacks associated with HLA-B44 and -DR2.[110,122]

c. MHC Class II and Class III Associations in Asians

HLA-DR2 has been associated with SLE in both Chinese[123] and Japanese.[124,125] However, as in other groups, C4A null alleles have (at least in Chinese) been associated with SLE, although not associated with HLA-DR3 haplotypes.[126]

d. Autoantibody Subsets and HLA Class II Associations

The function of HLA class II antigens is in the presentation of processed antigens to the T cell receptor (TCR). Thus, many have proposed that HLA-DR or -DQ associations with SLE are better explained by autoantibody subsets (Figure 3).

The anti-Ro/SSA and anti-La/SSB autoantibody responses — The anti-Ro autoantibody response (with or without anti-La) is present in about 40 to 50% of patients with SLE and has been associated with vasculitis, sicca symptoms, photosensitive skin rashes, and greater serologic reactivity in the setting of SLE. Other ''variants'' of SLE

Table 2 **HLA-DR Specificities in Systemic Lupus Erythematosus Patients and Controls in Different Racial and Ethnic Groups**

Study	Racial or Ethnic Group	Location	HLA-DR Association	Frequency in Patients (%)	Frequency in Controls (%)	Odds Ratio
So et al.[104]	Whites	England	DR3[a]	51	25	3.1
Dunckley et al.[103]	Whites	Australia	DR3[a]	54	36	2.1
Gomez-Reino et al.[270]	Whites	Spain	DR3	45	27	2.2
Lulli et al.[271]	Whites	Rome	DR3	32	12	3.4
Hartung et al.[107]	Whites	Germany	DR2[b]	44	29	2.0
Reveille et al.[105]	Whites	Alabama	DR3[a]	52	29	2.6
Ahearn et al.[100]	Whites	Baltimore	DR2[b]	40	28	1.7
Fronek et al.[272]	Whites	California	DR2	46	20	2.7
Barron et al.[196]	American blacks	Southern U.S.	DR2	49	28	2.5
Doherty et al.[273]	Chinese	Malaysia	DR2	52	18	4.8
Hashimoto et al.[124]	Japanese	Japan	DR2	47	28	2.2

[a]HLA-DR3 associations found to be associated with the presence of C4A gene deletions. [b]HLA-DR3 was also increased in these groups, associated with a C4A gene deletion.

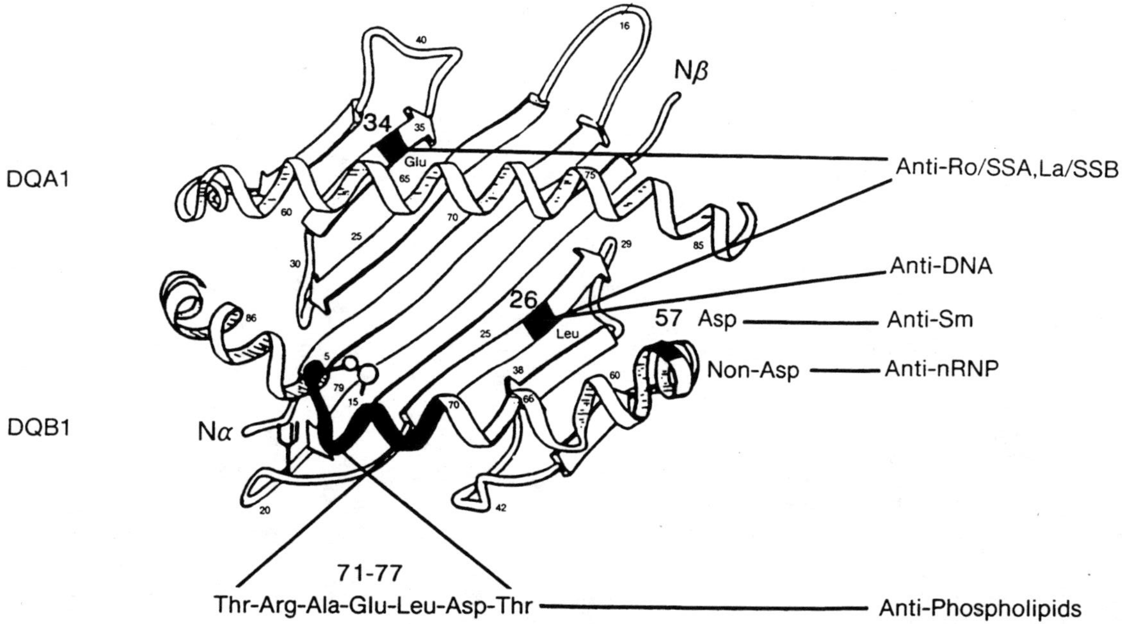

Figure 3 Schematic representation of a proposed model of the MHC or HLA class II molecule, here representing HLA-DQ. The position of amino acid residues implicated in specific autoantibody responses in SLE are indicated in black, such as *Thr-Arg-Ala-Glu-Leu-Asp-Thr (TRAELDT),* spanning residues 71 to 77 of the HLA-DQB1 outermost domain, and the anti-phospholipid (lupus anticoagulant) response. Also shown are the associations of a *glutamine* at position 34 (*Gln*-34) of the HLA-DQA1 outermost domain and a *leucine* at position 26 (*Leu*-26) of the HLA-DQB1 chain and the anti-Ro/La autoantibody responses, the latter and the anti-DNA autoantibody response, and the presence or absence of an *aspartic acid* residue at position 57 of the HLA-DQB1 chain for the anti-Sm vs anti-RNP autoantibody responses, respectively.

associated with anti-Ro and -La autoantibodies include neonatal LE, an inflammatory disorder of neonates characterized by transient cutaneous lesions and/or congenital heart block,[127] as well as the lupus-like syndrome associated with congenital C2 deficiency[128] and subacute cutaneous LE.[129] Previous studies have correlated anti-Ro and -La with HLA-DR3.[100] The highest levels of anti-Ro have been found in those who are heterozygous for the broad serologic specificities HLA-DQw1 and -DQw2.[130] More recently, using RFLP analysis, heterozygosity for specific subtypes of HLA-DQw1 and DQw2, namely HLA-DQw2.1 and -DQw6, was most highly associated with the anti-Ro/La autoantibody responses in both Caucasians and American blacks.[131] A subsequent study of oligotyping for HLA-DRB1, -DQA1, and -DQB1 alleles was able to account for all patients with these autoantibody responses by the presence of a *glutamine* at position 34 of the DQA1 and a *leucine* at position 26 of the DQB1 outermost domains.[132]

Anti-Sm, U1 RNP — The genetics of the U1-RNP and anti-Sm (the latter highly specific for SLE) autoantibody responses has been less well defined. Serologic and RFLP typing have suggested associations of anti-U1-RNP (especially its 70-kDa component) with HLA-DR4.[105,133-135] Work from our own group has suggested anti-Sm to be most closely associated with HLA-DQB1*0602 and -DQA1*0102, which comprise HLA-DQw6 on many -DR2 haplotypes.[136]

The lupus anticoagulant and anti-cardiolipin antibodies — This autoantibody response has been linked in SLE patients with arterial or venous thrombosis, miscarriages, thrombocytopenia, and cardiac valvular disease.[137] Serologic typing data have reported associations of anti-cardiolipin antibodies (associated with the lupus anticoagulant) with HLA-DR4, -DR7, and -DRw53.[138-140] One recent study using RFLP analysis correlated the presence of the lupus anticoagulant with HLA-DQw7.[141]

3. Sjögren's Syndrome

a. Serologic Typing in Different Ethnic Groups

Evidence that genetic factors are operative in predisposition to Sjögren's syndrome (SS) include: (1) numerous reports of familial aggregation, as well as (2) the finding of an increased frequency of other autoimmune diseases and autoantibodies in family members of SS patients (summarized in Reference 142). The original studies of HLA class II antigen frequencies in Caucasian patients with SS showed associations with HLA-DR3 in primary SS and -DR4 in patients with SS associated with RA.[143-145] Subsequent studies reported associations in different groups with HLA-DR2[146] and DRw52.[147] Fewer studies have been carried out in other ethnic groups, although one in a limited number of American blacks also showed an increased frequency of HLA-DR3[147] and another in Greek SS patients showed HLA-DR5.[148] Finally, studies in Japanese patients with both primary and RA-associated SS have suggested the HLA-DRB4 allele DRw53 (DRB4*0101) to be the strongest risk factor in that population.[149] Thus, studies from different ethnic groups have yielded inconsistent results.

b. Molecular Genetic Analyses of Autoantibody Subsets of SS

However, as in SLE, examination of autoantibody subsets in SS allows a different and more consistent interpretation of the SS-HLA associations. Specifically, the anti-Ro/La autoantibody responses occur in the majority of SS patients, and are associated in SS with the presence of vasculitis, cytopenias, hyperglobulinemia, and rheumatoid factor.[150] In SS, like in SLE, the anti-Ro/La autoantibody response is associated with HLA-DR3

(DRw17), DRw52a, DQw2.1 haplotypes, and even more specifically with heterozygosity for HLA-DQw2.1/DQw6.[150,151] In fact, primary SS patients lacking these autoantibodies show similar frequencies of these HLA specificities to controls.[150] Moreover, the presence of these autoantibodies is entirely explained by the presence of HLA-DQA1 and -DQB1 containing the *glutamine*-34 and *leucine*-26 residues described above. Thus, in SS, as in SLE, the HLA class II associations can be better explained by autoantibody subsets of the disease.

4. Progressive Systemic Sclerosis (PSS)

a. Associations of Class I, II, and III Specificities with PSS

Progressive systemic sclerosis (PSS) encompasses a spectrum of diseases characterized by skin thickening (scleroderma), frequently accompanied by widespread visceral fibrosis with sometimes critical pulmonary, cardiac, gastrointestinal, and renal involvement. The cause of PSS is unknown, although both environmental and genetic factors have been implicated in pathogenesis. A variety of studies have reported PSS associations with class I MHC specificities, including HLA-A9,[152,153] -B8,[154,155] and -B35.[156] Class II associations thus far reported include HLA-DR1, -DR3,[155,157] and -DR5.[156,158,159] Two reports also noted class III MHC associations, specifically with C4 null alleles.[157,160] These associations have generally been weak and inconsistent between different centers, with some reports failing to find any significant HLA association with PSS.[161-165]

b. Autoantibody Subsets of PSS

Given the putative role of class II MHC heterodimers in the presentation of processed antigen to the TCR, it would not be surprising to find that autoantibody subsets of PSS showed stronger and more consistent associations with class II MHC polymorphisms (Figure 4).

Anti-centromere antibodies (ACA) — The ACA response has been associated with limited skin and visceral involvement, including the CREST variant of PSS (subcutaneous *C*alcinosis, *R*aynaud's phenomenon, *E*sophageal dysmotility, *S*clerodactyly, and *T*elangiectasia), and usually portends a better prognosis.[166,167] An increased frequency of HLA-DR1 has been found in PSS patients with ACA in some reports using serologic typing.[167,168] The latter of these two reports also reported ACA to be associated with DR4 and DRw8.[168] Another study, determining HLA alleles by RFLP analysis, found ACA to be associated with HLA-DR5 (DRw11) and DQw7.[169] More recent data, however, using oligotyping have reported the ACA response to be entirely explained by the presence of HLA-DQB1 alleles having a polar *glycine* or *tyrosine* at position 26 of the first domain (including HLA-DQB1*0301, *0501–*0503, *0601, and *0402), suggesting this to form the candidate epitope for the ACA response.[170]

Anti-topoisomerase I (anti-Scl-70) — This autoantibody response, highly specific for PSS, has been correlated with widespread cutaneous involvement, is more common in non-Caucasians,[171] and has been associated with the serologically defined HLA-DR2[165] and -DR5.[168] A recent study using DNA typing has linked this autoantibody response primarily to the broad specificity HLA-DQw3.[172]

Anti-nucleolar (anti-PM-Scl) — Anti-nucleolar antibodies occurring in about 15% of patients with PSS encompass encompasses a heterogeneous group of autoantibodies directed against different nucleolar antigens. The best-described of these, anti-PM-Scl, had been linked to myositis occurring in the setting of PSS[173] and has a 100% association with HLA-DR3.[168]

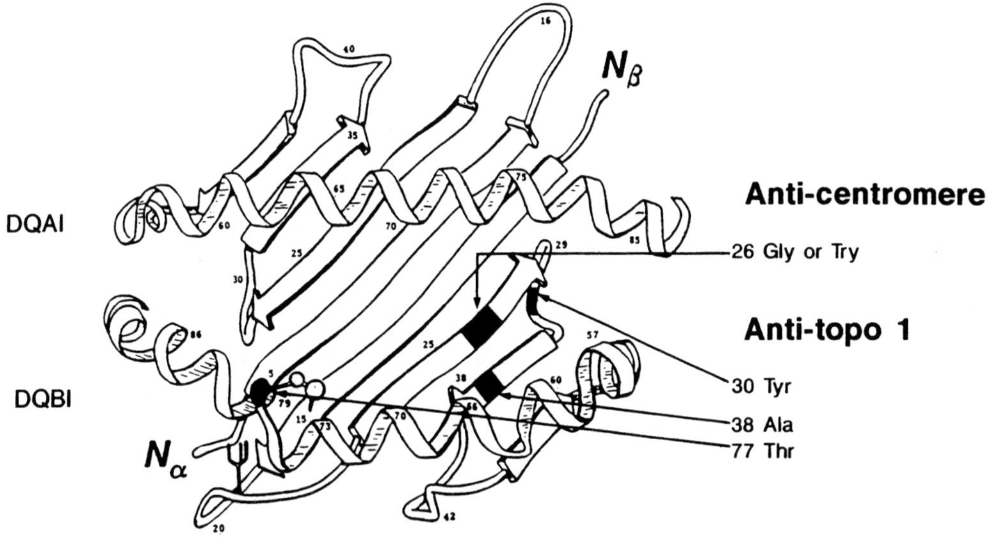

Figure 4 Schematic representation of a proposed model of the MHC or HLA class II molecule, here representing HLA-DQ. The position of amino acid residues implicated in specific autoantibody responses in systemic sclerosis, such as the anti-centromere antibody (ACA) response, is associated with the presence of a polar amino acid residue at position 26 of the HLA-DQB1 chain. The anti-topoisomerase autoantibody response is associated with the presence of a *tyrosine* at position 30 or the *Thr-Arg-Ala-Glu-Leu-Asp-Thr* (*TRAELDT*) sequence spanning positions 71 to 77 of the HLA-DQB1 outermost domain. (Modified after References 168 and 171.)

5. Dermato/Polymyositis (DM/PM)

Like the other systemic connective tissue diseases the inflammatory myopathies comprise a heterogeneous group of disorders. The most widely used of the current classifications is that of Bohan and Peter,[174] in which five groups have been proposed.

a. Dermatomyositis in Adults

HLA studies in this disorder thus far have been inconclusive, with data in Caucasians ranging from no HLA associations at all[175] to HLA-DR3.[176]

b. Polymyositis (PM)

The most consistent association has been with HLA-DR3 (DRw17),[175,176] although even these data have lacked consistency between different groups studied.[176] More consistency emerged when autoantibody subsets of PM were considered. Studies over the past decade have suggested that the presence of specific autoantibodies in PM may have clinical significance, such as the association of the aminoacyl tRNA synthetase antibodies (especially anti-Jo-1 (histidyl tRNA synthetase)) with interstitial lung disease and arthritis occurring in the setting of PM.[177-184] Previous studies, using serologic typing, suggested that the HLA-DR3 association with PM was better explained by the more specific correlation with anti-Jo-1 autoantibodies.[185] A more recent study, using RFLP typing and studying Caucasians and American blacks, found the presence of the amino acid sequence EYSTS in codons 9–13 of the HLA-DRB1 outermost domain to be present in 100% of those with anti-Jo-1 autoantibodies.[186] This sequence is found in HLA-DR3, -DR5, and -DRw6 specificities. An even more recent study using oligotyping has suggested that HLA-DQA1*0501 may be the class II allele most highly correlated with these autoantibodies in PM.[187]

c. Dermato/Polymyositis in Children

After early studies suggested in an association with HLA-DR3, juvenile DM/PM has more recently likewise been associated with HLA-DQA1*0501,[188] which is found on HLA-DR3, and most -DR5-bearing haplotypes.

d. DM/PM Associated with Malignancy

This rare subset has not been convincingly studied regarding HLA-associations.

e. DM/PM Occurring in the Presence of Another Connective Tissue Disease (CTD)

Inflammatory myopathy occurring in CTDs, such as SLE or PSS, usually is associated with specific autoantibodies, such as anti-U1-RNP and anti-PM-Scl, discussed above.

6. Juvenile Rheumatoid Arthritis (JRA)

This actually comprises a heterogeneous group of diseases, subclassified by clinical and laboratory characteristics such as the number of joints involved, the presence of systemic features, the age at disease onset, sex, the presence of anti-nuclear antibodies (ANA) and/or serum rheumatoid factor.[189] Pauciarticular JRA, often associated with ANA and occasionally with iridocyclitis, has been associated with HLA-DR5 (DRw11), -DRw8 (DRB1*0801), and DPw2.1 (DPB1*0201).[190-194] Polyarticular JRA, seronegative for rheumatoid arthritis, has been associated with DRw8 (DRB1*0801), DQw4, and DPw3 (DPB1*0301).[195-197] Polyarticular JRA, seropositive for rheumatoid factor, is associated with the same HLA-DR4 subtypes as in adult RA (DRB1*0401, *D404, *0408).[196,197]

B. ENDOCRINE DISEASES

Insulin-dependent diabetes mellitus (IDDM) — Also known as type I diabetes mellitus or, classically (and inaccurately), juvenile-onset diabetes mellitus, IDDM is postulated as an autoimmune disease on the basis of immune-mediated destruction of the beta cells in the islets of Langerhans and the presence of anti-beta cell antibodies.[198,199] The association of IDDM with HLA antigens has been an evolving story, reflecting the growth of knowledge of the complexity of the MHC. HLA-DR3 and/or -DR4 have been implicated in studies from most ethnic groups.[200-207] HLA-DR2 has been found to confer protection against IDDM.[208,209] Moreover, heterozygosity for HLA-DR3/DR4 markedly increases the risk for this disease.[210,211] But the finding that these two DR specificities share no unique sequences, the growing awareness of the rich polymorphism at the HLA-DQα and DQβ loci and the availability of molecular typing has implicated position 57 in the third hypervariable region of the HLA-DQB1 and position 52 in the third hypervariable region of the HLA-DQA1 outermost domains in susceptibility to IDDM,[212,213] an association that crosses racial and ethnic lines.[214]

C. NEUROLOGIC DISEASES

Myasthenia gravis — This autoimmune disease, characterized by muscle weakness and anti-acetylcholine receptor antibodies, has been consistently associated in Caucasians with HLA-B8, -DR3 haplotypes.[215-218] More recent studies in Chinese have found associations with HLA-Bw46, -DR9 haplotypes.[219,220]

Narcolepsy — This disorder, in which any possible autoimmune role in pathogenesis is unclear, has been consistently associated with HLA-DR2 (DRB1*1501) in Caucasians,[221-225] American blacks,[226] and Japanese.[227]

Multiple sclerosis (MS) — In studies of Caucasians from the U.S. and Europe MS has consistently been associated with HLA-DR2.[226,228-236] Other reports from Israel,[237] Japan,[238] and southern China[239] have shown this association not to cross further racial and ethnic lines. Furthermore, family studies and sib pair analysis have not shown the susceptibility to MS to consistently segregate with HLA haplotypes. Thus, the role of HLA specificities in predisposition to MS remains to be defined.

D. DERMATOLOGIC DISEASE

Pemphigus vulgaris and foliaceus — Pemphigus is an autoimmune disease of the skin characterized by bullae and weeping erosions and associated with circulating autoantibodies against the intracellular substances of the epidermis. It is most common in middle-aged persons of Jewish descent, as well as Brazilians and Japanese. Two types of pemphigus have been studied immunogenetically. Pemphigus vulgaris (PV), the more common type and associated with significant mortality, is associated with HLA-DR4 in Jewish and Japanese patients.[240,241] Studies in Jewish patients have most specifically implicated the HLA-DRB1*0402 subtype of -DR4.[242] Among non-Jewish Caucasians, the DRB1*1401 subtype of DRw6 is increased in frequency.[242] More recent data have suggested the HLA-DQB1 locus alleles might be more highly associated with PV,[242,243] specifically HLA-DQw7 (DQB1*0301) and -DQw5. Another study in Japanese patients found PV to be also associated with HLA-DRw12 and -DQw7 and negatively associated with -DR2.[244] Pemphigus foliaceus (PF) is characterized by more superficial bullae and a better prognosis. In Brazilian patients with PF it has been associated with the DRB1*0102 subtype of HLA-DR1, which differs from other -DR1 alleles at position 86 in the third hypervariable region.[245] It is noteworthy, however, that HLA-DR1 is in linkage disequilibrium with HLA-DQw5. Among Japanese PF patients, HLA-DRw6, -DQw5 haplotypes were increased.[240]

Alopecia areata (AA) — AA is a dermatologic disorder characterized by either limited patchy hair loss (alopecia areata), loss of all scalp hair (alopecia totalis), or of all body hair (alopecia universalis). It is postulated to be an autoimmune disorder on the basis of being associated with other autoimmune diseases[246] and because there is an inflammatory infiltrate of activated T cells surrounding the hair follicles.[247] Reports using serologic typing,[248-250] RFLP typing,[251] and primed lymphocyte testing[252] have shown increased frequencies of HLA-DR4, -DR5 (DRw11), and -DPw4. One of these suggested that HLA-DR4 and -DR5, which share no common unique sequences, are increased in frequency in AA patients only because of the near-absence of HLA-DRw52a (DRB3*0101) and that the latter may confer protection against AA.[251]

Dermatitis herpetiformis — This disorder has been, in Caucasians, most consistently associated with HLA-DR3, particularly on HLA-A1, -B8, -DR3, -DQw2 haplotypes.[253-257]

Vitiligo — Vitiligo is an acquired idiopathic loss of pigmentation (hypomelanosis) characterized by pale white macules that usually enlarge over time. It is felt to have an autoimmune etiology by many on the basis of: (1) the increased frequency in patients with autoimmune disease (8 to 15%), compared to the general population (1%), and the increased frequency of autoantibodies in vitiligo patients. Vitiligo has been associated with HLA-B13 in French patients[258] and Moroccan Jews,[259] -B35 in Yemenite Jews,[260] and, more recently, with HLA-DR4 in American blacks[261] and Caucasians.[261] More recently, it was proposed that extended HLA haplotypes may mark a different age at vitiligo onset, including HLA-DR5 (DRw11), -DQw3, *BfS; *C4A3, C4B1 haplotypes in those with pediatric onset and HLA-DR7, -DQw2, *BfS, *C4A3, *C4B1 in those with adult onset vitiligo.[262]

Epidermolysis bullosa acquisita (EBA) — This is a rare, chronic blistering disease characterized by circulating and tissue-bound IgG autoantibodies against the basement membrane zone of stratified squamous epithelium. The EBA autoantibody has also been described in patients with bullous lupus erythematosus. HLA-DR2 has been associated with EBA autoantibodies in Caucasians and American blacks.[263]

E. CELIAC DISEASE

Most studies of HLA antigens in celiac disease (gluten-sensitive enteropathy) have shown association with HLA-DR3, particularly on HLA-A1, -B8, -DR3 haplotypes.[257,264-267] Some of these have secondarily implicated HLA-DR7[265,266] (usually in combination with -DR3 or -DR5), including some showing HLA-DR3/DR7 heterozygotes having the highest risk. It is noteworthy that HLA-DR3 and DR7 are both linked to HLA-DQB1. In fact more recent studies have implicated the HLA-DQA1*0501, DQB1*0201 heterodimer as most important in susceptibility to celiac disease,[267] whether encoded in cis (from the same chromosome), such as on an HLA-DR3, -DQw2.1 haplotype, or in trans (from different chromosomes), such as from an individual heterozygous for HLA-DR5, -DQw7 (contributing the DQA1*0501) and HLA-DR7, -DQw2.2 (contributing the DQB1*0201 allele). HLA-DPB1 alleles have also been implicated,[268,269] but this finding could not be confirmed in other studies.

F. TYPING FOR CLASS II MHC ALLELES IN CLINICAL PRACTICE

The potential clinical usefulness of typing for HLA-B27, albeit limited, has already been discussed. There are, likewise, few indications to type for MHC class II or class III alleles in clinical practice. The main exception is in rheumatoid arthritis, where the determination of homozygosity for HLA-DR4, or more specifically, for the so-called "rheumatoid epitope" may indeed impact on therapy. Since homozygous RA patients seem to be at risk for more aggressive disease, earlier and more aggressive disease-modulating or immunosuppressive therapy may be in order in such individuals. Another possible application of class II typing would be in the confirmation of a diagnosis of narcolepsy, given the 100% association with HLA-DR2. But given the 20 to 25% frequency of this specificity in Caucasian controls, even this would be of limited value.

IV. CONCLUSION

The story of HLA and disease associations is rapidly evolving, and the very near future should clarify some of these situations where the disease association is less easy to explain, as well as to clarify situations that are more straightforward, as function, polymorphism, and disease associations of some of the more recently described MHC genes that have only recently been discovered become clear (such as HLA-E, -F, and -G in the class I region or the transport assisting proteins [TAP] or large-molecular-weight proteasome [LMP] in the class II region or, in the class III region, the heat shock protein 70 [HSP], RD or the B-associated transcript [BAT] genes).

Finally, with the precise characterization of the specific contribution to disease pathogenesis provided by each MHC gene family, more rational approaches to therapy could be attempted. For example, with the determination of the crucial amino acids involved in the binding of the antigenic fragment in the peptide groove in class I and II molecules, attempts at blocking (using monoclonal antibodies) or, in other instances, promoting this binding could be designed that might attenuate disease expression in an HLA-B27-positive individual with a spondyloarthropathy, or the production of anti-Ro antibodies in a pregnant mother with a history of a previous child with neonatal lupus, or anti-cardiolipin antibodies in a patient with recurrent arterial or venous thromboses. In the approximately 20 years that have passed since the original definitive descriptions of HLA and disease association we have come a long way. What lies ahead appears exciting indeed.

REFERENCES

1. **Schlosstein, L., Terasaki, P. I., Bluestone, R., and Pearson, C. M.M.,** High association of an HL-A antigen, W27, with ankylosing spondylitis, *N. Engl. J. Med.*, 288, 704, 1973.
2. **Brewerton, D. A., Hart, F. D., Nichols, A., Caffrey, M., James, D. C. O., and Sturrock, R. D.,** Ankylosing spondylitis and HL-A27, *Lancet*, I, 904, 1973.
3. **McClusky, O. E., Lordon, R. E., and Arnett, F. C., Jr.,** HL-A 27 in Reiter's syndrome and psoriatic arthritis: a genetic factor in disease susceptibility and expression, *J. Rheumatol.*, 1, 263, 1974.
4. **Chan, S. H., Satkunananthan, K., Wee, G. B., Seinivan, N., and Chacha, P.,** HLA-B27 and Chinese ankylosing spondylitis, *Singapore Med. J.*, 21, 710, 1980.

5. **Sengupta, S., Sehgal, S., Aikat, B. K., Deodhar, S. D., and James, D. C.,** HLA-B27 in ankylosing spondylitis in India, *Lancet,* I, 1209, 1977.
6. **Al-Rawi, Z. S., Al-Shakarchi, H. A., Hasan, F., and Thewaini, A. J.,** Ankylosing spondylitis and its association with the histocompatibility antigen HLA-B27: an epidemiological and clinical study, *Rheumatol. Rehabil.,* 17, 72, 1978.
7. **Davatchi, F., Nikbin, B., and Ala, F.,** Histocompatibility antigen (HLA) in rheumatic diseases in Iran, *J. Rheumatol.,* 3(Suppl. 4), 36, 1977.
8. **Brautbar, C., Porat, S., Nelken, D., Gabriel, K. R., and Cohen, T.,** HLA-B27 and ankylosing spondylitis in the Israeli population, *J. Rheumatol.,* 4(Suppl. 3), 24, 1977.
9. **Fraga, A., Gorodezky, C., Lavalle, C., Castro-Escobar, L. E., Magana, L., and Escobar-Guiterrez, A.,** HLA-B27 in Mexican patients with ankylosing spondylitis, *Arthritis Rheum.,* 22, 302, 1979.
10. **Arnett, F. C., Jr., Schacter, B. Z., Hochberg, M. C., Hsu, S. H., and Bias, W. B.,** Homozygosity for HLA-B27. Impact on rheumatic disease expression in two families, *Arthritis Rheum.,* 20, 797, 1977.
11. **Arnett, F. C., Jr., Hochbert, M. C., and Bias, W. B.,** Cross-reactive HLA antigens in B27-negative Reiter's syndrome and sacroiliitis, *Johns Hopkins Med. J.,* 141, 193, 1977.
12. **Edmonds, J., Bashir, H., Thomson, G., and Carbonara, A. O.,** HLA-B27-negative ankylosing spondylitis, in *Histocompatibility Testing,* Albert, E. D., Ed., Springer-Verlag, Berlin, 1984, 388.
13. **Robinson, H. S., Gofton, J. P., and Price, G. E.,** A study of rheumatic disease in a Canadian Indian population, *Ann. Rheum. Dis.,* 22, 232, 1963.
14. **Gofton, J. P., Chalmers, A., Price, G. E., and Reeve, C. E.,** HL-A27 and ankylosing spondylitis in B. C. Indians, *J. Rheumatol.,* 2, 314, 1975.
15. **Sonozaki, H., Seki, H., Chang, S., Okuyama, M., and Juji, T.,** Human lymphocyte antigen, HL-A27, in Japanese patients with ankylosing spondylitis, *Tissue Antigens,* 5, 131, 1975.
16. **Tsujimoto, M.,** Epidemiological research on the prevalence of ankylosing spondylitis, *Med. J. Osaka Univ.,* 28, 363, 1978.
17. **Chalmers, I. M.,** Ankylosing spondylitis in African blacks, *Arthritis Rheum.,* 23, 1366, 1980.
18. **Hill, A. V. S., Allsopp, C. E. M., Kwiatkowski, D., Anstey, N. M., Greenwood, B. M., and McMichael, A. J.,** HLA class I typing by PCR: HLA-B27 and an African B27 subtype, *Lancet,* 337, 640, 1991.
19. **Payne, R., Feldman, M., Cann, H., and Bodmer, J. G.,** A comparison of HLA data of the North American black with North American caucasoid populations, *Tissue Antigens,* 9, 135, 1977.
20. **Baum, J. and Ziff, M.,** The rarity of ankylosing spondylitis in the black race, *Arthritis Rheum.,* 14, 12, 1971.
21. **Khan, M. A., Braun, W. E., Kushner, I., Grecek, D. E., Muir, W. A., and Steinberg, A. G.,** HLA B27 in ankylosing spondylitis: differences in frequency and relative risk in American Blacks and Caucasians, *J. Rheumatol.,* 4, 39, 1977.
22. **Good, A. E., Kawanishi, H., and Schultz, J. S.,** HLA B27 in blacks with ankylosing spondylitis or Reiter's syndrome, *N. Engl. J. Med.,* 294, 166, 1976.
23. **Lawrence, J. S.,** Epidemiologie de la polyarthrite rhumatoide, *Rev. Med.,* 10, 1, 1963.

24. **van der Linden, S. M., Valkenburg, H. A., deJongh, B. M., and Cats, A.,** The risk of developing ankylosing spondylitis in HLA-B27 positive individuals. A comparison of relatives of spondylitis patients with the general population, *Arthritis Rheum.*, 27, 241, 1984.
25. **Suarez-Almazor, M. E., Russell, A. S., and LeClercq, S.,** Ankylosing spondylitis in families with two distinct B27 haplotypes: a selective association, *Arthritis Rheum.*, 29, 1510, 1986.
26. **McDaniel, D. O., Acton, R. T., Barger, B. O., Koopman, W. J., and Reveille, J. D.,** Association of a 9.2-kilobase PvuII class I major histocompatibility complex restriction fragment length polymorphism with ankylosing spondylitis, *Arthritis Rheum.*, 30, 894, 1987.
27. **Reveille, J. D., Koopman, W. J., Barger, B. O., Acton, R. T., and McDaniel, D. O.,** Restriction fragment length polymorphism analysis in ankylosing spondylitis, *Am. J. Med.*, 85(Suppl.), 48, 1988.
28. **Ahearn, J. M., Calomiris, J. J., Wigley, F. M., Jabs, D. A., and Bias, W. B.,** Characterization of the class I 9.2 kb PvuII restriction fragment length polymorphism (RFLP): linkage to HLA-A and lack of disease association, *Arthritis Rheum.*, 320, 870, 1989.
29. **Durand, J. P. and Taurog, J. D.,** Association between AS and a 9.2 kb PvuII class I HLA DNA restriction fragment, *J. Rheumatol.*, 115, 1119, 1988.
30. **Hammer, R. E., Maika, S. D., Richardson, J. A., Tang, J.-P., and Taurog, J. D.,** Spontaneous inflammatory disease in transgenic rats expressing HLA-B27 and human beta2m: an animal model of HLA-B27-associated human disorders, *Cell,* 63, 1099, 1990.
31. **Yu, D. T. Y., Choo, S. Y., and Schaack, T.,** Molecular mimicry in HLA-B27 related arthritis, *Ann. Intern. Med.*, 111, 581, 1989.
32. **Inman, R. D., Chiu, B., Johnston, M. E. A., Vas, S., and Falk, J.,** HLA-class I-related impairment of IL-2 production and lymphocyte response to microbial antigens in reactive arthritis, *J. Immunol.*, 142, 4256, 1989.
33. **Ishikawa, H., Ohno, O., Yamasaki, K., Ikuta, S., and Hirohata, K.,** Arthritis presumably caused by Chlamydia in Reiter's syndrome, *J. Bone Jt. Surg.*, 68, 777, 1986.
34. **Keat, A., Dixey, J., Sonnex, C., Thomas, B., Osborne, M., and Taylor-Robinson, D.,** Chlamydia trachomatis and reactive arthritis: the missing link, *Lancet,* i, 72, 1987.
35. **Granfors, K., Jalkanen, S., VonEssen, R., Lahesmaa-Rantala, R., Isomaki, O., Pekkola-Heinoi, K., Merilahti-Palo, R., Saario, R., Isomaki, H., and Toivanen, A.,** Yersinia antigens in synovial fluid cells from patients with reactive arthritis, *N. Engl. J. Med.*, 320, 216, 1989.
36. **Granfors, K., Jalkanen, S., Lindberg, A. A., Maki-Ikola, O., VanEssen, R., Lahesmaa-Rantala, R., Isomaki, H., Saario, R., Arnold, W. J., and Toivanen, A.,** Salmonella lipopolysaccharide in synovial cells from patients with reactive arthritis, *Lancet,* 335, 685, 1990.
37. **Schwimmbeck, P. L., Yu, D. T. Y., and Oldstone, M. B. A.,** Autoantibodies to HLA-B27 in sera of HLA-B27 patients with ankylosing spondylitis and Reiter's syndrome, *J. Exp. Med.*, 166, 173, 1987.
38. **Steiglitz, H., Fosmire, S., and Lipsky, P.,** Identification of a 2-Md plasmid from Shigella flexneri associated with reactive arthritis, *Arthritis Rheum.*, 32, 937, 1989.

39. **Madden, D. R., Gorga, J. C., Strominger, J. L., and Wiley, D. C.,** The structure of HLA-B27 reveals nonamer self-peptides bound in an extended conformation, *Nature,* 353, 321, 1991.
40. **Jardetzky, T. S., Lane, W. S., Robinson, R. A., Madden, D. R., and Wiley, D. C.,** Identification of self peptides bound to purified HLA-B27, *Nature,* 353, 326, 1991.
41. **Matsumura, M., Fremont, D. H., Peterson, P. A., and Wilson, I. A.,** Emerging principles for the emerging recognition of peptide antigens by MHC class I molecules, *Science,* 257, 927, 1992.
42. **Benjamin, R. and Parham, P.,** Guilt by association: HLA-B27 and ankylosing spondylitis, *Immunol. Today,* 11, 137, 1990.
43. **Choo, S. Y., Fan, L. A., and Hansen, J. A.,** A novel HLA-B27 allele maps B27 allospecificity to the region around position 70 in the alpha 1 domain, *J. Immunol.,* 147, 174, 1991.
44. **MacLean, L.,** HLA-B27 subtypes: implications for the spondyloarthropathies, *Ann. Rheum. Dis.,* 51, 929, 1992.
45. **Rojo, S., Aparicio, P., Choo, S. Y., Hansen, J. A., and Lopez de Castro, J. A.,** Structural analysis of an HLA-B27 population variant: B27f: multiple patterns of amino acid changes within a single polypeptide segment generate polymorphism in HLA-B27, *J. Immunol.,* 139, 831, 1987.

45a. **Choo, S. Y.,** personal communication.

46. **Russel, J. J., Schultes, L. M., and Kuben, D. J.,** Histocompatibility (HLA) antigens associated with psoriasis, *N. Engl. J. Med.,* 287, 738, 1972.
47. **White, S. H., Newcomer, V. D., Mickey, M. R., and Terasaki, P. I.,** Disturbance of HL-A antigen frequency in psoriasis, *N. Engl. J. Med.,* 287, 740, 1972.
48. **Svejgaard, A., Staub-Nielsen, L., Svejgaard, E., Kissmeyer-Nielsen, F., Hjortshoj, A., and Zachariae, H.,** HL-A in psoriasis vulgaris and pustular psoriasis — population and family studies, *Br. J. Dermatol.,* 91, 145, 1974.
49. **Benevolenskaia, L. I., Erdes, S. H., Iakovleva, D. B., and Groppa, L. P.,** Antigeny gistosovmestimosti pri psoriaticheskum seronegativnom revmatoidnom artritakh, *Ter. Arkh.,* 58, 17, 1986.
50. **Pitchappan, R. M., Koteeswaran, A., Kakkaniah, V. N., Manickasundari, M., Rajaram, V., Muthuveeralakshmi, P., Mahendran, V., and Brahmajothibai, V.,** HLA Bw57 and DR7 association with psoriasis vulgaris in south India, *Tissue Antigens,* 34, 133, 1989.
51. **Sasuzuki, T., Maksushita, S., Nakamizo, Y. et al.,** HLA and psoriasis in Asian Population. Joint report in HLA, in *Asia-Oceania,* Aizawa, M., Ed., Hokkaido University Press, Sapporo, 1986, 349.
52. **Tilikainen, A., Lassus, A., Karuonen, J., Vartiainen, P., and Julin, M.,** Psoriasis and Cw6, *Br. J. Dermatol.,* 102, 179, 1980.
53. **Marcusson, J. A., Johannesson, A., and Moller, E.,** HLA A,B,C and DR antigens in psoriasis, *Tissue Antigens,* 17, 525, 1981.
54. **Batchelor, J. R. and Morris, P. J.,** HLA and disease. Joint report, in *Histocompatibility Testing 1977,* Bodmer, W. F., Ed., Munksgaard, Copenhagen, 1977, 230.
55. **Murray, C., Mann, D. L., Gerber, L. N., Barth, W., Perlmann, S., Decker, J. L., and Nigra, T. P.,** Histocompatibility alloantigens in psoriasis and psoriatic arthritis, *J. Clin. Invest.,* 66, 670, 1980.

56. **Nakagawa, H., Asahina, A., Akazaki, S., Tokunaga, K., Matsuki, K., Ishibashi, Y., and Juji, T.,** Association of Cw11 in Japanese patients with psoriasis vulgaris, *Tissue Antigens,* 36, 241, 1990.
57. **Asahina, A., Akazaki, S., Nakagawa, H., Kuwata, S., Tokunaga, K., Ishibashi, Y., and Juji, T.,** Specific nucleotide sequence of HLA-C is strongly associated with psoriasis vulgaris, *J. Invest. Dermatol.,* 97, 254, 1991.
58. **Espinoza, L. R., Vasey, F. B., Oh, J. H., Wilkinson, R., and Osterland, C. K.,** Association between HLA-BW38 and peripheral psoriatic arthritis, *Arthritis Rheum.,* 21, 72, 1978.
59. **Metzger, A. L., Morris, R. I., Bluestone, R., and Terasaki, P. I.,** HL-A W27 in psoriatic arthropathy, *Arthritis Rheum.,* 18, 111, 1975.
60. **Reveille, J. D., Conant, M. A., and Duvic, M.,** HIV-associated psoriasis, psoriatic arthritis and Reiter's syndrome: a disease continuum?, *Arthritis Rheum.,* 33, 1574, 1990.
61. **Woodrow, J. C., Mapstone, R., Anderson, J., and Usher, N.,** HL-A27 and anterior uveitis, *Tissue Antigens,* 6, 116, 1975.
62. **Dekker-Saeys, B. J., Meuwissen, S. G. M., Van Den Berg-Loonen, E. M., DeHaas, W. H. D., Meijers, K. A. F., and Tytgat, G. N. J.,** Clinical characteristics and results of histocompatibility typing (HLA B27) in 50 patients with both ankylosing spondylitis and inflammatory bowel disease, *Ann. Rheum. Dis.,* 37, 36, 1978.
63. **Russell, A. S.,** Arthritis, inflammatory bowel disease, and histocompatibility antigens, *Ann. Intern. Med.,* 86, 820, 1977.
64. **Baricordi, O. R., Sensi, A., Pivetti-Pezzi, P., Perrone, S., Balboni, A., Catarinelli, G., Filippi, F., Melchiorri, L., Moncada, A., and Mattiuz, P. L.,** Behcet's disease associated with HLA-B51 and DRw52 antigens in Italians, *Hum. Immunol.,* 17, 297, 1986.
65. **Chajek-Shaul, T., Pisanty, S., Knobler, H., Matzner, Y., Glick, M., Ron, N., Rosenman, E., and Brautbar, C.,** HLA-B51 may serve as an immunogenetic marker for a subgroup of patients with Behcet's syndrome, *Am. J. Med.,* 83, 666, 1987.
66. **Ohno, S., Anasuma, T., Sugiura, S., Wakisaka, A., and Aizawa, M.,** HLA-B51 and Behcet's disease, *JAMA,* 240, 529, 1978.
67. **Chung, Y. M., Tsai, S. T., Liao, F., and Liu, J. H.,** A genetic study of Behcet's disease in Taiwan Chinese, *Tissue Antigens,* 30, 68, 1987.
68. **Isohisa, I., Numano, F., Maezawa, H., and Sasazuki, T.,** HLA-Bw52 in Takayasu disease, *Tissue Antigens,* 12, 246, 1978.
69. **Sasazuki, T., Ohta, N., Isohisa, I., Numano, F., and Maezawa, H.,** Association between Takayasu disease and HLA-DHO, *Tissue Antigens,* 14, 177, 1979.
70. **Moriuchi, J., Wakisaka, A., and Aizawa, M.,** HLA-linked susceptibility gene of Takayasu disease, *Hum. Immunol.,* 4, 87, 1982.
71. **Numano, F., Namba, K., Susuki, K., and Matsumoto, H.,** Hereditary factors in Takayasu disease. III. Polymorphism of human complements, *Exp. Clin. Immunogenet.,* 6, 236, 1989.
72. **Dong, R. P., Kimuar, A., Numano, F., Yajima, M., Hashimoto, Y., Kishi, Y., Nishimura, Y., and Sasazuki, T.,** HLA-DP antigen and Takayasu arteritis, *Tissue Antigens,* 39, 106, 1992.
73. **Khraishi, M. M., Gladman, D. D., Dagenais, P., Fam, A. G., and Keystone, E. G.,** HLA antigens in North American patients with Takayasu arteritis, *Arthritis Rheum.,* 35, 573, 1992.

74. **Stastny, P.,** Mixed lymphocyte cultures in rheumatoid arthritis, *J. Clin. Invest.,* 57, 1148, 1976.
75. **Panayi, G. S., Wooley, P., and Batchelor, J. P.,** Genetic basis of rheumatoid disease: HLA antigens, disease manifestations, and toxic reactions to drugs, *Br. Med. J.,* 2, 1326, 1978.
76. **Roitt, I. M., Corbett, M., Festenstein, H., Jaraquemada, D., Papasteriadis, C., Hay, F. C., and Nineham, L. J.,** HLA-DRw4 and prognosis in rheumatoid arthritis, *Lancet,* 1, 990, 1978.
77. **Karr, R. W., Rodey, G. E., Lee, T., and Schwartz, B. D.,** Association of HLA-DRw4 with rheumatoid arthritis in black and white patients, *Arthritis Rheum.,* 23, 1241, 1980.
78. **Ohta, N., Nishimura, Y. K., Tanimoto, K., Horiuchi, Y., Abe, C., Shiokawa, Y., Abe, T., Katagiri, M., Yoshiki, T., and Sasazuki, T.,** Association between HLA and Japanese patients with rheumatoid arthritis, *Hum. Immunol.,* 5, 123, 1982.
79. **Malaviya, A. N., Mehra, N. K., Dasgupta, B., Khan, K. M., Rao, V. R. K., Agarwal, A., and Tiwari, S. C.,** Clinical and immunogenetic studies in rheumatoid arthritis from northern India, *Rheumatol. Int.,* 3, 105, 1983.
80. **Schiff, B., Mizrachi, Y., Orgad, S., and Giazit, E.,** Association of HLA-Aw31 and HLA-DR1 with adult rheumatoid arthritis, *Ann. Rheum. Dis.,* 41, 403, 1982.
81. **Nichol, F. E. and Woodrwo, J. C.,** HLA-DR antigens in Indian patients with rheumatoid arthritis, *Lancet,* I, 220, 1981.
82. **Wilkens, R. F., Nepom, G. T., Marks, J., Nettles, J. W., and Nepom, B. S.,** Association of HLA Dw16 in Yakima Indians: further evidence for the shared epitope hypothesis, *Arthritis Rheum.,* 34, 43, 1991.
83. **Gregersen, P. K., Silver, J., and Winchester, R. J.,** The shared epitope hypothesis. An approach to understanding the molecular genetics of susceptibility to rheumatoid arthritis, *Arthritis Rheum.,* 30, 1205, 1987.
84. **Gao, X., Brautbar, C., Gazit, E., Segal, R., Naparstok, Y., Livneh, A., and Stastny, P.,** A variant to HLA-DR4 determines susceptibility to rheumatoid arthritis in a subset of Israeli Jews, *Arthritis Rheum.,* 34, 547, 1991.
85. **Sanchez, B., Moreno, I., Magarino, R., Garzon, M., Gonzalez, M. F., Garcia, A., and Nunez-Roldan, A.,** HLA-DRw10 confers the highest susceptibility to rheumatoid arthritis in a Spanish population, *Tissue Antigens,* 36, 174, 1990.
86. **Ollier, W. E. R., Stephens, C. S., Awod, J., Carthy, D., Gupten, A., Perry, D., Javad, A., and Festenstein, H.,** Is rheumatoid arthritis associated with HLA antigens sharing a DRB1 epitope?, *Ann. Rheum. Dis.,* 50, 295, 1991.
87. **Gregersen, P. K., Shen, M., Song, Q. L., Merryman, P., Degar, S., Seki, T., Maccari, J., Goldberg, D., Murphy, H., Schwenger, J., Want, C. Y., Winchester, R. J., Nepom, G. T., and Silver, J.,** Molecular diversity of HLA-DR4 haplotypes, *Proc. Natl. Acad. Sci. U.S.A.,* 83, 2642, 1986.
88. **Albani, S., Tuckwell, J. E., Esparza, L., Carson, D. A., and Roudier, J.,** The susceptibility sequence to rheumatoid arthritis is a cross-reactive B cell epitope shared by the Escherichia coli heat shock protein dnaJ and the histocompatibility leukocyte antigen DRB10401 molecule, *J. Clin. Invest.,* 89, 327, 1992.
89. **Roudier, J., Petersen, J., Rhodes, G., Luka, J., and Carson, D.,** Susceptibility to rheumatoid arthritis maps to a T cell epitope shared by the HLA Dw4 DR beta 1 chain and the Epstein Barr virus glycoprotein gp110, *Proc. Natl. Acad. Sci. U.S.A.,* 86, 5104, 1989.

90. **Salmon, M.,** The immunogenetic component of susceptibility to rheumatoid arthritis, *Current Opin. Rheumatol.*, 4, 342, 1992.
91. **Deighton, C. M., Walker, D. J., Griffiths, I. D., and Roberts, D. F.,** The contribution of HLA to rheumatoid arthritis, *Clin. Genet.*, 36, 178, 1989.
92. **Wordsworth, B. P., Lanchbury, J. S. S., Sakkas, L. I., Welsh, K. I., Panayi, G. S., and Bell, J. I.,** HLA-DR4 subtype frequency in rheumatoid arthritis indicates that DRB1 is the major susceptibility locus within the human leucocyte antigen class II region, *Proc. Natl. Acad. Sci. U.S.A.*, 86, 10049, 1989.
93. **deJongh, B. M., Van Romunde, L. K. J., Valkenberge, H. A., De Lange, G. G., and Van Rood, J. J.,** Epidemiological study of HLA and Gm in rheumatoid arthritis and related syndromes in an open Dutch population, *Ann. Rheum. Dis.*, 13, 613, 1984.
94. **Van Zeben, D., Hazes, J. M. W., Zwinderman, A. H., Cats, A., Schreuder, G. M. T., d'Amaro, J., and Breedfeld, F. C.,** Association of HLA-DR4 with a more progressive disease course in patients with rheumatoid arthritis, *Arthritis Rheum.*, 43, 822, 1991.
95. **Weyand, C., Hicok, K., Conn, D., and Goronzy, J.,** The role of homozygosity at the HLA-DRB1 locus in determining disease severity in rheumatoid arthritis, *Arthritis Rheum.*, 34(Suppl.), S33, 1991.
96. **Nepom, B. S., Palmer, J., Kim, S. J., Hansen, J. A., Holbeck, J. A., and Nepom, G. T.,** Specific genomic markers of the HLA-DQ subregion discriminate between DR4+ insulin-dependent diabetes mellitus and DR4+ seropositive rheumatoid arthritis, *J. Exp. Med.*, 164, 345, 1986.
97. **Lanchburg, J. S. S., Jaeger, E. E. M., Sansom, D. M., Hall, M. A., Wordsworth, B. P., Stedeford, J., Bell, J. I., and Panayi, G. S.,** Strong primary selection for the Dw4 subtype of DR4 accounts for the HLA-DQw7 association with Felty's syndrome, *Hum. Immunol.*, 32, 56, 1991.
98. **Reinertsen, J. L., Klippel, J. H., Johnston, A. H., Steinberg, A. D., Decker, J. L., and Mann, D. L.,** B-lymphocyte alloantigens associated with systemic lupus erythematosus, *N. Engl. J. Med.*, 299, 1978.
99. **Gibofsky, A. M., Winchester, R. J., Patarroyo, M., Fotino, M., and Kunkel, H. G.,** Disease association of the Ia-like human alloantigens: contrasting patterns in rheumatoid arthritis and systemic lupus erythematosus, *J. Exp. Med.*, 148, 1728, 1978.
100. **Ahearn, J. M., Provost, T. T., Dorsch, C. A., Stevens, M. B., Bias, W. B., and Arnett, F. C.,** The interrelationships of HLA-DR, MB and MT phenotypes, autoantibody expression and clinical features in systemic lupus erythematosus, *Arthritis Rheum.*, 25, 1031, 1982.
101. **Scherak, O., Smolen, J. S., and Mayr, W. R.,** Prevalence of HLA-DRw2 not increased in systemic lupus erythematosus, *N. Engl. J. Med.*, 301, 612, 1979.
102. **Bell, D. A. and Maddison, P. J.,** Serologic subsets in systemic lupus erythematosus: an examination of autoantibodies in relationship to clinical features of disease and HLA antigens, *Arthritis Rheum.*, 23, 1268, 1980.
103. **Dunckley, H., Gatenby, P. A., and Serjeantson, S. W.,** DNA typing of HLA-DR antigens in systemic lupus erythematosus, *Immunogenet,* 24, 158, 1986.
104. **So, A. K. L., Fielder, A. H. L., Warner, C. A., Isenberg, D. A., Batchelor, J. R., and Walport, M. J.,** DNA polymorphism of major histocompatibility complex class II and class III genes in systemic lupus erythematosus, *Tissue Antigens,* 35, 144, 1990.

105. **Reveille, J. D., Anderson, K. L., Schrohenloher, R. E., Acton, R. T., and Barger, B. O.,** Restriction fragment length polymorphism analysis of HLA-DR, DQ, DP and C4 alleles in Caucasians with systemic lupus erythematosus, *J. Rheumatol.*, 18, 14, 1991.
106. **Whittingham, S., Matthews, J. D., Schanfield, M. S., Tait, B. D., and Mackay, I. R.,** HLA and Gm Genes in systemic lupus erythematosus, *Tissue Antigens,* 21, 50, 1983.
107. **Hartung, K., Baur, M. P., Coldewey, R., Fricke, M., Kalden, J. R., Lakomek, H. J., Peter, H. H., Schendel, D., Schneider, P. M., Seuchter, S. A., Stangel, W., and Deicher, H. R. G.,** Major histocompatibility complex haplotypes and complement C4 alleles in systemic lupus erythematosus, *J. Clin. Invest.*, 90, 1346, 1992.
108. **Fielder, A. H. L., Walport, M. J., Batchelor, J. R., Rynes, R. I., Black, C. M., Dodi, I. A., and Hughes, G. R. V.,** Family study of the major histocompatibility complex in patients with systemic lupus erythematosus: importance of null alleles of C4A and C4B in determining disease susceptibility, *Br. J. Med.*, 286, 425, 1983.
109. **Reveille, J. D., Arnett, F. C., Wilson, R. W., Bias, W. B., and McLean, R. H.,** Null alleles of the fourth component of complement and HLA haplotypes in familial systemic lupus erythematosus, *Immunogenet,* 21, 299, 1985.
110. **Howard, P. F., Hochberg, M. C., Bias, W. B., Arnett, F. C., and McLean, R. H.,** Relationship between C4 null genes, HLA-D region antigens, and genetic susceptibilities to systemic lupus erythematosus in Caucasians and black Americans, *Am. J. Med.*, 81, 187, 1986.
111. **Christiansen, F. T., Dawkins, R. L., Uko, G., McCluskey, J., Kay, P. H., and Zilko, P. J.,** Complement allotyping in SLE: association with C4A null, *Aust. NZ J. Med.*, 13, 483, 1983.
112. **Kemp, M. E., Atkinson, J. P., Skanes, V. M., Levine, R. P., and Chaplin, D. D.,** Deletion of C4A genes in patients with systemic lupus erythematosus, *Arthritis Rheum.*, 30, 1015, 1987.
113. **Goldstein, R., Arnett, F. C., McLean, R. H., Bias, W. B., and Duvic, M.,** Molecular heterogeneity of complement component C4-null and 21-hydroxylase genes in systemic lupus erythematosus, *Arthritis Rheum.*, 31, 736, 1988.
114. **Alarif, L. I., Ruppert, G. B., Wilson, R., Jr., and Varth, W. F.,** HLA-DR antigens in blacks with rheumatoid arthritis and systemic lupus erythematosus, *J. Rheumatol.*, 10, 297, 1983.
115. **Kachru, R. B., Sequeira, W., Mittal, K. K., Siegel, M. E., and Telischi, M.,** A significant increase of HLA-DR3 and DR2 in systemic lupus erythematosus among blacks, *J. Rheumatol.*, 11, 471, 1984.
116. **Wilson, W. A., Scopelitis, E., and Mikalski, J. P.,** Association of HLA-DR7 with both antibody to SSA(Ro) and disease susceptibility in blacks with systemic lupus erythematosus, *J. Rheumatol.*, 11, 653, 1985.
117. **Hochberg, M. C., Boyd, R. E., Ahearn, J. M., Arnett, F. C., Bias, W. B., Provost, T. T., and Stevens, M. B.,** Systemic lupus erythematosus: a review of clinico-laboratory features and immunogenetic markers in 150 patients, with emphasis on demographic subsets, *Medicine,* 64, 285, 1985.
118. **Reveille, J. D., Schrohenloher, R. E., Acton, R. T., and Barger, B. O.,** DNA analysis of HLA-DR and DQ genes in American blacks with systemic lupus erythematosus, *Arthritis Rheum.*, 32, 1243, 1989.

119. **Reveille, J. D., Barger, B. O., and Hodge, T. W.,** HLA-DR2-DRB1 allele frequencies in DR-positive black Americans with and without systemic lupus erythematosus, *Tissue Antigens,* 38, 178, 1991.
120. **Demopulos, J. T., Hodge, T. W., Wooten, W., and Acton, R. T.,** A novel DRB1 allele in DR2-positive American blacks, *Hum. Immunol.,* 30, 41, 1991.
121. **Barron, K. S., Silverman, E. D., Gonzales, J., Arnett, F. C., and Reveille, J. D.,** Childhood-onset systemic lupus erythematosus (SLE): a clinical, serologic and immunogenetic analysis, *Arthritis Rheum.,* in press.
122. **Olsen, M. L., Goldstein, R., Arnett, F. C., Duvic, M., Pollack, M., and Reveille, J. R.,** C4A gene deletion and HLA associations in black Americans with systemic lupus erythematosus, *Immunogenet,* 30, 27, 1989.
123. **Hawkins, B. R., Wong, K. L., Wong, R. W. S., Chan, K. H., Dunckley, H., and Serjeantson, S. W.,** Strong association between the major histocompatibility complex and systemic lupus erythematosus in Southern Chinese, *J. Rheumatol.,* 14, 1128, 1987.
124. **Hashimoto, H., Tsuda, H., Matsumoto, T., Nasu, H., Takasaki, Y., Shokawa, Y., Hirose, S., Terasaki, P. I., and Iwaki, Y.,** HLA antigens associated with systemic lupus erythematosus in Japan, *J. Rheumatol.,* 12, 919, 1985.
125. **Hirose, S., Ogawa, S., Nishimura, H., Hashimoto, H., and Shirai, T.,** Association of HLA-DR2/DR4 heterozygosity with systemic lupus erythematosus in Japanese patients, *J. Rheumatol.,* 15, 1489, 1988.
126. **Dunckley, H., Gatenby, P. A., Hawkins, B., Naito, S., and Serjeantson, S. W.,** Deficiency of C4A is a genetic determinant of systemic lupus erythematosus in three ethnic groups, *J. Immunogenet.,* 14, 209, 1987.
127. **Watson, R. M., Lane, A. T., Barnett, N. K., Bias, W. B., Arnett, F. C., and Provost, T. T.,** Neonatal lupus erythematosus: a clinical, serological and immunogenetic study with review of the literature, *Medicine,* 63, 362, 1984.
128. **Provost, T. T., Arnett, F. C., and Reichlin, M.,** Homozygous C2 deficiency, lupus erythematosus, and anti-Ro (SSA) antibodies, *Arthritis Rheum.,* 26, 1279, 1983.
129. **Sontheimer, R. D., Maddison, P. J., Reichlin, M., Jordon, R. E., Stasny, P., and Gilliam, J. N.,** Serologic and HLA associations in subacute cutaneous lupus erythematosus: a clinical subset of lupus erythematosus, *Ann. Int. Med.,* 97, 664, 1982.
130. **Hamilton, R. G., Harley, J. B., Bias, W. B., Roebber, M., Reichlin, M., Hochberg, M. C., and Arnett, F. C.,** Two Ro (SS-A) autoantibody responses in systemic lupus erythematosus: correlation of HLA-DR/DQ specificities with quantitative expression of Ro (SS-A) autoantibody, *Arthritis Rheum.,* 31, 496, 1988.
131. **Arnett, F. C., Bias, W. B., and Reveille, J. D.,** Genetic studies in Sjogren's syndrome and systemic lupus erythematosus, *J. Autoimmun.,* 2, 403, 1989.
132. **Reveille, J. D., MacLeod, M. J., Whittington, K., and Arnett, F. C.,** Specific amino acid residues in the second hypervariable region of HLA-DQA1 and DQB1 chain genes promote the Ro (SS-A)/La (SS-B) autoantibody responses, *J. Immunol.,* 146, 3871, 1991.
133. **Smolen, J. S., Klippel, J. H., Penner, E., Reichlin, M., Steinberg, A. D., Chused, T. M., Scherak, O., Grainger, W., Hartter, E., Zielinski, C. C., Wolf, A., Davey, R. J., Mann, D. L., and Mayr, W. R.,** HLA-DR antigens in systemic lupus erythematosus: association with specificity of autoantibody responses to nuclear antigens, *Ann. Rheum. Dis.,* 46, 457, 1987.

134. **Hoffman, R. W., Rettenmaier, L. J., Takeda, Y., Hewett, J. E., Pettersson, I., Nyman, U., Luger, A. M., and Sharp, G. C.,** Human autoantibodies against the 70-kd polypeptide of U1 small nuclear RNP are associated with HLA-DR4 among connective tissue disease patients, *Arthritis Rheum.*, 33, 666, 1990.
135. **Kaneoka, H., Hsu, K. C., Takeda, Y., Sharp, G. C., and Hoffman, R. W.,** Molecular genetic analysis of HLA-DR and HLA-DQ genes among anti-U1-70 kd autoantibody positive connective tissue disease patients, *Arthritis Rheum.*, 35, 83, 1992.
136. **Olsen, M. L., Arnett, F. C., and Reveille, J. D.,** Anti-Sm and anti-RNP antibodies are associated with distinct and different HLA-DQ alpha and DQ beta chain genes, *Arthritis Rheum.*, 33(Suppl.), S100, 1990.
137. **Love, P. E. and Santoro, S. A.,** Antiphospholipid antibodies: anticardiolipin and the lupus anticoagulant in systemic lupus erythematosus (SLE) and in non-SLE disorders. Prevalence and clinical significance, *Ann. Intern. Med.*, 112, 682, 1990.
138. **Savi, M., Ferraccioli, G. F., Neri, T. M., Zanelli, P., Dall'Aglio, P. P., Tincani, A., Balestriere, G., Carella, G., and Cattaneo, R.,** HLA-DR antigens and anticardiolipin antibodies in Northern Italian systemic lupus erythematosus patients, *Arthritis Rheum.*, 31, 1568, 1988.
139. **McHugh, N. J. and Maddison, P. J.,** HLA-DR antigens and anticardiolipin antibodies in patients with systemic lupus erythematosus, *Arthritis Rheum.*, 32, 1623, 1989.
140. **McNeil, H. P., Gavaghan, T. P., Krilis, S. A., Geczy, A. F., and Chesteman, C. N.,** HLA-DR antigens and anticardiolipin antibodies, *Clin. Exp. Rheumatol.*, 8, 425, 1990.
141. **Arnett, F. C., Olsen, M. L., Anderson, K. L., and Reveille, J. D.,** Molecular analysis of major histocompatibility complex alleles associated with the lupus anticoagulant, *J. Clin. Invest.*, 87, 1490, 1991.
142. **Reveille, J. D., Wilson, R. W., Provost, T. T., Bias, W. B., and Arnett, F. C.,** Primary Sjogren's syndrome and other autoimmune diseases in families. Prevalence and immunogenetic studies in six kindreds, *Ann. Intern. Med.*, 101, 748, 1984.
143. **Hinzova, E., Ivanyi, D., Sula, K., Horejs, J., Dostal, C., and Drizhal, I.,** HLA-Dw3 in Sjogren's syndrome, *Tissue Antigens*, 37, 10, 1977.
144. **Chused, T. M., Kassan, S. S., Opelz, G., Moutsopoulus, H. M., and Terasaki, P. I.,** Sjogren's syndrome associated with Dw3, *N. Engl. J. Med.*, 296, 895, 1977.
145. **Moutsopoulos, H., Mann, D. L., Johnson, A. H., and Chused, T. M.,** Genetic differences between primary and secondary sicca syndrome, *N. Engl. J. Med.*, 301, 761, 1979.
146. **Manthorpe, R., Morling, N., Platz, P., Ryder, L. P., Svejgaard, A., and Thomsen, M.,** HLA-D antigen frequencies in Sjogren's syndrome, *Scand. J. Rheumatol.*, 10, 124, 1981.
147. **Wilson, R. W., Provost, T. T., Bias, W. B., Alexander, E. L., Edlow, D. W., Hochberg, M. C., Stevens, M. B., and Arnett, F. C.,** Sjogren's syndrome. Influence of multiple HLA-D region alloantigens on clinical and serologic expression, *Arthritis Rheum.*, 27, 1245, 1984.
148. **Papasteriades, C., Skopouli, F. N., Drosos, A. A., Andonopoulos, A. P., and Moutsopoulos, H. M.,** HLA alloantigen associations in Greek patients with Sjogren's syndrome, *J. Autoimmun.*, 1, 85, 1988.

149. **Moriuchi, J., Ichikawa, Y., Takaya, M., Shimizu, H., Uehigama, M., Sato, K., Tsuji, K., and Arimori, S.,** Association between HLA and Sjogren's syndrome in Japanese patients, *Arthritis Rheum.*, 29, 1518, 1986.
150. **Reveille, J. D. and Arnett, F. C.,** The immunogenetics of Sjogren's syndrome, in *Rheumatic Disease Clinics of North America,* Fox, R. I., Ed., W. B. Saunders, Philadelphia, 1992, 539.
151. **Longster, G. and Giles, C. M.,** A new antibody specificity, anti-Rg[a], reacting with a red cell and serum antigen, *Vox Sang.*, 30, 175, 1976.
152. **Clements, P. J., Opelz, G., Terasaki, P. I., Mickey, M. R., and Furst, D.,** Association of HLA antigen A9 with progressive systemic sclerosis (scleroderma), *Tissue Antigens,* 11, 357, 1978.
153. **Ercilla, M. G., Arriaga, F., Gratacos, M. R., Coll, J., Lecha, V., Vives, J., and Castillo, R.,** HLA antigens and scleroderma, *Arch. Dermatol. Res.*, 271, 381, 1981.
154. **Hughes, P., Gelsthorpe, K., Doughty, R. W., Rowell, N. R., Rosenthal, F. D., and Sneddon, I. B.,** The association of HLA-B8 with visceral disease in systemic sclerosis, *Clin. Exp. Immunol.*, 31, 351, 1978.
155. **Kallenberg, C. G. M., van der Voort-Beelen, J. M., d'Amaro, J., and The, T. H.,** Increased frequency of B8/DR3 in scleroderma and association with impaired cellular immune response, *Clin. Exp. Immunol.*, 43, 478, 1981.
156. **Lynch, C. J., Singh, G., Whiteside, T. L., Rodnan, G. P., Medsger, T. A., and Rabin, B. S.,** Histocompatibility antigens in progressive systemic sclerosis (PSS; scleroderma), *J. Clin. Immunol.*, 2, 314, 1982.
157. **Briggs, D. C., Welsh, K., Pereira, R. S., and Black, C. M.,** A strong association between null alleles at the C4A locus in the major histocompatibility complex and systemic sclerosis, *Arthritis Rheum.*, 29, 1274, 1986.
158. **DiBartolomeo, A. G., Rabin, B. S., and Rodnan, G. P.,** HLA-D antigens in progressive systemic sclerosis (scleroderma), *Immunol. Commun.*, 10, 733, 1981.
159. **Black, C. M., Welsh, K. I., Maddison, P. J., Jayson, M. I. V., and Berstein, R. M.,** HLA antigens, autoantibodies and clinical subsets in scleroderma, *J. Rheumatol.*, 23, 267, 1984.
160. **Mollenhauer, E. R., Schmidt, R., Heinrichs, M., and Rittner, C.,** Scleroderma: possible significance of silent alleles at the C4B locus, *Arthritis Rheum.*, 27, 711, 1984.
161. **Rabin, B. S., Rodn, G. P., Bassion, S., and Gill, T. J.,** HLA antigens in progressive systemic sclerosis (scleroderma), *Arthritis Rheum.*, 18, 381, 1975.
162. **Crouzet, J., Marbach, M. C., Camus, J. P., Godeau, P., Herreman, G., Richier, D., Hors, J., and Dausset, J.,** Recherche d'une association entre antigens HL-A et sclerodermie systemique, *Presse Med.*, 4, 2489, 1975.
163. **Birnbaum, N. S., Rodnan, G. P., Rabin, B. S., and Bassion, S.,** Histocompatibility antigens in progressive systemic sclerosis (scleroderma), *J. Rheumatol.*, 4, 425, 1977.
164. **Niks, M., Rovensky, J., Nyulassy, J., Buc, M., Stefanovic, J., and Zitnan, D.,** Lack of association of HLA-DR antigens with progressive systemic sclerosis (scleroderma), *Tissue Antigens,* 19, 238, 1982.
165. **Livington, J. Z., Scott, T. E., Wigley, F. M., Anhalt, G. J., Bias, W. B., McLean, R. H., and Hochberg, M. C.,** Systemic sclerosis (scleroderma): clinical, genetic and serologic subsets, *J. Rheumatol.*, 14, 512, 1987.

166. **Fritzler, M. J., Kinsella, J. D., and Garbutt, E.,** The CREST syndrome: a distinct serologic entity with anticentromere antibodies, *Am. J. Med.,* 69, 520, 1980.

167. **Steen, V. D., Powell, D. L., and Medsger, T. A., Jr.,** Clinical correlations and prognosis based on serum autoantibodies in patients with progressive systemic sclerosis, *Arthritis Rheum.,* 31, 196, 1988.

168. **Genth, E., Mierau, R., Genetzky, P., von Muhlen, C. A., Kaufman, S., von Wilmowsky, H., Meurer, M., Krieg, T., Pollman, H. J., and Hartl, P. W.,** Immunogenetic associations of scleroderma-related antinuclear antibodies, *Arthritis Rheum.,* 33, 657, 1990.

169. **Dunckley, H., Jazwinska, E. C., Gatenby, P. A., and Serjeantson, S. W.,** DNA-DR typing shows HLA-DRw11 RFLPs are increased in frequency in both progressive systemic sclerosis and CREST variants of scleroderma, *Tissue Antigens,* 33, 418, 1989.

170. **Reveille, J. D., Owerbach, D., Goldstein, R., Moreda, R., Isern, R. A., and Arnett, F. C.,** Association of polar amino acids at position 26 of the HLA-DQB1 first domain with the anticentromere autoantibody response in systemic sclerosis (scleroderma), *J. Clin. Invest.,* 89, 1208, 1992.

171. **Reveille, J. D., Durban, E., Goldstein, R., Moreda, R., and Arnett, F. C.,** Racial differences of scleroderma-related autoantibodies, *Arthritis Rheum.,* 35, 216, 1992.

172. **Reveille, J. D., Durban, E., MacLeod, M. J., Goldstein, R., Moreda, R., Altman, R. D., and Arnett, F. C.,** Association of amino acid sequences in the HLA-DQB1 first domain with the anti-topoisomerase I autoantibody response in scleroderma (progressive systemic sclerosis), *J. Clin. Invest.,* 90, 973, 1992.

173. **Reimer, G., Steen, V. D., Penning, C. A., Medsger, T. A., Jr., and Tan, E. M.,** Correlates between autoantibodies to nucleolar antigens and clinical features in patients with systemic sclerosis (scleroderma), *Arthritis Rheum.,* 31, 525, 1988.

174. **Bohan, A. and Peter, J. B.,** Polymyositis and dermatomyositis (Pts. 1 and 2), *N. Engl. J. Med.,* 292, 344, 1975.

175. **Hirsch, T. J., Enlow, R. W., Bias, W. B., and Arnett, F. C.,** HLA-D related (DR) antigens in various kinds of myositis, *Hum. Immunol.,* 3, 181, 1981.

176. **Love, L. A., Leff, R. L., Fraser, D. D., Targoff, I. N., Dalakas, M., Plotz, P. H., and Miller, F. W.,** A new approach to the classification of idiopathic inflammatory myopathy: myositis-specific autoantibodies define useful homogeneous patient groups, *Medicine,* 70, 360, 1991.

177. **Wasisek, C. A., Reichlin, M., Montes, M., and Raghu, G.,** Polymyositis and interstitial lung disease in a patient with anti-Jo-1 prototype, *Am. J. Med.,* 76, 538, 1984.

178. **Mathews, M. B. and Bernstein, R. M.,** Myositis autoantibody inhibits histidyl-tRNA synthetase: a model for autoimmunity, *Nature,* 304, 177, 1983.

179. **Mathews, M. B., Reichlin, M., Hughes, G. R., and Bernstein, R. M.,** Anti-threonyl tRNA synthetase, a second myositis-related autoantibody, *J. Exp. Med.,* 160, 420, 1984.

180. **Bonn, C. C., Bernstein, R. M., and Mathews, M. B.,** Autoantibodies against alanyl-tRNA synthetase and tRNA (ALA) coexist and are associated with myositis, *J. Exp. Med.,* 163, 1281, 1986.

181. **Targoff, I. N.,** Autoantibodies to aminoacyl-transfer RNA synthetases for isoleucine and glycine. Two additional synthetases are antigenic in myositis, *J. Immunol.,* 144, 1737, 1990.

182. **Hochberg, M. C., Feldman, D., Stevens, M. B., Arnett, F. C., and Reichlin, M.,** Antibody to Jo-1 in polymyositis/dermatomyositis: association with interstitial pulmonary disease, *J. Rheumatol.,* 11, 663, 1984.
183. **Oddis, C. V., Medsger, T. A., and Cooperstein, L. A.,** A subluxing arthropathy associated with the anti-Jo-1 antibody in polymyositis/dermatomyositis, *Arthritis Rheum.,* 33, 1640, 1990.
184. **Targoff, I. N. and Arnett, F. C.,** Clinical manifestations in patients with antibody to PL-12 antigen (alanyl-tRNA synthetase), *Am. J. Med.,* 88, 241, 1990.
185. **Arnett, F. C., Hirsch, T. J., Bias, W. B., Nishikai, M., and Reichlin, M.,** The Jo-1 antibody system in myositis relationships to clinical features and HLA, *J. Rheumatol.,* 8, 925, 1981.
186. **Goldstein, R., Duvic, M., Targoff, I. N., Reichlin, M., McMenemy, A. M., Reveille, J. D., Warner, N. B., Pollack, M. S., and Arnett, F. C.,** HLA-D region genes associated with autoantibody responses to histidyl-transfer RNA synthetase (Jo-1) and other translation-relation factors in myositis, *Arthritis Rheum.,* 33, 1240, 1990.
187. **Gurley, R. C., Love, L. A., Targoff, I. N., Leff, R. L., Plotz, P. H., and Miller, F. W.,** Association among myositis-specific autoantibodies (MSA) and HLA-DQA1 alleles, *Arthritis Rheum.,* 34(Suppl.), S137, 1991.
188. **Reed, A. M., Pachman, L., and Ober, C.,** Molecular genetic studies of major histocompatibility complex genes in children with juvenile dermatomyositis: increased risk associated with HLA-DQA1*0501, *Hum. Immunol.,* 32, 235, 1991.
189. **Cassidy, J. T., Levinson, J. E., and Brewer, E. J., Jr.,** The development of classification criteria for children with juvenile rheumatoid arthritis, *Bull. Rheum. Dis.,* 38, 1, 1989.
190. **Begovich, A. B., Bugawan, T. L., Nepom, B. S., Klitz, W., Nepom, G. T., and Erlich, H. A.,** A specific HLA-DPB allele is associated with pauciarticular juvenile rheumatoid arthritis but not adult rheumatoid arthritis, *Proc. Natl. Acad. Sci. U.S.A.,* 88, 9489, 1989.
191. **Barron, K. S., Joseph, A., MacLeod, M., Owerbach, D., and Reveille, J. D.,** DNA analysis of HLA-DR, DQ and DP genes in pauciarticular juvenile rheumatoid arthritis, *J. Rheumatol.,* 18, 1723, 1991.
192. **Fernandez-Vina, M. A., Fink, C. W., and Stastny, P.,** HLA antigens in juvenile arthritis. Pauciarticular and polyarticular juvenile arthritis are immunogenetically distinct, *Arthritis Rheum.,* 33, 1787, 1990.
193. **Glass, D., Litvin, D., Wallace, K., Chylack, L., Garovoy, M., Carpenter, C. B., and Schur, P. H.,** Early onset pauciarticular juvenile rheumatoid arthritis associated with human leukocyte antigen: DRw5, iritis and antinuclear antibody, *J. Clin. Invest.,* 66, 426, 1980.
194. **Arnaiz-Villena, A., Gomez-Reino, J. J., Gamin, M. L., Regueiro, J. R., Vicario, J. L., Gomez-Reino, F. J., Alonso, A., Fernandez-Dapica, M. P., Irigoyen, M. V., Mateo, I., and Zea, A.,** DR, C4 and Bf allotypes in juvenile rheumatoid arthritis, *Arthritis Rheum.,* 27, 1281, 1984.
195. **Trowsdale, J., Ragoussis, J., and Campbell, R. D.,** Map of the human major histocompatibility complex, *Immunol. Today,* 12, 443, 1991.
196. **Barron, K. S., Silverman, E. D., Gonzalez, J. C., Owerbach, D., and Reveille, J. D.,** DNA analysis of HLA-DR, DQ, and DP alleles in children with polyarticular juvenile rheumatoid arthritis, *J. Rheumatol.,* 19, 1611, 1992.

197. **Vehe, R. K., Begovich, A. B., and Nepom, B. S.,** HLA susceptibility genes in rheumatoid factor positive juvenile rheumatoid arthritis, *J. Rheumatol.,* 17(Suppl. 26), 11, 1990.
198. **MacCuish, A. C., Barnes, E. W., Irvine, W. J., and Duncan, L. J. P.,** Antibodies to pancreatic islet cell in insulin-dependent diabetes with coexistent autoimmune disease, *Lancet,* 2, 1529, 1974.
199. **Bottazzo, G. F., Dean, B. M., McNally, J. M., Mackay, E. H., Swift, P. G., and Gamble, D. R.,** In situ characterization of autoimmune phenomena and expression of HLA molecules in the pancreas in diabetes mellitus, *N. Engl. J. Med.,* 313, 353, 1985.
200. **Thomsen, M., Platz, P., Andersen, O. O., Christy, M., Lyngsoe, J., Nerup, J., Rasmusen, K., Ryder, L. P., Staub-Nielsen, L., and Svejgaard, A.,** MLC typing in juvenile diabetes mellitus and idiopathic Addison's disease, *Transplant. Rev.,* 22, 125, 1975.
201. **Reitnauer, P. J., Roseman, J. M., Barger, B. O., Murphy, C. C., Kirk, K. A., and Acton, R. T.,** HLA associations with insulin-dependent diabetes mellitus in a sample of the American black population, *Tissue Antigens,* 17, 286, 1981.
202. **Wolf, E., Spencer, K. M., and Cudworth, A. G.,** The genetic susceptibility to type I (insulin-dependent) diabetes; analysis of HLA-DR association, *Diabetologia,* 24, 224, 1983.
203. **Christy, M., Mandrup-Poulsen, T., and Nerup, J.,** Genetic markers in insulin-dependent (type I) diabetes mellitus, *Ann. Clin. Res.,* 16, 53, 1984.
204. **Cambon-de Mouzon, A., Ohayon, E., Hauptmann, G., Sevin, A., Abbal, M., Sommer, E., Vergnes, H., and Ducus, J.,** HLA-A, B, C, DR antigens, Bf, C4 and glyoxylase I (GLO) polymorphisms in French Basques with insulin dependent diabetes mellitus (IDDM), *Tissue Antigens,* 19, 366, 1982.
205. **Partanen, J., Koskimies, S., Ilonen, J., and Knip, M.,** HLA antigens and complotypes in insulin-dependent diabetes mellitus, *Tissue Antigens,* 27, 291, 1986.
206. **Behbehani, K., Richens, E. R., Abdella, N., Jayyab, A. K., Shaltout, A., Al-Saffar, M., and Siboo, R.,** HLA associations in an Arab type I diabetes population, *Dis. Markers,* 5, 165, 1987.
207. **Pinelli, L., Drei, F., Gonfiantini, E., Visentin, A., Roata, C., Ciaffoni, S., and Maffeis, C.,** Insulin dependent diabetes mellitus epidemiology: HLA genotype study in 12 north eastern Italian families with two sibships affected by type I diabetes, *Eur. J. Epidemiol.,* 5, 456, 1989.
208. **Svejgaard, A., Platz, P., and Ryder, L. P.,** HLA and disease, 1982 — a survey, *Immunol. Rev.,* 70, 193, 1983.
209. **Cohen, D., Cohen, O., Marcadet, A., Massart, C., Lathrup, M., Deschamps, I., Hors, J., Schuller, E., and Dausset, J.,** Class II HLA-DC beta chain DNA restriction fragments differentiate among HLA-DR2 individuals in insulin-dependent diabetes and multiple sclerosis, *Proc. Natl. Acad. Sci. U.S.A.,* 81, 1774, 1984.
210. **Johnston, C., Pyke, D. A., Cudworth, A. G., and Wolf, E.,** HLA-DR typing in identical twins with insulin-dependent diabetes mellitus: difference between concordant and discordant pairs, *Br. Med. J.,* 286, 253, 1983.
211. **Contu, L., Deschamps, I., Lestradet, H., Hors, J., Schmid, M., Busson, M., Benajam, A., Barge-Marcelli, A., and Dausset, J.,** HLA haplotype study of 53 juvenile insulin-dependent diabetic (I.D.D.) families, *Tissue Antigens,* 20, 123, 1982.

212. **Todd, J. A., Bell, J. I., and McDevitt, H. O.,** HLA-DQ beta chain contributes susceptibility and resistance to insulin-dependent diabetes mellitus, *Nature,* 329, 599, 1987.
213. **Khalil, I., d'Auriol, L., Gobet, M., Morin, L., Lepage, V., Deschamps, I., Park, M. S., Degos, L., Galibert, F., and Hors, J.,** A combination of HLA-DQ beta Asp57-negative and HLA-DQ alpha Arg52 confers susceptibility to insulin dependent diabetes mellitus, *J. Clin. Invest.,* 85, 1315, 1990.
214. **Mijovic, C. H., Barnett, A. H., and Todd, J. A.,** Genetics of diabetes. Transracial gene mapping studies, *Clin. Endocrinol. Metab.,* 5, 321, 1991.
215. **Naeim, F., Keesey, J. C., Hermann, C., Jr., Lindstrom, J., Zeller, E., and Walford, R. L.,** Association of HLA-B8 DRw3, and anti-acetylecholine receptor antibodies in myasthenia gravis, *Tissue Antigens,* 12, 381, 1978.
216. **Behan, P. O.,** Immune disease and HLA association with myasthenia gravis, *J. Neurol. Neurosurg. Psychiatry,* 43, 611, 1980.
217. **Dawkins, R. L., Christiansen, F. T., and Garlepp, M. J.,** Autoantibodies and HLA antigens in ocular, generalized and penicillamine-induced myasthenia gravis, *Ann. NY Acad. Sci.,* 377, 372, 1981.
218. **Matej, H., Nowakowska, B., Kaamarz, M., Paradowski, B., Podemski, R., and Brzecki, A.,** HLA antigens and susceptibility to myasthenia gravis, *Arch. Immunol. Ther. Exp.,* 35, 795, 1987.
219. **Thajeb, P., Chee, C. Y., and Huang, C. C.,** The distribution of HLA-A, B, DR antigens in Chinese myasthenia gravis, *Tissue Antigens,* 29, 273, 1987.
220. **Chiu, H. C., Hsieh, R. P., and Hsieh, K. H.,** Association of HLA antigens with myasthenia gravis in Chinese on Taiwan, *Chung Hua Min Kuo Wei Shang Wu Chi Mien I Hsueh Tsa Chih,* 23, 12, 1990.
221. **Langdon, N., Welsh, K. I., van Dam, M., Vaughan, R. W., and Parkes, D.,** Genetic markers in narcolepsy, *Lancet,* 2, 1178, 1984.
222. **Billiard, M. and Cadilhac, J.,** Narcolepsy, *Rev. Neurol.,* 141, 515, 1985.
223. **Seignalet, J.,** HLA and narcolepsy, *Pathol. Biol.,* 34, 741, 1986.
224. **Mueller-Eckhardt, G., Meier-Ewert, K., Schendel, D. J., Reinecker, F. B., Multhoff, G., and Mueller-Eckhardt, C.,** HLA and narcolepsy in a German population, *Tissue Antigens,* 28, 163, 1986.
225. **Neely, S., Rosenberg, R., Spire, J. P., Antel, J., and Arnason, B. G.,** HLA antigens in narcolepsy, *Neurology,* 37, 1858, 1987.
226. **Roth, B., Nevsimalova, S., Sonka, K., Docekaly, P., Schulz, H., Geisler, P., Pollmacher, T., Andreas-Zietz, A., Keller, E., and Scholz, S.,** A study of the occurrence of HLA-DR2 in 124 narcoleptics: clinical aspects, *Schweiz. Arch. Neurol. Psychiatry,* 139, 41, 1988.
227. **Juji, T., Satake, M., Honda, Y., and Doi, Y.,** HLA antigens in Japanese patients with narcolepsy. All the patients were DR2 positive, *Tissue Antigens,* 24, 316, 1984.
228. **Compston, D. A. S., Batchelor, J. R., and McDonald, W. I.,** B-lymphocyte alloantigens associated with multiple sclerosis, *Lancet,* 2, 1261, 1976.
229. **Terasaki, P. I., Park, M. S., Opelz, G., and Ting, A.,** Multiple sclerosis and high incidence of a B lymphocyte antigen, *Science,* 193, 1245, 1976.
230. **Paty, D. W., Cousin, H. K., Stiller, C. R., Boucher, D. W., Furesz, J., Warren, K. G., Marchuk, L., and Dossetor, J. B.,** HLA-D typing with an association of Dw2 and absent immune responses toward herpes simplex (type I) antigen in multiple sclerosis, *Transplant. Proc.,* 9, 1845, 1977.

231. **Poskanzer, D. C., Terasaki, P. I., Prenney, L. B., Sheridan, J. L., and Park, M. S.,** Multiple sclerosis in the Orkney and Shetland Islands. III. Histocompatibility determinants, *J. Epidemiol. Community Health,* 34, 253, 1980.
232. **Poser, S., Ritter, G., Bauer, H. J., Gross-Wilde, H., Kuwert, E. K., and Raun, N. E.,** HLA antigens and the prognosis of multiple sclerosis, *J. Neurol.,* 225, 219, 1981.
233. **Govaerts, A., Gony, J., Martin-Mondiere, C., Poirer, J. C., Schmid, M., Schuller, E., Degos, J. D., and Dausset, J.,** HLA and multiple sclerosis: population and families study, *Tissue Antigens,* 25, 187, 1985.
234. **Clerici, N., Hernandez, M., Fernandez, M., Rosique, J., and Alvarez-Cermeno, J.,** Multiple sclerosis is associated with HLA-DR2 antigen in Spain, *Tissue Antigens,* 34, 309, 1989.
235. **Cassetta, I., Granieri, E., Conighi, C., Grappa, M. T., Tola, M. R., Govoni, V., Paolino, E., Mattiuz, P. L., and Carrera, M.,** HLA antigens and multiple sclerosis in the Province of Ferrara, Northern Italy: a community based study, *Rev. Neurol.,* 61, 12, 1991.
236. **Elian, M., Alonso, A., Awad, J., Dean, G., Okoye, R., Sachs, J., Savettieri, G., Vassallo, L., and Festenstein, H.,** HLA associations with multiple sclerosis in Sicily and Malta, *Dis. Markers,* 5, 89, 1987.
237. **Brautbar, C., Cohen, I., Alter, M., Jorgensen, F., and Lamm, L.,** Histocompatibility determinants in Israeli Jewish patients with multiple sclerosis, *Tissue Antigens,* 10, 291, 1977.
238. **Naito, S., Kuroiwa, Y., Itoyama, T., Tsubaki, T., Horikawa, A., Sasazuki, T., Noguchi, S., Ohtsuki, S., Tokuomi, H., Miyatake, T., Takahata, N., and Kawanami, S.,** HLA and Japanese MS, *Tissue Antigens,* 12, 19, 1978.
239. **Hawkins, B. R., Yu, Y. L., Woo, E., and Huang, C. Y.,** No apparent association between HLA and multiple sclerosis in southern Chinese, *J. Neurol. Neurosurg. Psychiatry,* 51, 443, 1988.
240. **Matsuyama, M., Hashimoto, K., Yamasaki, Y., Shirakura, R., Higuchi, R., Miyajima, T., and Amemiya, H.,** HLA-DR antigens in pemphigus among Japanese, *Tissue Antigens,* 17, 238, 1981.
241. **Park, M. S., Terasaki, P. I., Ahmed, A. R., and Tiwari, J. L.,** HLA-DRW4 in 91% of Jewish pemphigus vulgaris patients, *Lancet,* 2, 441, 1979.
242. **Scharf, S. J., Friedmann, A., Steinman, L., Brautbar, C., and Erlich, H. A.,** Specific HLA-DQB and HLA-DRB1 alleles confer susceptibility to pemphigus vulgaris, *Proc. Natl. Acad. Sci. U.S.A.,* 86, 6215, 1989.
243. **Scharf, S. J., Long, C. M., and Erlich, H. A.,** Sequence analysis of the HLA-DR beta and HLA-DQ beta loci from three pemphigus vulgaris patients, *Hum. Immunol.,* 22, 61, 1988.
244. **Niizeki, H., Inoko, H., Narimatsu, H., Takata, H., Sonoda, A., Tadakuma, T., Ando, A., Tsuji, K., Hashimoto, T., and Nishikawa, T.,** HLA class II antigens are associated with Japanese pemphigus patients, *Hum. Immunol.,* 31, 246, 1991.
245. **Moraes, J. R., Moraes, M. E., Fernandez-Vina, M., Diaz, L. A., Friedman, H., Campbell, I. T., Alvarez, R. R., Sampaio, S. A., Rivitti, E. A., and Stastny, P.,** HLA antigens and risk for development of pemphigus foliaceus (fogo selvagem) in endemic areas of Brazil, *Immunogenet,* 33, 388, 1991.
246. **Cunliffe, W. J., Hall, R., Stevenson, C. J., and Weightman, D.,** Alopecia areata, thyroid disease and autoimmunity, *Br. J. Dermatol.,* 81, 877, 1969.

247. **Thiers, B. H. and Galbraith, G. M. P.,** Alopecia areata, in *Pathogenesis of Skin Disease,* Thiers, B. H. and Dobson, R. L., Eds., Churchill Livingstone, New York, 1986, 57.
248. **Mikesell, J. F., Bergfold, W. F., and Braun, W. E.,** HLA-DR antigens in alopecia areata: preliminary report, *Cleveland Clin. Q.,* 53, 189, 1986.
249. **Orecchia, G., Belvedere, M. D., Martinetti, M., Capelli, E., and Rabbiosi, G.,** Human leukocyte antigen region involvement in the genetic predisposition to alopecia areata, *Diabetologia,* 175, 10, 1987.
250. **Frentz, G., Thomsen, K., Jacobsen, B. K., and Svejgaard, A.,** HLA-DR4 in alopecia areata, *J. Am. Acad. Dermatol.,* 14, 129, 1986.
251. **Duvic, M., Hordinsky, M. K., Fiedler, V. C., O'Brien, W. R., Young, R., and Reveille, J. D.,** HLA-D locus associations in alopecia areata: DRw52a may confer disease resistance, *Arch. Dermatol.,* 127, 64, 1991.
252. **Odum, N., Morling, N., Georgsen, J., Jakobsen, B. K., Frentz, G., Jensen, G. F., Fugger, L., and Svejgaard, A.,** HLA-DP antigens in patients with alopecia areata, *Tissue Antigens,* 35, 114, 1990.
253. **Richiardi, P., Borelli, I., Malavesi, F., Curtoni, E. S., Berti, E., Gianotti, F., and Giannetti, A.,** HLA antigens in juvenile dermatitis herpetiformis, *Acta Dermatol. Venereol.,* 61, 241, 1981.
254. **Hall, R. P., Lawley, T. J., and Katz, S. I.,** Dermatitis herpetiformis, *Springer Semin. Immunopathol.,* 4, 33, 1981.
255. **Buckley, D. B., English, J., Molloy, W., Doyle, C. T., and Whelton, M. J.,** Dermatitis herpetiformis: a review of 119 cases, *Clin. Exp. Dermatol.,* 8, 477, 1983.
256. **Karpati, S., Kosnai, I., Verkasalo, M., Kuitunen, P., Simon, Z., Kosminies, S., Reunale, T., Gyodi, E., and Torok, E.,** HLA antigens, jejunal morphology and associated diseases in children with dermatitis herpetiformis, *Acta Paediatr. Scand.,* 75, 297, 1986.
257. **Hall, R. P. and Otley, C.,** Immunogenetics of dermatitis herpetiformis, *Semin. Dermatol.,* 10, 240, 1991.
258. **Retornaz, G., Betuel, H., Ortonne, J. P., and Thivolet, J.,** HL-A antigens and vitiligo, *Br. J. Dermatol.,* 95, 173, 1976.
259. **Metzker, A., Zamir, R., Gazit, E., David, M., and Feuerman, E. J.,** Vitiligo and the HLA system, *Diabetologia,* 160, 100, 1980.
260. **Foley, L. M., Lowe, N. J., Misheloff, E., and Tiwari, J. L.,** Association of HLA-DR4 with vitiligo, *J. Am. Acad. Dermatol.,* 8, 39, 1983.
261. **Dunston, G. M. and Halder, R. M.,** Vitiligo is associated with HLA-DR4 in Black patients. A preliminary report, *Arch. Dermatol.,* 126, 56, 1990.
262. **Finco, O., Cuccia, M., Martinetti, M., Ruberto, G., Orecchia, G., and Rabbiosi, G.,** Age of onset in vitiligo: relationship with HLA supratypes, *Clin. Genet.,* 39, 48, 1991.
263. **Gammon, W. R., Heise, E. R., Burke, W. A., Fine, J. D., and Woodley, D. T.,** Increased frequency of HLA-DR2 in patients with autoantibodies to epidermolysis bullosa acquisita antigen: evidence that the expression of autoimmunity to type VII collagen is HLA class II allele associated, *J. Invest. Dermatol.,* 91, 228, 1988.
264. **Tiwari, J. L. and Terasaki, P. I.,** *HLA and Disease Associations,* Springer-Verlag, New York, 1985.

265. **Mearin, M. L., Biemond, I., Pena, A. S., Polanco, I., Vasquez, G., Schreuder, Th. M., de Vries, R. R. P., and van Roud, J. J.**, HLA-DR phenotypes in Spanish coeliac children; their contribution to the understanding of the genetics of the disease, *Gut,* 24, 532, 1983.
266. **Morellini, M., Trabace, S., Mazzilli, M. C., Lulli, P., Capellacci, S., Bonamico, M., Margarit, I., and Gandini, E.**, A study of HLA class II antigens in an Italian pediatric population with coeliac disease, *Dis. Markers,* 6, 23, 1988.
267. **Thorsby, E., Lundin, K. E. A., Ronningen, K. S., Sollid, L. M., and Vartdal, F.**, Molecular basis and functional importance of some disease-associated HLA polymorphisms, *Tissue Antigens,* 34, 39, 1989.
268. **Niven, M. J., Caffrey, C., Sachs, J. A., Cassell, P. G., Gallagher, R. B., Kumar, P., and Hitman, G. A.**, Susceptibility to celiac disease involves genes in HLA-DP region, *Lancet,* II, 805, 1987.
269. **Howell, M. D., Smith, J. R., Austin, R. K., Kelleher, D., Nepom, G. T., Volk, B., and Kagnoff, M. F.**, An extended HLA-D region haplotype associated with celiac disease, *Proc. Natl. Acad. Sci. U.S.A.,* 85, 222, 1988.
270. **Gomez-Reino, J. J., Martinez-Laso, J., Vicario, J. L., paz-Artal, E., Aragon, A., Martin-Villa, J. M., DeJuan, M. D., Perez-Aciego, P., and Arnaiz-Villena, A.**, Immunogenetics of systemic lupus erythematosus in Spanish patients: differential HLA markers, *Immunobiology,* 182, 465, 1991.
271. **Lulli, P., Sebastiani, G. D., Trabace, S., Passiu, G., Cappellacci, S., Porzio, F., Morellini, M., Cutrupi, F., and Galeazzi, M.**, HLA antigens in Italian patients with systemic lupus erythematosus: evidence for the association of DQw2 with the autoantibody response to extractable nuclear antigens, *Clin. Exp. Rheumatol.,* 9, 475, 1991.
272. **Fronek, Z., Timmerman, L. A., Alper, C. A., Hahn, B. H., Kalunian, K., Peterlin, B. M., and McDevitt, H. O.**, Major histocompatibility complex genes and susceptibility to systemic lupus erythematosus, *Arthritis Rheum.,* 33, 1542, 1990.
273. **Doherty, D. G., Ireland, R., Demaine, A. G., Wang, F., Veerapan, K., Welsh, K. I., and Vergani, D.**, Major histocompatibility complex genes and susceptibility to systemic lupus erythematosus in southern Chinese, *Arthritis Rheum.,* 35, 641, 1992.

Appendix

APPENDIX

The table contains reagents and materials used to perform the tests described in this book. The commercial suppliers are selected based on the personal experience of the editors and is not meant to be complete.

Material	Source	Comments
General Information	Linscott Directory of Immunological and Biological Reagents 4877 Grand Road, Santa Rosa, CA 95404 Tel: 707-544-9555	A guide for reagents kits and services
ELISA kits for rheumatology/immunology laboratories: autoantibodies	Diamedix Corp. 2140 Miami Avenue Miami, Fl 33127 Tel: 800-327-4565	Kits for individual antibodies
	TheraTest Laboratories Inc. 2201 W. Campbell Park Dr., Chicago, IL 60612 Tel: 800-441-0771	Kits formated for individual antibodies and as panels of multitest simultaneous runs
	Kalestead Diagnostics Sanofi Diagnostics Pastuer, Inc. 1000 Lake Hazeltine Dr. Chaska, MN 55318-1084 Tel: 800-666-5111	Kits for individual antibodies
	Whittaker Bioproducts 8830 Biggs Ford Rd. A08 Walkersville, MD 21793-0127 Tel: 800-638-8174	Kits for individual antibodies
	INOVA Diagnostics, Inc. 10451 Roselle Street San Diego, CA 92121 Tel: 800-545-9495	
	Helix Diagnostics 3148 Industrial Blvd West Sacramento, CA 95691 Tel: 800-345-1545	ANA screening test

	Wampole Laboratories Half Acre Road Cranbury, NJ 08512-0181 Tel: 800-257-9525	F-ANA test
Cytokine kits	Cistron Biotechnology, Inc. 10 Bloomfield Ave. Pine Brook, NJ 07058 Tel: 800-642-0167	
	Cytokine Sciences, Inc. 25 Harvard St. Boston, MA 02111 Tel: 617-742-6528	
	Genzyme Corp. One Kendall Square Cambridge, MA 02139-1562 Tel: 800-332-1042	Cytokine kits, cytokines and monoclonal antibodies
Complement assays	Quidel 10165 McKellar Court San Diego, CA 92121 Tel: 619-552-1100	ELISA tests for complement fragments
	Beckman Instruments, Inc. Diagnostic Systems Group Brea, CA 92621-6209 Tel: 800-526-3821	Nephelometry
	See Tables in Chapter 9	
	Behring Diagnostics Inc. 17 Chubb Way Somerville, NJ 08876 Tel: 908-707-3800	Nephelometry, turbidimetry, radial diffusion
Services specialized in tests for rheumatology	Rheumatology Diagnostics 1538 20th Street Santa Monica, CA 90404 Tel: 800-338-1918	Tests by ELISA and other methods, anti-nuclear, anti-cardiolipin, complement
	Speciality Laboratories, Inc. 2211 Michigan Ave Santa Monica, CA 90404 Tel: 800-421-7110	Tests by various methods, Farr assay for anti-DNA, anti-nuclear antibodies, anti-cardiolipin, complement fragments, and null alleles

	TheraTest Laboratories Inc. 2201 W. Campbell Park Dr., Chicago, IL 60612 Tel: 800-441-0771	Anti-nuclear antibodies (ELISA) Rhematoid factor IgM, IgG, IgA Anti-cardiolipin
	Antiphospholipid Standardization Laboratory 511 S. Floyd Street, Rm 615 Louisville, KY 40220 Tel: 502-588-7874	Anti-cardiolipin
Nuclear and other antigens	Worthington Biochemical Corp. P.O. Box 5003 Halls Mill Rd. Freehold, NJ 07728 Tel: 800-445-9603	Histones
	Sigma Chemical Co. P.O. Box 14508 St. Louis, MO 63178 Tel: 800-521-8956	DNA, cardiolipin, histones
	Immunovision Inc. 1506 Ford Ave Springdale, AR 72764 Tel: 800-541-0960	Immunoaffinity-purified nuclear antigens
	Fisher Scientific Headquarters Pittsburgh 711 Forbes Ave Pittsburgh, PA 15219-4785 Tel: 800-766-7000	Calf thymus and bacteriophage DNA
	Pharmacia Biotech Inc. 800 Centennial Ave Piscataway, NJ 08854 Tel: 800-526-3593	Calf thymus and bacteriophage DNA
ELISA readers, robotics	Bio-Tek Instruments, Inc. P.O. Box 998 Highland Park Winooski, VT 05404-0998	
	Dynatech Laboratories Inc. Tel: 800-336-4543	Readers and robotics

	Tecan SLT Instruments P.O. Box 8101 Hillsborough, NC 27278 Tel: 800-338-3226	
	Bio-Rad Laboratories, Inc. Life Science Group 2000 Alfred Nobel Drive Hercules, CA 94547 Tel: 800-424-6723	
	Cambridge Technology, Inc. (Readers and Washers) 23 Elm Street Watertown, MA 02172	
	Beckman Instruments, Inc. Diagnostic Systems Group Brea, CA 92621-6209 Tel: 800-526-3821	Robotics
	Hyperion, Inc. 14100 S.W. 136th Street Miami, FL 33186 Tel: 305-238-3020	Automated ELISA
	ICN Biomedicals (Also Pipettes) 3300 Hyland Avenue Costa Mesa, CA 92626 Tel: 800-854-0530	
Plate washers	Danley Instruments Inc. Tel: 800-836-5391	
	Perkin-Elmer Corporation (Washers) Mail Station 12 761 Main Ave Norwalk, CT 06856-9966 Tel: 800-762-4000	
	Bio-Tek Instruments, Inc. P.O. Box 998 Highland Park Winooski, VT 05404-0998	

	Bio-Rad Laboratories, Inc. Life Science Group 2000 Alfred Nobel Drive Hercules, CA 94547 Tel: 800-424-6723	
Standards and control sera	Centers for Disease Control, Immunology Branch, 1600 Clifton Road, 1-1202 A25, Atlanta, Georgia	Controls are limited to once a year for each laboratory
	Central Laboratory Netherlands Red Cross Blood Transfusion Service Department of Immune and Blood Groups Reagents P.O. Box 9190 1006 AD Amsterdam The Netherlands Tel: 3120-5123246	One sample per laboratory for each standard; internal standards are prepared to match
	Antiphospholipid Standardization Laboratory 511 S. Floyd Street, Room 615 Louisville, KY 40220 Tel: 502-588-7874	For anti-cardiolipin antibody standards
Control plasma and sera	Biomedical Resources 31 North York Road Hatboro, PA 19040 Tel: 215-672-7587	Bulk plasma with various autoantibody specificities
	PlasmaLab International 3128 Norton Ave Everett, WA 98201 Tel: 206-258-3653	Bulk plasma with various autoantibody specificities
Computer programs for ELISA	TheraTest Laboratories Inc. 2201 W. Campbell Park Dr., Chicago, IL 60612 Tel: 800-441-0771	Patient data analysis and graphic display; interface with most popular reader
	J. Peterman 301-949-7127	

	Bio-Tek Instruments, Inc. P.O. Box 998 Highland Park Winooski, VT 05404-0998	Kinetics analysis
	Bio-Rad Laboratories, Inc. Life Science Group 2000 Alfred Nobel Drive Hercules, CA 94547 Tel: 800-424-6723	
	Dynatech Laboratories, Inc. 14340 Sullyfield Circle Chantilly, VA 22021 Tel: 800-336-4543	
	Extensive listing in *Immunochemistry of Solid Phase Immunoassays,* J.E. Butler, Ed., CRC Press, Boca Raton, 1991, page 293.	Information regarding specific functions; check with software manufacturers for reader compatibility
Multichannel pipettors	VWR Scientific P.O. Box 66929 O'Hare AMF Chicago, IL 60666 Tel: 800-932-5000	
	Fisher Scientific Headquarters Pittsburgh 711 Forbes Ave Pittsburgh, PA 15219-4785 Tel: 800-766-7000	
	Baxter Diagnostics Inc. Scientific Products 1210 Waukegan Road McGaw Park, IL 60085 Tel: 708-689-8410	
Plastic accessories	Denville Scientific, Inc. P.O. Box 304 Denville, NJ 07834 Tel: 201-328-0822	Minitubes, 1.2 ml racked in 96-well format, cubetubes (2 ml)

	Fisher Scientific Headquarters Pittsburgh 711 Forbes Ave Pittsburgh, PA 15219-4785 Tel: 800-766-7000	Minitubes, 1.2 ml racked in 96-well format, cubetubes (2 ml)
	Midwest Scientific P.O. Box 458 228 Meramec Station Road Valley Park, MO 63088 Tel: 800-227-9997	Pipette tips, racks of tubes in 96-well format
Microtiter plates	Dynatech Laboratories, Inc. 14340 Sullyfield Circle Chantilly, VA 22021 Tel: 800-336-4543	
	Costar Corp. One Alewife Center Cambridge, MA 02140 Tel: 800-492-1110	
	Nunc, Inc. 2000 North Avenue Naperville, IL 60563 Tel: 800-288-6862	
	Denly Instruments 4905 Pine Cone Dr. Suite 3 Durham, NC 27707 Tel: 919-493-8026	
Enzyme-conjugated antibodies and substrates	Jackson ImmunoResearch Labs, Inc. P.O. Box 9 West Grove, PA 19390 Tel: 800-367-5296	Immunoaffinity-purified antibodies
	Kirkegaard & Perry Labs Inc. 2 Cessna Court Gaithersburg, MD 20879 Tel: 800-638-3167	TMB substrate in one two solutions; various substrates

Bio-Rad Laboratories, Inc. Life Science Group 2000 Alfred Nobel Drive Hercules, CA 94547 Tel: 800-424-6723	Various substrates
Sigma Chemical Co. P.O. Box 14508 St. Louis, MO 63178 Tel: 800-521-8956	

Index

INDEX

A

B

C

D

E

F

G

H

N

O

P

Q

R

S

T

U

V

W

Y